Advanced Practice in Nursing and the Allied Health Professions

Third Edition

Edited by

Paula McGee

WILEY-BLACKWELL

A John Wiley & Sons, Ltd., Publication

This edition first published 2009
© 2009 by Blackwell Publishing Ltd

Blackwell Publishing was acquired by John Wiley & Sons in February 2007. Blackwell's publishing program has been merged with Wiley's global Scientific, Technical, and Medical business to form Wiley-Blackwell.

Registered office
John Wiley & Sons Ltd, The Atrium, Southern Gate, Chichester, West Sussex, PO19 8SQ, United Kingdom

Editorial Offices
9600 Garsington Road, Oxford, OX4 2DQ, United Kingdom
2121 State Avenue, Ames, Iowa 50014-8300, USA

For details of our global editorial offices, for customer services and for information about how to apply for permission to reuse the copyright material in this book please see our website at www.wiley.com/wiley-blackwell.

Library of Congress Cataloging-in-Publication Data

Advanced practice in nursing and the allied health professions / edited by Paula McGee.—3rd ed.
    p. ; cm.
  Rev. ed. of: Advanced nursing practice / edited by Paula McGee and George Castledine. 2nd ed. 2003.
  Includes bibliographical references and index.
  ISBN 978-1-4051-6239-5 (pbk. : alk. paper) 1. Nurse practitioners—Great Britain. 2. Nursing—Great Britain. I. McGee, Paula. II. Advanced nursing practice.
  [DNLM: 1. Nurse Clinicians—trends—Great Britain. 2. Allied Health Personnel—trends—Great Britain. 3. Nurse Practitioners—trends—Great Britain. WY 128 A2435 2009]
  RT82.8.A365 2009
  610.73′60941—dc22

                           2009008239

A catalogue record for this book is available from the British Library.

Set in 10/12.5 pt Palatino by Laserwords Pvt Ltd, Chennai, India
Printed and bound in Malaysia by KHL Printing Co Sdn Bhd

1 2009

Advanced Practice in Nursing and the Allied Health Professions

Thir<

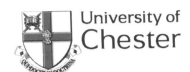

University of Chester

CLÄTTERBRIDGE LIBRARY

Contents

8 Advanced Practice in Occupational Therapy **97**
Lynne Frith and Janette Walsh

9 Working as an Advanced Nurse Practitioner **107**
Mark Radford

Contributors

David Cole, Senior Lecturer, Faculty of Health, Birmingham City University.

Lynne Frith, Occupational Therapist, Stoke on Trent Primary Care Trust.

Kate Gee, Nurse Consultant, Cardiology, University Hospital, Birmingham NHS Foundation Trust.

Katharine Hardware, Senior Lecturer, Birmingham City University.

Alistair Hewison, Director of Postgraduate Studies, School of Health Sciences, University of Birmingham.

Linda Hindle, Consultant Dietitian in Obesity, Birmingham East and North Primary Care Trust.

Chris Inman, Senior Lecturer, Faculty of Health, Birmingham City University.

Paula McGee, Professor or Nursing, Faculty of Health, Birmingham City University.

Mark Radford, Nurse Consultant (Perioperative Emergency Care) and Associate Deputy Director of Nursing, Heart of England NHS Foundation Trust.

Madrean Schober, Senior Visiting Fellow, Alice Lee Centre for Nursing Studies, National University of Singapore.

Sally Shaw, Former Director of the ICN Leadership for Change programme.

Sue Shortland, Advanced Nurse Practitioner, Langton Medical Centre, Lichfield.

Janette Walsh, Occupational Therapist, Stoke on Trent Primary Care Trust.

Introduction

Advanced practice is an approach to health care that enables practitioners to meet the everyday needs of their patients in whatever setting these arise. Advanced practitioners may be found in any health profession. Their enhanced knowledge and skills complement those of medicine and, therefore, increase both access to and the availability of health care. Advanced practice represents a reconceptualisation of professional roles in health care: a move away from the traditional approach, in which medicine was pre-eminent, towards a more collegiate model in which the strengths of each profession can be fully utilised. This reconceptualisation requires health professions, societies and governments to recognise the increased complexities of modern health care and to find the best ways of addressing these. In other words, modern health care leads people to ask what sort of a health-care practitioner will best meet their needs, what type of doctor, nurse or physiotherapist is needed and what they should be able to do.

Nursing provides an example of this reconceptualisation. In countries as diverse as Botswana and the United Kingdom, nurses make up by far the largest part of the health-care workforce. They are, therefore, an important resource through which health care is delivered, especially to vulnerable and socially marginalised populations (World Health Organisation 2000). It is appropriate that governments should attempt to make good and better use of this resource. One example can be seen in the United Kingdom. The NHS Plan introduced a wide-ranging reform of the health service that had implications for all health professions including nursing. New roles would allow nurse-led services to be developed. These would enable nurses to admit and discharge certain patients, manage caseloads, prescribe and treat patients. They would also be trained to perform certain types of surgery, triage patients and carry out resuscitation procedures (DH 2000). These plans facilitated the development of advanced nursing practice, allowing it the freedom to develop new approaches to care and treatment. They also provided a basis from which advanced nurses could function as clinical and professional leaders (DH 2000).

Advanced nursing practice now has many different forms, both in the United Kingdom and worldwide. In remote areas and developing countries, primary care providers and advanced nurse practitioners are well placed to promote health, assess, diagnose and treat common ailments. In secondary care, they are able to extend their role, taking responsibility for aspects of patient care that might previously have required medical attention, for example, the management of patients with long-term conditions. In all settings, advanced practitioners are able to apply their knowledge and skills to the development of innovative approaches to care that meet the health needs of local people (Schober and Affara 2006).

Alongside this development is a trend towards comparable changes in allied health professions. In the United Kingdom, for example, the NHS Plan introduced new roles for pharmacists in managing repeat prescribing and other aspects of care, especially for patients with long-term conditions. Other allied health professionals were also given the opportunity to develop their roles and pioneer new ways of working. Physiotherapists, occupational therapists, speech therapists and many other professionals could become consultant practitioners working closely 'with senior hospital doctors, nurses and midwives in drawing up local clinical and referral protocols alongside primary care colleagues' (DH 2000, p. 86). Medical practice was also to be reconfigured to ease pressure on general practitioner (GP) services and allow hospital consultants to develop new ways of working (DH 2000).

Inherent in these developments is a huge cultural shift away from traditional modes of operation towards a patient-centred system of health care. This cultural shift has required changes in the initial preparation of practitioners, equipping them to work more in partnership with patients and reduce health inequalities by ensuring that everyone can access and use services. Post-registration education has also changed to enable practitioners to further enhance their professional knowledge and skills and take the lead in working with certain patient groups. Advanced practitioners are, therefore, prepared as versatile professionals, able to provide both direct care to patients and leadership to colleagues.

This climate of professional and organisational change has provided many opportunities for advanced practitioners to combine their traditional expertise with new health knowledge and technologies. Such combinations exemplify the growing confidence of practitioners in testing out and adopting new roles, even if these mean taking on work previously the preserve of other professionals. This does not mean that advanced practitioners are becoming doctors. Their roles are meant to complement, rather than replace medical practice, leaving doctors free to develop their own work in new ways that better meet the needs of patients. Nevertheless, there is a risk that advanced practitioners may leave too much of their traditional work to assistant practitioners in order to take on tasks that they regard as more exciting or prestigious. It is a matter of balance. Patients still need to be washed, fed and made comfortable; they still need help with mobility problems, speech and mental health difficulties. However, they also need expert care from practitioners who are able to draw on the latest authoritative evidence and competently implement new health technologies.

The aim of this book

This new edition is based on the view that, in health professions, there is a form of practice, which exceeds that achieved by initial registration and which is distinguishable by definable characteristics. This is referred to, throughout this book, as *advanced practice*. This book aims to clarify these characteristics across different professional fields with the intention of

- presenting an account of developments in different professions with a view to the possible future establishment of parity between advanced practitioners, regardless of their particular origins;
- examining the ways in which advanced practice is conceptualised both theoretically and in response to health policies;
- demonstrating the actual and potential contributions of advanced practice to direct patient care;
- examining the influence of advanced practitioners as professional and clinical leaders;
- reflecting on the preparation required for advanced practice and the ways in which practitioners are currently developing their careers;
- developing an agenda for future research and development in advanced practice.

Key features of this new edition

This third edition has been substantially revised to include both nursing and allied health professions. As in previous editions the key questions are presented at the end of each chapter. It is hoped that these will help readers to continue to debate the many issues raised in this book and contribute towards the further development of advanced practice in health professions.

The book begins with an overview of the development of advanced nursing practice in the United Kingdom. This allows continuity with previous editions, which, together with this chapter, form what is probably the only account of how advanced nursing practice developed. The chapter highlights several issues that are further discussed as the book unfolds: the influence of health policy, the role of professional bodies and the interface with medicine. The chapter shows that advanced nursing practice has not developed in an orderly or predictable fashion. Rather, development seems to be a piecemeal affair with many disparate elements that do not necessarily fit neatly together partly because so many different factors and factions have been involved and also because no one thought to maintain a running record of events; the result is an incomplete account of developments.

In Chapter 2, Alistair Hewison takes up and expands upon the issue of health policies in the United Kingdom. As he points out, this is no easy task given that the NHS seems to be in a constant process of reform and change. This chapter presents an accessible explanation of these reforms and their implications for advanced nursing practice as a new role through which the changing health-care needs of the population can be accommodated. As this chapter points out, one of the main problems with advanced nursing practice is that, in the United Kingdom at least, the profession seems unable to make up its mind about what it should be. Consequently, advanced or higher-level nursing is not clearly defined.

Nursing and health policy provide a basis for introducing advanced practice in allied health professions. Chapter 3 begins by examining the implications of health policy and reforms in terms of the introduction of consultant practitioners and the subsequent pathways taken by professional bodies. This is followed by an overview of developments in physiotherapy, a profession that has, so far, relied heavily on nursing research, particularly that of Benner (1984). Benner (1984) proposed that nurses developed through several stages, beginning as novices and gradually progressing to become experts. Occupational therapy has also drawn on Benner's (1984) work in developing post-registration roles and levels of practice. The one allied health profession that appears to be out of step with this reliance is radiography. In this instance, health policy and the example of nursing do not seem to have been driving forces. Instead, as David Cole explains, advanced roles in radiography have developed in response to direct pressure, on NHS trusts, to improve pay and careers. This pressure came directly from practitioners and this chapter presents the first published account of their efforts that appear to have resulted in a sonography role that is very similar to advanced roles in other professions.

Changes in health policy, new developments in treatment and care and the rise of advanced practice in allied health professions necessitated a reappraisal of the conceptualisation of advanced practice put forward in the last edition (McGee and Castledine 2003). Chapter 4 presents an updated view of the three elements first described in the previous edition: *professional maturity, challenging professional boundaries* and *pioneering new practice*. These elements are discussed in a broader way that explains their applicability to allied health professions and the ways in which emergent advanced roles may interface with medicine. This discussion puts forward the view that direct practice and engagement with patients, together with interpersonal skills, form the core of advanced practice irrespective of the professional discipline involved. To be considered advanced, the practitioner must spend a significant amount of time in practice; without this, individuals cannot be considered to be advanced, no matter how competent they are in other ways. The next two chapters expand on the key activities of assessment, diagnosis, treatment and care within advanced roles. Chapter 5 presents a discussion of the different types of assessment that an advanced practitioner may employ. In Chapter 6, Sue Shortland and Katharine Hardware present an overview of the regulations and governance issues concerning the prescription of medication.

Chapters 7 to 10 present, for the first time, views of advanced practice from differing professional perspectives. In Chapter 7, Linda Hindle describes her work in dietetics and, in particular, in helping obese people to manage their weight more effectively. In Chapter 8, Lynne Frith and Janette Walsh discuss specialist and consultant roles in occupational therapy. These have been slow to develop but it is anticipated that further developments will take place as the profession develops a clearer career structure. Chapters 9 and 10 see a return to nursing. In Chapter 9, Mark Radford discusses his views as an advanced nurse practitioner. This is followed by Kate Gee's account of her work in cardiology, based on a model devised by Zubialde *et al.* (2005).

The next three chapters address other aspects of advanced practice. These may be part of direct interaction with patients but can also apply in working with colleagues and other staff. Chapter 11 examines the importance of cultural competence. As senior members of their professions, advanced practitioners should be skilled in working with patients and colleagues from diverse backgrounds. Moreover, they should be able to promote cultural competence within the organisation as a whole ensuring an ethical environment in which patients and staff are treated equitably. In Chapter 12, Sally Shaw addresses the role of the advanced practitioner as a professional and clinical leader. The indicators of successful leadership are deliberately set out as checklists to provide a tool to help practitioners and their managers to determine progress. The topic of management is taken up by Paula McGee and Mark Radford in Chapter 13. This chapter sets out the key points that concern managers, including strategic planning in the light of current health service priorities, and examines the implications of these for the advanced practitioner as both a clinical expert and a manager. The chapter also addresses issues in managing advanced practice posts and the need to evaluate their impact.

Chapters 14 and 15 address the preparation and careers of advanced practitioners. Chapter 14 examines the issue of competence and the types of expertise required by advanced practitioners. These competences fall into two groups: generic and specialist. The chapter proposes that generic competences could be common to all advanced roles; specialist competencies could be generated by the individual practitioner's specific field and profession. Chapter 15 focuses on career development and presents, for the first time, the outcomes of a survey, by Chris Inman and Paula McGee, of graduates from an MSc advanced nursing practice course. This survey reinforces earlier statements about the piecemeal development of advanced nursing practice in the United Kingdom and the need for progress on matters relating to employment, work activities and long-term career prospects.

The final two chapters present two different aspects of advanced practice. In Chapter 16, Madrean Schober discusses the factors that have contributed to the international development of advanced nursing practice and highlights the different approaches adopted by various countries. It is hoped that, in future, this chapter may be complemented by a similar account of developments in allied health professions. However, there is still much to be done before this can happen. Chapter 17 draws the book to a close by setting out an agenda for further work based around direct practice, collaboration with service users, inclusivity, professional regulation and control, education and assessment. These ideas take account of the recommendations set out in the most recent health service review that provide many exciting opportunities for advanced practitioners in nursing and allied health professions (DH 2008).

Paula McGee

References

Benner, P. (1984) *From Novice to Expert: Excellence and Power in Clinical Nursing Practice*. Menlo Park, California, Addison Wesley.

Department of Health (2000) *The NHS Plan. A Plan for Investment. A Plan for Reform*. Wetherby, DH.

Department of Health (2008) *High Quality Care for All. NHS Next Stage Review Final Report*. London, DH.

McGee, P. and Castledine, G. (2003) *Advanced Practice*, 2nd edn. Oxford, Blackwell Publishing.

Schober, M. and Affara, F. (2006) *International Council of Nurses, Advanced Nursing Practice*. Oxford, Blackwell Publishing.

World Health Organisation (2000) *Global Advisory Group on Nursing and Midwifery. Report of the 6th Meeting*. Available at www.who.org.

Zubialde, J.P., Shannon, K. and Devenger, N. (2005) The quadrants of care model for health services planning. *Families, Systems and Health* **23** (2), 172–85.

Chapter 1

The Development of Advanced Nursing Practice in the United Kingdom

Paula McGee

Introduction

The United Kingdom Central Council (UKCC) defined advanced practice as 'adjusting the boundaries for the development of future practice, pioneering and developing new roles responsive to changing needs and with advancing clinical practice, research and education enrich professional practice as a whole' (UKCC 1994:20). To a certain extent, this definition can be taken to represent the culmination of years of work and debate in which individual nurses explored and experimented with new ideas and roles that might enable them to provide both better patient care and meaningful professional activity. In this context, the Council can be seen as trying to bring some sort of order to the patchwork of established and emerging roles beyond registration by issuing a statement about the form these roles should take. Alternatively, the definition can be regarded as the beginning of a thorough examination of the nature of post-qualifying nursing practice, about what patients, the profession and society as a whole want from nursing and the impact this might have on other health professions, especially medicine.

One of the difficulties in both analyses is that the Council never quite made clear how the definition of advanced practice would apply to the realities of daily life in practice. Consequently, there was a great deal of confusion among nurses, managers, employers and other health professionals as to what the Council intended. This confusion created a fertile ground for debate, both useful and acrimonious, as nurses and other health professionals tried to determine the most appropriate way forward; there was quite a lot of research, some of which helped illuminate the path. In practice, there was a proliferation of posts and roles that were labelled as *advanced* but that were never formally scrutinised to ascertain whether they conformed to the Council's ideas (RCN 2008).

In spite of, or maybe because of, the fluidity of this situation, some consensus has emerged in which there appears to be an agreement that advanced practice should contain a clinical component, set the pace for changing practice and be underpinned by formal preparation that is beyond the level of initial registration. There is also an acceptance that practice is not static and that nursing must continue to move forward. However, there is far less agreement about the nature of this clinical practice, how that move forward should be made or even the direction it should take.

This chapter presents an examination of the main issues and influences that have contributed to the current state of advanced practice in the United Kingdom and the further developments anticipated. The chapter closes with some key questions to prompt further discussion.

Health policies and reforms

The health policies and reforms instigated by the Labour government during the late 1990s and early 2000s have had a marked effect on the development of advanced practice by creating opportunities for innovation both in the development of nursing roles and in clinical practice. The reforms were intended to improve the quality of health services by ensuring that they were tailored to meet local needs and reduce health inequalities (Box 1.1). The reforms were also aimed at valuing staff and developing a more transparent approach to both the management of information and the decision-making process (DH 1997, 2000, 2001a). The strategy for nursing that accompanied the introduction of these policies and reforms made clear that the profession had an essential role to play because nurses were seen as ideally placed to promote health, particularly in community settings such as schools and places of work (Box 1.2). Their skills and expertise could be directed towards early identification and treatment of health problems and the provision of support for those with long-term conditions, especially during periods of crisis. Such nurse-led activity could offset the need for more expensive services including admission to hospital. Where such admission was necessary, nurses could use their skills to develop care pathways, promote continuity of care and address specific problems such as infection control (DH 1999).

Box 1.1   Core principles of health policy reforms

Provision of a health service that covers all clinical needs is available to
    everyone and is free at the point of delivery
Development of individual packages of care and services that are accessible by,
    and which meet the needs of, local populations instead of a *one-size-fits-all*
    approach
Improvements in the quality of care and greater transparency about what is
    happening in health-care organisations, both locally and nationally
Creation of a better working environment for staff
Patient and public involvement in service design and delivery
New ways of working, better interprofessional and multi-agency working
Promotion of health and the reduction of health inequalities

Source: Adapted from Department of Health (2000) *The NHS Plan. A Plan for Investment.
A Plan for Reform.* Wetherby, DH.

Box 1.2   The role of nursing in health policy reforms

Promoting health in ways that meet local needs
Reducing health inequalities, especially among members of marginalised
    groups
Instigating nurse-led initiatives to provide faster access to services and
    treatment
Expanding roles in primary care settings to reduce hospital admissions and
    enable people with long-term conditions to remain at home
Independently prescribing medicines
Expanding roles in secondary care and collaborating with other professionals
    to provide specialist care, develop care pathways and promote
    evidence-based practice
Providing intermediate care and promoting independence for those with
    complex needs
Tackling specific problems such as infection control
Promoting seamless care and inter-agency working

Sources: Summarised from Department of Health (2005) *Supporting People with Long
Term Conditions: Liberating the Talents of Nurses Who Care for People with Long Term
Conditions.* London, DH.
Department of Health (1999) *Making a Difference. Strengthening the Nursing, Midwifery and
Health Visiting Contribution to Health and Healthcare.* London, DH.

The UKCC and *higher-level* practice

The Council recognised the growing concern about the lack of understanding and agreement regarding forms of practice beyond registration, both within the profession and among employers. There was a lack of clarity about the terms *advanced, specialist, specialism and speciality* as used within the Council's statements about practice after registration, and practitioners had difficulty in distinguishing between them, especially with regard to the differences between working in a *speciality* and being a *specialist*. Similarly, distinctions between the roles, responsibilities and preparation of both *advanced* and *specialist* nurses were unclear. This lack of clarity had the potential to erode public confidence in nursing (Waller 1998).

In response to these concerns, the Council entered into consultation with the nursing, midwifery and health visiting professions, including practitioners, stakeholders and professional organisations, about forms of practice beyond registration; after much deliberation, the Council accepted that these forms were actually levels of practice but carefully avoided associating these with the term *advanced* (UKCC 1999). From this consultation emerged the concept of *higher-level practice*, which the Council explained as applying to those nurses who were clinical experts and were able to apply their extensive knowledge, skills and expertise to develop practice and improve patient care (UKCC 1999). Following this consultation, the Council pressed forward with plans to develop *higher-level practice*, further assisted by 700 volunteer nurses, midwives and health visitors, from across all four countries of the United Kingdom. The result was a standard for *higher-level practice*, incorporating seven domains that were later taken up by employers to facilitate the development of nurse consultant posts. The final report from the Council's working group made 15 recommendations that were then referred to the then newly constituted Nursing and Midwifery Council (NMC) in 2002 (UKCC 2002, Castledine 2003).

One of the many problems with the concept of *higher-level practice* was the inexact use of terminology; words such as *expert* require some clarification. There are varying opinions on what it takes to be an *expert*, none of which seems to provide a completely satisfactory explanation (Table 1.1). The Council itself did not venture to explain what it regarded as an *expert*, and gradually *higher-level practice, expert* and *advanced practice* were used interchangeably. The Council's decision to award all the volunteers who met the higher-level standard the status of advanced practitioners compounded the situation and subsequently there has been no serious consideration of what these terms mean for advanced nursing.

The interface with medicine

The introduction of the New Deal and the Working Time (Statutory Instrument 2002) Regulations 2002 created opportunities for advanced nursing by altering the working lives of doctors through reducing their contracted hours and improving their training (NHSE 1991). In August 2007 the junior doctors' contracts stipulated a maximum working week of 56 hours. This will be reduced to 48 hours by August 2009

Table 1.1 Perspectives on expert practice.

Author	Definitions	Comments
Benner (1984)	An *expert* is one who is able to intuit the essence of a situation and to focus accurately on a clinical problem; is not distracted by irrelevancies	Benner's work focuses on clinical practice. The *higher-level practice* standard incorporates domains that are not necessarily associated with direct practice. It is not clear whether her views of an expert performance would apply
Hamric (2005)	Clinical practice is the focus of *advanced practice* but there are other competencies which are also essential. These include acting as a consultant for others. The advanced practitioner is described as an *expert*	The term *expert* is not examined in depth but *expert* clinical practice is only a part of advanced practice. Thus a nurse may be highly proficient in one sphere but not *advanced*
Jasper (1994)	The *expert* must possess a specialised body of knowledge, extensive experience, be able to generate new knowledge and be recognised as an *expert*	Jasper does not elaborate on how nurses acquire such knowledge the nature of that knowledge, and whether or how *expert* knowledge differs from that of others. The deeper knowledge of the *higher-level* practitioner must be recognised by others
Zukav (1979, pp. 34–5)	The *expert* is someone who 'started before you did' and 'always begins at the centre, at the heart of the matter' with the enthusiasm of acting for the first time	Zukav's *expert* has a store of knowledge on which to draw and thus may be said to be dealing with what is known. In pioneering new roles the *advanced* practitioner is entering into the unknown

Sources: Benner, P. (1984) *From Novice to Expert: Excellence and Power in Clinical Nursing Practice.* Menlo Park, California, Addison Wesley.
Hamric, A., Spross, J. and Hanson, C. (eds) (2005) *Advanced Nursing Practice. An Integrative Approach*, 3rd edn. St Louis, Elsevier Saunders.
Jasper, M. (1994) Expert: a discussion of the implications of the concept as used in nursing. *Journal of Advanced Nursing.*
Zukav, G. (1991) *The Dancing Wu Li Masters.* London, Rider.

(DH 2007). Alongside these contractual changes is a move away form the traditional apprenticeship system for training junior doctors towards a new, competency-based scheme. All junior doctors now enter a 2-year foundation programme that equips them with *'basic practical skills and competencies in medicine and will include: clinical skills; effective relationships with patients; high standards in clinical governance and safety; the use of evidence and data; communication, team working, multiprofessional practice, time management and decision-making and an effective understanding of the different settings in which medicine is practised'* (DH 2004a, p. 8). Those who successfully complete the foundation programme may enter a further programme to become either a general practitioner (GP) or a hospital specialist. Inevitably, implementing these programmes has affected the amount of day-to-day work that junior doctors are able to do, a situation that has been complicated by the number of senior practitioners who are approaching retirement. A flexible retirement scheme was introduced to encourage hospital consultants to continue in post beyond the age of 65 and financial incentives were offered to GPs for each additional year that they deferred retirement (The Lords Hansard 2002).

The implications of the reduction in the availability of doctors were not lost on the British Medical Association (BMA), which proposed that, in primary care, nurse practitioners (NPs) could act as the first point of contact for most patients and refer them on to doctors or other health professionals if necessary. Similarly, in hospitals, specialist nurses could act as care coordinators (BMA 2002a, b). Even prescribing by nurses and pharmacists was accepted provided that it was 'limited and in line with the individual's training and experience' (BMA 2006). The BMA was thus supportive of new roles in nursing to the extent that its members expressed frustration at, as they saw it, the failure of both employers and the NMC to bring about a change, which resulted in 'the undermining and de-valuing of nurses with extended roles' (BMA 2004).

This justifiable criticism is not new. The history of advanced practice shows that some doctors have been very influential in spearheading new developments, often providing a vision of what could be achieved. For example, in 1957, in North Carolina, Dr Eugene Stead envisaged an NP's role that was between nursing and medicine and found a nurse to share this vision but was opposed by both the senior nurses in the local university and the National League for Nursing, which refused to accredit the necessary postgraduate training course because doctors would have had to teach much of the content. As a result of this failure, the university instituted a physicians' assistant (PA) course. In another example, Loretta Ford, one of the most well-known NPs, worked with Dr Silver setting up a postgraduate course in paediatric care for poor rural children in Colorado but the American Nurses Association would not support this, preferring to concentrate on preparing nurses for teaching or management. In both examples, the doctor provided or helped to provide a significant vision through which particular health needs might be met; it was nursing's professional bodies that appeared to have difficulties. Unsurprisingly, the doctors concerned lost interest and moved on (Dunphy *et al.* 2004).

Nursing theorists are keen to point out that advanced practice is about developing nursing and not about taking over medical work, but the interface between the two professions is not clear cut. Advanced NPs diagnose and treat illness – activities that are perceived by patients to be part of the doctor's repertoire of skills. There is certainly an area of overlap between the two roles. For example, the advanced NP and the doctor may diagnose repeated and severe tonsillitis but it is the doctor who will have the skills required to perform a tonsillectomy and the nurse who will be best equipped to manage the post-operative period. Both will draw on the same research and use the same decision-making and problem management skills but in different ways (Hunsberger *et al.* 1992) (Figure 1.1). Thus the two roles are complementary

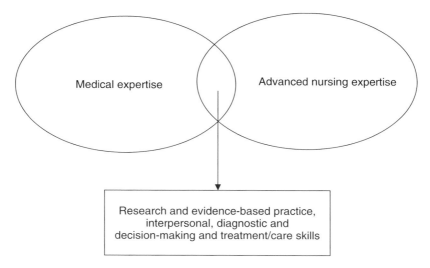

Fig. 1.1   The interface between advanced nursing and medicine (based on Hunsberger *et al.* 1992).

rather than competitive, allowing both to concentrate their efforts where they are most needed. Moreover, the holistic orientation of the advanced NP allows for greater consideration of factors that may impinge on the patient's recovery, for example, social circumstances or psychological problems. Patients often do not like to, as they see it, *bother the doctor with such details* but are likely to reveal them to an advanced nurse.

This notion of complementarity leads naturally to the idea that the two roles of advanced nurse and doctor meet as equals in the practice setting. While individual practitioners in both camps may agree with this, as a body, doctors clearly disagree. The BMA's support for advanced nursing roles was qualified by their capacity 'to improve the working lives of doctors' (BMA 2004). Nurses might extend their roles but only within 'a defined field answerable to a medically qualified doctor' (BMA 2005). The subordination of nursing to medical expertise was, therefore, to continue and there was strident protest when nurses attained positions in which this balance of power was overturned. Thus the BMA found it 'outrageous and totally unacceptable that a nurse consultant has been appointed as the lead clinician in occupational health and that she, with the assistant director of human resources, will perform the annual appraisal of the occupational health consultant' (BMA 2005).

It would seem, therefore, that the interface between advanced nursing and medicine is highly ambivalent. Individual practitioners may develop pioneering partnerships based on mutual regard for each other's expertise but formal relations between the two professions still require considerable effort on both sides. In practice, it is usually the advanced nurse who must make the first move, involving medical staff from the start of any initiative so that they understand what is happening and the reasons for it and can begin to see the potential that advanced nursing practice can bring to their own sphere of work.

The introduction of new roles

Modern matrons

The managerial roles of matrons were introduced in hospitals as part of a range of initiatives to improve the quality of service. Other initiatives included tackling standards of cleanliness, improving the quality of hospital food, the introduction of the Patient Advisory Liaison Service and benchmarking. The title of *matron* emerged following public consultation that revealed a preference for the presence of a clearly identified and authoritative presence, in each setting, to whom patients and relatives could turn for help, advice and to complain. Matrons were to take charge of a group of wards and resources to ensure that patients received the best possible care and that support services fulfilled their responsibilities to the highest standard and to provide leadership (NHSE 1999, DH 2001b).

More recently, matrons' roles have been exported to primary care settings as part of the strategy for supporting patients with long-term conditions (DH 2005). The intention is to enable patients to receive the help they need from primary care services and, therefore, reduce the number of admissions to hospital. Community matrons were intended to use case management strategies to identify patients' needs and formulate care plans based on multi-professional working to enable patients to become as independent as possible (DH 2005).

The managerial orientation of matrons' roles tends to place them outside the advanced nursing sphere. Advanced nurses are primarily practitioners engaged in direct patient care; their roles do not include responsibility for managerial issues such as staffing, budgeting or resources. Matrons, on the other hand, are concerned with precisely these factors as a means of creating environments in which patients can be given the best possible care. It is possible that there may be some areas of overlap between the two roles and research is needed to examine this unexplored territory. What is certain is that, to be effective, the advanced nurse, like the matron, must have the status, power and authority to act and to direct others when necessary. Consequently, the advanced practitioner must ensure that these issues are clearly addressed in the development of any new post.

Nurse consultants

The idea of nurse consultants is not new. In the 1970s, it was envisaged that the development of a consultant's role would provide clinical leadership but would be free from the demands of managerial responsibilities (Ashworth 1975). The health service reforms introduced in the late 1990s facilitated the introduction of nurse consultant posts (DH 1999, 2000, 2001c, NHSE 1999). Consultants were expected to be clinical experts who spent at least half their working time in practice, working directly with patients and acting as focal points for professional advice, education and research, activities similar to those required by advanced practitioners. Many of the attributes of advanced nursing practice can be found within the consultant's role and a number of advanced practitioners have gravitated towards nurse consultant posts.

The introduction of nurse consultant posts was of considerable significance because, for the first time, nurses seeking to develop their careers did not have to leave the practice setting. Previous generations of nurses had been faced with two options, management or education, both of which meant leaving practice. The opportunity to remain in the practice setting not only offered satisfaction to those nurses who took it up but also ensured that the much-needed expertise remained in patient care.

Physicians' assistants

This is a separate, non-nursing role that developed in the United States. A PA trains at undergraduate level for at least 2 years and is able to assess patients, diagnose and treat common ailments, undertake routine laboratory work, minor surgical procedures and administrative matters such as billing insurance companies. PAs work within a medical framework and *for* a doctor (Castledine 1998). However, their roles may at times overlap with those of other health-care professionals.

In Britain, a small number of nurses began working as PAs in the 1990s. The first to do so was Suzanne Holmes who was employed to conduct vein harvesting and other procedures at the Oxford Heart Centre. The development of these posts was quite haphazard and many were initially not paid as nurses but as medical technicians. The PA's role was eventually formalised as that of '*a* new health-care professional who, while not a doctor, works to the medical model, with the attitudes, skills and knowledge base to deliver holistic care and treatment within the general medical and/or general practice team under defined levels of supervision' (DH 2006, p. 3). Those wishing to become PAs must now gain a recognised qualification based on a degree-level course, located in a medical school, of at least 90 weeks, followed by a year of supervised practice. It is anticipated that a professional register will be opened.

The PA's role is open to anyone with the appropriate entry qualifications, which include a first degree in a relevant science. The work involves activities, which, in some ways, appear broadly similar to those of the advanced practitioner: assessing patients and formulating diagnoses, requesting appropriate investigations, formulating treatment plans and prescribing medication (DH 2006). The main difference is that the PA is not a professional in his or her own right; a PA works *for* and is supervised *by* a doctor even though, on a day-to-day basis, a fair degree of apparent autonomy may be allowed. In contrast, an advanced nurse practitioner is a member of a recognised profession and is responsible and accountable for all aspects of the care she or he delivers to patients. Nevertheless, it is probable that, as PAs become more widely available in the National Health Service (NHS), patients will have some difficulty in distinguishing them from advanced nurse practitioners and, possibly, other roles. Advanced nurse practitioners will, therefore, need to explore ways of conveying the nature of their role to patients.

Nurse practitioners and the Royal College of Nursing

Nurse practitioners were introduced, by the Department of Health (DH), in the early 1990s as part of the strategies to reduce junior doctors' working hours. There was no overall plan regarding their role and consequently several parallel developments took place. A survey of the North Thames Region identified four categories of NPs in hospitals: those who performed specified procedures, those in charge of pre-admission clinics, designated posts in accident and emergency departments or minor injuries units and nurses who had extended their skills in order to perform certain tasks for their caseload of patients (Kendall *et al.* 1997). In contrast, a study of NPs in primary care showed them acting as the first point of contact with the health service and thus having assessment and diagnostic responsibilities similar to prototype NPs' roles in the 1980s (Burke-Masters 1986, Stillwell *et al.* 1987, Ashburner *et al.* 1997). The huge variety of posts was reflected in employment conditions. There was no national agreement about grading and in primary care NPs were initially employed by GPs rather than by the NHS.

A recent postal survey by the Royal College of Nursing (RCN) for the Nurse Practitioner Association (NPA) showed that NPs ($n = 1021$) are typically women in their mid-forties; two-thirds work in primary care; are highly qualified – 35% at Masters level – and view the core elements of their role as making autonomous decisions, assessing the health needs of patients, undertaking physical examinations, making new/initial diagnoses and formulating a diagnosis. The grading of posts varied from F to H, bands 6–8. Of the NPs, 44% reported that referrals to other clinicians and for X-rays were refused. The numbers were higher among those working in general practices. They reported feeling that their jobs were under threat, especially those who worked in hospitals. This feeling was fuelled by the introduction of the PA's role (Ball 2006).

In response to widespread concern about the employment of NPs and the roles that they were expected to fulfil, the RCN began to investigate what was happening from both a trade union and a professional perspective. The College drew on the expertise of members and a wide range of other sources, which included the National Organisation of Nurse Practitioner Faculties (NONPF), to develop a definition of an NP as 'a registered nurse who has undertaken a specific course of study of at least first degree (honours) level' and who practised in seven core domains each of which was accompanied by a set of competencies (NONPF 1995, RCN 2002). In 2008, the College revised and updated its position. The definition issued in 2002 was applied to advanced practice. Thus, according to the College, an advanced NP is 'a registered nurse who has undertaken a specific course of study of at least first degree (honours) level' (Box 1.3) (RCN 2008, p. 3). The College went on to identify seven domains for advanced nurse practitioner practice, each of which was accompanied by a set of competencies to be achieved. For example, the first domain, *assessment and management of patient health/illness status*, has 32 competencies that include critical thinking, assessing and intervening to assist patients in complex, urgent or emergency situations, performing and interpreting common screening and diagnostic tests (RCN 2008). Finally, the College set out 15 standards and criteria for courses that prepare nurses for advanced practice. These standards and criteria form the basis of a system of accreditation that enables educational institutions to ensure that their courses are 'up-to-date, of the highest quality, effective in educating nurses and the wider health care family, and to promote best practice' (RCN 2008, p. 21).

Box 1.3   Characteristics of the advanced NP

Professional autonomy and accountability over one's caseload
Diagnostic skills that include the ability and authority to initiate investigations
    and referrals to other agencies
Collaborative working with patients, other professionals and disciplines
Extended knowledge and skill base for providing treatment and care
Counselling and health education
Clinical and professional leadership

Source: Summarised from Royal College of Nursing (2008) *Advanced Nurse Practitioners. An
RCN Guide to the Advanced Nurse Practitioner Role, Competencies and Programme Accreditation.*
p 3, London, RCN.

The Nursing and Midwifery Council

The NMC received the work of the UKCC's *higher-level practice* project but made
little progress on the issue of advanced practice for some years. Finally, the Council
undertook its own consultation about a post-registration nursing framework and was
able to state that 'advanced nurse practitioners are highly experienced, knowledgeable
and educated members of the care team who are able to diagnose and treat your health
care needs or refer you to an appropriate specialist' and who carried out a specific
range of activities (NMC 2005, p. 3) (Box 1.4). Furthermore, the Council agreed that
advanced practitioners should be registered and that the role should be defined in a
way that was meaningful for patients and the public. Advanced competencies were
to be mapped against the Knowledge and Skills Framework (DH 2004b). The Council
also agreed that a policy was needed to accommodate nurses thought to be already
working as advanced practitioners (NMC 2005, p. 3).

Box 1.4   The NMC's first view of advanced nursing practice

Advanced NPs are highly skilled nurses, with extended skills and knowledge,
    who can do the following:
Examine patients physically, initiate investigations and diagnose health
    problems.
Initiate and make decisions about treatment and care, prescribe medication or
    refer patients to other sources of help.
Evaluate and alter treatment and care as appropriate.
Provide leadership and ensure that patients receive high standards of treatment
    and care.

Source: Summarised from Nursing and Midwifery Council (2005) *Implementation of a
Framework for the Standard of Post Registration Nursing Agendum 27.1 C/05/160.* December
2005. Available at http://www.nmc-uk.org.

In 2006, the NMC tried to obtain approval from the Privy Council to open a further sub-part of the nurses' part of the register in order to register advanced NPs. A letter was sent to the Privy Council in December 2005 with additional information being sent in January 2006. The Privy Council has been seeking the views of the Department of Health (England), which takes the lead on regulatory matters relating to health-care professions across the NMC (2006). In 2007, some slight progress was evident in the White Paper Trust, Assurance and Safety – the Regulation of Health Professionals in the 21st Century, which stated that 'the Department with ask the Council for Healthcare Regulatory Excellence to work with regulators, the professions and those working on European and international standards to ... the development of standards for higher levels of practice in nursing, AHPs and healthcare scientists' (NMC 2007). However, at the time of writing, no further progress has been made and the situation remains unresolved.

Conclusion

This chapter has presented a discussion of the main influences on the development of advanced practice in the United Kingdom. This development has been rather haphazard, with new roles introduced to expedite the achievement of particular policies, such as the reduction in junior doctors' working hours or as a response to public opinion about how the NHS should function. The lack of an overarching plan can be seen as providing an opportunity for experimentation but it has also served to hinder the coherent development of advanced practice and to differentiate it from other new roles. There is an urgent need for progress to allow the title of advanced practitioner to be protected and to ensure that only those who have the appropriate qualifications and experience are allowed to use it. The following key questions are intended to promote discussion about potential ways forward.

 Key questions for Chapter 1

In your field of practice:
(1) What strategies might be useful in educating the public about the advanced nursing role?
(2) How might you explain the advanced nursing role, as opposed to that of doctor, matron or PA, to patients?
(3) Assuming that the NMC will be able to register advanced practitioners, what further action, if any, should the Council take and why?

References

Ashburner, L., Birch, K., Latimer, J. and Scrivens, E. (1997) *Nurse Practitioners in Primary Care. The Extent of Practice and Research.* Keele University, Centre for Health Planning and Management.

Ashworth, P. (1975) The clinical nurse consultant. *Nursing Times* **17** (15) 574–77.

Ball, J. (2006) *Nurse Practitioners 2006. The Results of a Survey of Nurse Practitioners Conducted on Behalf of the RCN Nurse Practitioner Association*. Hove, Employment Research Ltd.

British Medical Association (2002a) *The Future Healthcare Workforce*. HPERU Discussion Paper No. 9. Available at http://www.bma.org.uk.

British Medical Association (2002b) *BMA Response to Consultation on Unfinished Business*. Available at http://www.bma.org.uk.

British Medical Association (2004) Junior Doctors' Policy Group. Available at http://www.bma.org.uk/bmapolicies.

British Medical Association (2005) *Annual Representative Meeting Policies*. Available at http://www.bma.org.uk.

British Medical Association (2006) Policy Group. *Annual Representative Meeting Policies*. Available at http://www.bma.org.uk/bmapolicies.

Burke-Masters, B. (1986) The autonomous nurse practitioner: an answer to the chronic problem of primary care. *The Lancet* **1** 1266.

Castledine, G. (1998) Clinical specialists in nursing in the UK: 1980s to the present day. Chapter 2 in *Advanced and Specialist Nursing Practice*, (eds G. Castledine and P. McGee), pp 33–54. Oxford, Blackwell Science.

Castledine, G. (2003) The development of advanced practice in the UK. Chapter 2 in *Advanced Nursing Practice*, (eds P. McGee and G. Castledine), 2nd edn. pp 8–16 Oxford, Blackwell Science.

Department of Health (1997) *The New NHS: Modern, Dependable*. London, DH.

Department of Health (1999) *Making a Difference. Strengthening the Nursing, Midwifery and Health Visiting Contribution to Health and Healthcare*. London, DH.

Department of Health (2000) *The NHS Plan. A Plan for Investment. A Plan for Reform*. Wetherby, DH.

Department of Health (2001a) *Involving Patients and the Public in Healthcare. A Discussion Document*. London, DH. Available at http://www.dh.gov.uk.

Department of Health (2001b) *Implementing the NHS Plan – Modern Matrons. Strengthening the Role of Ward Sisters and Introducing Senior Sisters*. Health Service Circular 2001/10 April. Available at http://www.dh.gov.uk/hsc.htm.

Department of Health (2001c) *More NHS Nurse Consultants*. News Desk. 10.9.01. Available at http://www.dh.gov.uk/newsdesk/archive.

Department of Health (2004a) *Modernising Medical Careers. The Next Steps. The Future Shape of Foundation, Specialist and General Practice Training Programmes*. Available at http://www.dh.gov.uk/en/PublicationsAndStatistics.

Department of Health (2004b). *The NHS Knowledge and Skills Framework and the Development Review Process*. Available at http://www.dh.gov.uk.

Department of Health (2005) *Supporting People with Long Term Conditions: Liberating the Talents of Nurses Who Care for People with Long Term Conditions*. London, DH.

Department of Health (2006) *The Competence and Curriculum Framework for the Physician Assistant*. London, DH.

Department of Health (2007) *European Working Time Directive*. Available at http://www.dh.gov.uk/en/Managingyourorganisation.

Department of Health (2007) *The White Paper Trust, assurance and safety: The regulation of health professionals*. London, DH.

Dunphy, L.M., Youngkin, E.Q. and Smith, N. (2004) Advanced practice nursing: doing what had to be done – radicals, renegades and rebels. Chapter 1 in *Advanced Practice Nursing. Essentials for Role Development*, (ed. L.A. Joel), pp 3–30. Philadelphia, F.A. Davis Co.

Hamric, A., Spross, J. and Hanson, C. (eds) (2005) *Advanced Nursing Practice. An Integrative Approach*, 3rd edn. St Louis, Elsevier Saunders.

Hunsberger, M., Mitchell, A., Blatz, S., *et al.* (1992) Definition of an advanced practice role in the NICU: the clinical nurse specialist/neonatal practitioner. *Clinical Nurse Specialist* **6** (2) 91–6.

Jasper, M. (1994) Expert: a discussion of the implications of the concept as used in nursing. *Journal of Advanced Nursing* **20** 769–76.

Kendall, S., Latter, S. and Rycroft-Malone, J. (1997) *Nursing's Hand in the New Deal. Nurse Practitioners and Secondary Health Care in North Thames.* Chalfont St. Giles, Buckinghamshire College.

The Lords Hansard (2002) *Doctors' Retirement Col.* 365–6. Available at http://www.publications.parliament.uk.pa.pahansard.

National Health Service Management Executive (1991) *Junior Doctors: The New Deal.* London, NHSME.

National Health Service Management Executive (1999) *Nurse, Midwife and Health Visitor Consultants.* Health Service Circular 1999/217 September 1999.

National Organisation of Nurse Practitioner Faculties (1995) *Advanced Nursing Practice: Curriculum Guidelines and Programme Standards for Nurse Practitioner Education.* Washington, DC, NONPF.

Nursing and Midwifery Council (2005) *Implementation of a Framework for the Standard of Post Registration Nursing Agendum 27.1 C/05/160.* December. Available at http://www.nmc-uk.org.

Nursing and Midwifery Council (2006) *Advanced Nursing Practice Update* 4 July 2006. Available at http://www.nmc-uk.org.

Nursing and Midwifery Council (2007) *Advanced Nursing Practice Update* 19 June 2007. Available at http://www.nmc-uk.org.

Royal College of Nursing (2002) *Nurse Practitioners. An RCN Guide to the Nurse Practitioner Role, Competencies and Programme Accreditation.* London, RCN.

Royal College of Nursing (2008) *Advanced Nurse Practitioners. An RCN Guide to the Advanced Nurse Practitioner Role, Competencies and Programme Accreditation.* London, RCN.

Statutory Instrument (2002) *The Working Time (Amendment) Regulations* No. 3128. Available at http://www.opsi.gov.uk/si/si2002/20023128.htm.

Stillwell, B., Greenfield, S., Drury, M. and Hull, F.M. (1987) A nurse practitioner in general nursing practice: working style and pattern of consultation. *Journal of the Royal College of General Practitioners* **37** 154–7.

United Kingdom Central Council for Nursing Midwifery and Health Visiting (1994) *The Future of Professional Practice – The Council's Standards for Education and Practice Following Registration.* London, UKCC.

United Kingdom Central Council for Nursing Midwifery and Health Visiting (1999) *A Higher Level of Practice. Report on the Consultation on the UKCC's Proposals for a Revised Regulatory Framework for Post-registration Clinical Practice.* London, UKCC.

United Kingdom Central Council for Nursing, Midwifery and Health Visiting (2002) *Report of the Higher Level of Practice Pilot and Project.* London, UKCC.

Waller, S. (1998) Clarifying the UKCC's position in relation to higher-level practice. *British Journal of Nursing, Specialist Nursing Supplement,* **7** (16) 960, 962–4.

The Working Time (Amendment) Regulations (2002) SI2002 no 3128. Available at http://www.opsi.gov.uk/si/si2002/20023128.htm.

Chapter 2

UK Health Policy and Health Service Reform

Alistair Hewison

Introduction

Nurses, midwives and health visitors make up the largest number of health profession-als and the biggest staff group in the National Health Service (NHS). Consequently, the nature of nursing work and the profession of nursing itself are fully intertwined with health and social policy development, particularly with regard to the development of advanced practice roles (Masterson 2001, p. 332). Advanced practice roles have arisen in response to, and been shaped by, a complex web of international, national and local health policies. In this context, the purpose of this chapter is to examine the UK health policy framework because without an understanding of policy and how it is developed and implemented, nurses cannot bring about change for their clients or for themselves (Maslin-Prothero and Masterson 1998).

However, examining policy is not a straightforward task. With at least five major structural reorganisations, an average of one every 5 years, along with numerous policy initiatives, the NHS has been in a state of 'permanent revolution' during its recent history (Hunter 2005, p. 209). Consequently, if a coherent and reasonably concise analysis of the overall direction of health policy is to be presented, it can, of necessity, only be selective. The approach adopted here is to take the election of the Labour government in 1997 as a starting point. This could be regarded as a somewhat arbitrary decision, because any policy initiative in health is introduced to a setting with a long and contested history (6P, Peck 2005), and so it could be argued that due attention should be given to that history. However, the scope and scale of health policy-making since 1997 provides more than enough material to work with, and ultimately the discussion has to start somewhere.

The chapter begins with a summary of the main elements of Labour's health policy. It then moves on to address the specific guidance, statements and circulars issued by bodies such as the Nursing and Midwifery Council (NMC), which relate to the introduction of advanced practice roles, as a means of tracing the process of policy implementation. The intention of doing this is not only to highlight the range of policy pressures that have influenced this area of care but also to suggest that engagement in the policy process can be considered a fundamental element of such roles. Indeed, the latest set of proposed competencies for advanced nursing practice includes a requirement that, as part of the leadership function, an approved practitioner 'participates in legislative and policy-making activities that influence an advanced level of nursing practice and the health of communities' (NMC 2005, p. 8).

An additional consideration at this point is the continuing confusion regarding the meaning, scope of and preparation for these advanced roles (Daly and Carnwell 2003). This means that in many instances their successful introduction into the organisation is dependent on the policy acumen or policy literacy of the post holder, particularly as nurses are involved in all aspects of health-care delivery and must bring their levels of knowledge and experience to influence policy decisions affecting the delivery of care to the public (Greipp 2002). The aim of this chapter is to provide some fresh insights on these important aspects of practice and to demonstrate how the notions of policy acumen and policy competence are central to advanced practice in the crowded UK health policy environment.

The policy process

Policy is not made in a vacuum and then introduced. Rather, it is the result of a complex process in which many different groups and individuals seek to exert influence to bring about change. Thus, the process of developing policy can involve pressure groups – the media, health professionals and the public – all of whom have varying levels of power to effect change. The policy development process is continuous with policy being made and adapted when it is implemented (Hanningan and Burnard 2000, Schofield 2004). There are concerns about what actually gets onto the agenda for policy development (Kingdon 1995) and/or what is necessary for policy to be implemented on the ground (6P, Peck 2005). Indeed, some suggest that to seek any notion of order or rationality in policy-making is inappropriate as it is the outcome of a messy process of 'muddling through' (Lindblom 1959, 1979), which results in decisions being made in a reactive, incremental way lacking any overall direction.

Hudson and Lowe (2004) suggest a schema for considering how policy is developed and implemented. They use a three-way classification to ensure that attention is given to the wide range of forces affecting the design of policy, as well as providing a series of vantage points that can inform its analysis. First, there are the *macro* forces that shape policy, such as globalisation and international influences. In the case of advanced practice, the importance of policy and practice from the United States is clearly of significance here. Second, the *meso-level* concerns the practice of the policy-making process itself and the institutions engaged in designing and seeing policy through to its delivery. This involves policy networks, professional bodies and other institutions and groups, which feed into the process. In terms of advanced practice, the role of the professional bodies, such as the United Kingdom Central Council for Nursing, Midwifery and Health Visiting (UKCC) and latterly the NMC, are clearly crucial players at this level of the process and can filter and change policy. Finally the *micro-level* concerns engagement between consumers and agencies, and individuals and personalities. In this context, the day-to-day interaction of advanced nurse practitioners with colleagues and clients is a crucial component of how policy is enacted. This brief summary indicates that to build a thorough understanding of the policy process, an awareness of the issues and perspectives involved is necessary (see, e.g. Hogwood and Gunn 1984, Hill and Bramley 1986, Hill 1997, Ham 2004).

Labour health policy since 1997

The Labour government, which came to power in 1997, began a process which more than doubled spending on the NHS from £33 billion in 1996–1997 to £67 billion in 2004–2005. The Labour government pledged to raise spending further to £90 billion in 2007–2008 (DH 2004). Although there has been a net overspend of £512 million in the year 2005–2006 (King's Fund 2006), by 2008 investment in the NHS as a whole was predicted to rise from £43.9 billion in 2000 to £92.6 billion (DH 2005). This increase in spending has been accompanied by a huge programme of change and modernisation. The range and scope of this activity can make it difficult to discern a clear direction of travel as the government was intent on addressing a series of issues at the same time.

The Labour government's policy since 1997 has been characterised as consisting of three *moments*, a term used to signify that policies come and go in a remarkably short space of time and are thus impossible to evaluate (Greener 2004):

1. the year 1997 based on a Fabian or socialist philosophy aimed at securing quality services
2. the year 2000 based on the 'Third Way' with a focus on performance
3. the year 2002 arising from a 'garbage' can model of policy-making emphasising choice

Terms such as *governance, choice* and *freedom* (Morrell 2006) have also been used to try and make sense of the array of policies and initiatives. An evaluation of Labour's approach to policy-making concluded that it relies on a mix of policy styles across a range of areas and that the nature of policy-making depends on both the stakeholders involved and the actual policy itself (Larsen *et al.* 2006). In other words, the nature of what is proposed and the people involved determine the approach taken. Larsen *et al.* (2006) characterise four categories of policy: service-orientated, the extension of government authority, ideologically driven and cost-intensive reforms. Clearly, these are not mutually exclusive, as they all have cost implications, but the style of implementation varies according to the content of the policy, which can be confusing for people working in and receiving health care. For example, in the case of policy relating to long-term care, agencies and patient groups outside the government had a crucial impact on the service delivery elements of the Health and Social Care Act (2001) but were largely ignored in the debate surrounding free personal care (Larsen *et al.* 2006). In many ways, this situation can be regarded as the outcome of an overall trend in the way policy is made, moving from a reliance on blueprints and central planning to manipulated emergence, which gives the impression of greater involvement in policy development by a wider group of contributors (Harrison and Wood 1999).

Thus, not only is policy development complex but it also involves ideology and incrementalism and is concerned with the art of the possible (Peckham 2000). In the current health-care environment, this has resulted in a constant stream of policies that can appear to lack coherence, leading some to regard it as a *hotchpotch* wanting an overarching strategy, reactive to events and media pressure (Greener 2004).

Within specific policy areas there have been particular challenges. Bate and Glenn (2006) report that eight policy paradoxes are associated with the introduction of National Health Service Treatment Centres (NHSTCs). For example, as NHSTCs are forced to close beds and reduce capacity in response to the introduction of independent treatment centres that have also been encouraged by the government, choice is reduced rather than increased (Bate and Glenn 2006). In another area of policy, Currie and Suhomlinova (2006) found that despite aspirations for the NHS to become a learning organisation with clear links between research and practice, the effect of using performance indicators for universities created barriers to cooperation and collaboration in research. In the context of patient choice, people without cars and those who are elderly or generally less mobile are not able to exercise as much choice, in terms of which provider to access, as others. This, in turn, may increase health inequalities rather than reduce them (Exworthy and Peckham 2006), with the effect that pursuing one policy strand undermines the aims of another. These examples illustrate that the interface between policy and practice is characterised by ambiguity of intent and unpredictability of response, making it both complex and problematic (Bergen and While 2005).

Thus, in addressing some aspects of its change agenda, such as reduction in waiting times and greater involvement of the private sector in provision, the government compromises another element such as increased choice. Similarly, in a study investigating the connection between NHS human resource policies and continuity of patient care, the conclusion was that there was simply too much happening, too quickly, with unrealistic time frames for implementation. In addition, doubts were expressed about the apparent lack of joined-up thinking between the various policy areas, which prevented the different objectives being achieved (Humphrey *et al.* 2003, p. 116).

Others are more optimistic, arguing that evidence can change the direction of policy and render it more rational (Cookson 2005). In contrast to some of the more bleak assessments presented earlier, the King's Fund (2005) argues that Labour's health reform programme has taken four main forms: clear targets and standards set nationally; regulatory inspection and assessment; central support of professionally led collaborations and market-style incentives (King's Fund 2005). The report concludes that in most areas where the government has focused policy development there have been improvements, resulting in more and better services. However, it is acknowledged that there is no evidence to show that the reforms have made a marked difference to health outcomes, particularly when considering the recent introduction of market incentives and regulation.

This brief discussion of recent trends in health policy in the United Kingdom locates the development of advanced nursing practice as just one policy strand within a vast programme of change in health care. The Labour government of the time wanted to make reform self-sustaining aimed to drive change through financial incentives and patient choice instead of targets and performance management (Ham 2006). These policies bear all the hallmarks of 'creative destruction' (Ham 2006, p. 985), that is, creating so much change and innovation that the system will ultimately adapt itself to changing circumstances instead of constantly being driven by the government (Ham 2006).

UK health policy and its implications for advanced nursing practice

The raft of policy emanating from the Department of Health (DH) and the Modernisation Agency (Bate and Glenn 2003) is part of an 'epidemic of health care reform' that has taken place over the last decade (Ham 2005, p. 192). The scope and scale of this programme of change is huge and it is not possible to examine it in detail here. Rather, examples have been drawn from key policy documents and initiatives, which illustrate how forces in policy development coalesced to create the conditions that have contributed to the development of advanced nursing practice.

A clear signal about advanced nursing practice can be found in the first major policy pronouncement after the Labour party came to power in 1997:

> The Government is particularly keen to extend the recent developments in the roles of nurses working in acute and community services. Expert nurses are taking on a leadership role, monitoring and educating nurses and other staff, managing care, developing nurse-led clinics and district-wide services. They work across organisational and professional boundaries ensuring continuity and integration of care. The Government is committed to encouraging and supporting the development of nursing practice in these ways. (DH 1997, section 6.11)

This pronouncement was carried forward into the *NHS Plan* (DH 2000) 3 years later where a little more detail was included:

> The new approach will shatter the old demarcations which have held back staff and slowed down care. NHS employers will be required to empower appropriately qualified nurses, midwives and therapists to undertake a wider range of clinical tasks including the right to make and receive referrals, admit and discharge patients, order investigations and diagnostic tests, run clinics and prescribe drugs. (DH 2000, p. 83)

Alongside this was a policy launched by the previous Conservative government to reduce the hours worked by junior doctors, which generated further impetus for considering how nursing roles could be changed (DH 1997a). For example, in a Health Service Circular from 1998, guidance is provided for NHS trusts on how to manage skill mix to facilitate the reduction. This suggested employing nurse practitioners, doctors' support workers and bed managers and indicated that there was scope for further sharing of certain clinical duties with nursing staff (HSC 1998). Later, there was a call for nursing to build on changes in roles it had already introduced (DH 1999), and more recent policy strands maintain this emphasis on changing roles, role expansion and innovation (DH 2005a, 2006).

This national and local focus on adapting nursing roles to meet the changing needs of the population and the service has continued as a result of developments in other areas of policy. The Modernisation Agency, which was established to bring about change in the NHS, was influential in this area (http://www.wise.nhs.uk/cmsWISE/Collaborate.htm). The Changing Workforce Programme, which ran from 2001 to 2005, was a national workforce modernisation programme aimed at creating new roles and moving tasks up and down the uni-disciplinary ladder. It supported health and social care organisations in implementing and evaluating role design (WISE 2006). This programme demonstrated that practitioners could function at higher or broader levels of responsibility and autonomy but, in order to do this, individuals must demonstrate that they have the requisite education, experience and competence (WISE 2006). Such outcomes are consistent with the aims of Agenda for Change (DH 2005b). This is the new pay spine for all staff in the NHS, except doctors and senior managers, which allows payment for advanced nurse practitioners at scales that equate to level 7 of the 9 bands in the new career framework (Skills for Health 2006). A job profile has also been developed (WISE 2006a). These measures provide a structure for advanced nursing practice and give an indication of how events may unfold. However, if the history of advanced nursing practice is considered, it is reasonable to conclude that there is still some way to go.

Advanced nursing practice

The enduring theme in the literature, which has examined the nature of advanced nursing practice, is the problem arising from the lack of clarity and definition concerning its nature and function (Manley 1997, Wilson-Barnett *et al.* 2000, Daly and Carnwell 2003, Bryant-Lukosius *et al.* 2004, Griffin and Melby 2006). This has been reflected in the absence of conceptual and policy consensus regarding an advanced or higher level for nurses in the United Kingdom (Atkins and Ersser 2000, p. 524). In many ways, this is not surprising. The emphasis in recent policy prescriptions on innovation and service development encourages the establishment of new roles to address specific patient and organisational needs. However, this results in a certain level of confusion because there is ambivalence on the part of the professional bodies towards the development of such roles; the post holders experience role ambiguity and there are problems in establishing effective working relationships with other personnel (Lloyd-Jones 2005). This pattern of internal contradiction is inherent in the broad sweep of current policy approaches. For example, the requirement to follow 'market principles' in the organisation of services, which will be rewarded in the form of 'payment by results' (DH 2005, p. 11), has been accompanied by the proliferation of *arms length* bodies that regulate the activities and performance of health-care professionals and NHS trusts (Crinson 2005). Thus, devolution of power to local trusts is, in reality, delegation of responsibility for administering national priorities (Lee and Woodward 2002).

In the light of this discussion, it is clear that there was a perceived need to create new roles for nurses, which would also advance the status and practice of nursing. This was strongly influenced by practice in the United States (Atkins and Ersser 2000) and has been underpinned by drives towards professionalisation and increased autonomy (Ketefian *et al.* 2001). Policy development did not occur in a planned or coordinated way and so roles were developed to meet local need, a situation that brought further confusion about titles, role boundaries and educational requirements (Daly and Carnwell 2003, Griffin and Melby 2006).

The reluctance of the UKCC, which preceded the NMC, to provide a clear policy direction in this area resulted in a prolonged period of uncertainty and lack of clarity for patients, practitioners and organisations. This was compounded by the differing views taken by the UKCC and the Royal College of Nursing concerning the nature and status of specialised and advanced practice (Scott 1998). This policy drift resulted in a situation, which, ironically, was summarised by the UKCC:

> A wide range of job titles, such as nurse practitioner, advanced midwife practitioner and clinical nurse specialist, are in common use across the United Kingdom to describe such developing roles but consumers, employers and the profession have expressed concern about what such titles mean. The titles are not protected and the UKCC has not set standards for the preparation of title holders. (UKCC 1999, p. 10)

However, this did not appear to discourage the creation of new roles, and recommendations on how to introduce them were produced (Woods 1998, Bryant-Lukosius *et al.* 2004). Interestingly, part of step 5 in Bryant-Lukosius and DiCenso's nine-stage model involves *defining the role*, indicating that questions relating to what the role actually is and what it is for persist; this in turn affects the way the role is managed.

When returning from programmes of preparation, many practitioners found that no consideration had been given to what they would do in their organisation (Daly and Carnwell 2003). In some areas of the United Kingdom, a regional approach was taken to address local need. For example, in the West Midlands, the Health Authority supported the development of programmes of preparation for advanced nursing practice, funding study and replacement costs for 225 students over 3 years (Dunn and Morgan 1998). Further funding was provided to evaluate this initiative (Wilson-Barnett *et al.* 1999, Carnwell *et al.* 2001). This indicated some general improvements in quality, although the difficulties associated with the integration of the roles into mainstream practice were reported as a significant issue. In a broader study of innovative roles, McKenna *et al.* (2006) found that the level of infrastructure support provided for new roles was not uniform.

This lack of clarity and support has further implications in that evaluating the effectiveness of advanced nursing practice is problematic because it is difficult to measure what direct impact it has on health outcomes (Daly and Carnwell 2003) or whether it provides value for money (McKenna *et al.* 2006). Clearly, the particular policy environment in the United Kingdom has shaped the development of advanced nursing practice. This can be demonstrated further if the approach taken in the Republic of Ireland is considered.

In contrast to the United Kingdom, Furlong and Smith (2005) report that in Ireland a clear national policy for the definition and introduction of advanced nurse and midwifery practice resulted in a smooth introduction. They concluded that an analysis of the policy demonstrates that it is unique in the international arena in terms of its clarity. This may not be the full account, as other work from Ireland indicates that problems persist, in the emergency care setting at least (Griffin and Melby 2006). However, there are clear benefits in having a coherent policy that incorporates a definition of the role.

This issue now appears to have been addressed in the United Kingdom with the NMC finally acknowledging that a definition is needed if the role is to be implemented widely (NMC 2005). The current definition is as follows:

> Advanced nurse practitioners are highly experienced, knowledgeable and educated members of the care team who are able to diagnose and treat your health care needs or refer you to an appropriate specialist if needed. (NMC 2005, p. 9)

Perhaps, most importantly, in policy terms there is a proposal to make advanced nurse practice a registerable qualification.

> Only nurses who have achieved the competencies set by the Nursing and Midwifery Council for a registered advanced nurse practitioner are permitted to call themselves by this title. The title will be protected through a registerable qualification on the Council's register. (NMC 2005, p. 3)

There have also been some attempts to achieve consistency across a range of policy areas. For example, the proposed NMC competencies for advanced nurse practice have been mapped against the Knowledge and Skills Framework, which is a central component of the Modernising Careers framework (NHS Modernisation Agency 2004).

More recently, the importance of locating advanced nursing practice in a broader plan to update nursing career choices and pathways has been identified in the report *Modernising Nursing Careers* (DH 2006a). A consultation exercise undertaken to garner views on the proposals put forward in this document found that

> Respondents supported regulation of advanced practice believing this to be a necessary step in enforcing compliance and investment in education in order to ensure the safety of the public. (DH 2008, p. 13)

This has been reinforced by the outcome of the 'Darzi review'. This is a report compiled by Lord Darzi, the parliamentary undersecretary of state for health, which drew on a wide-ranging process of consultation with patients, staff and the public to develop a vision of the health service for the twenty-first century (DH 2008a). In a supplementary report, focusing specifically on the workforce it is stated that

> In order to assure the quality of outcomes and to protect the public appropriately, clear nationally agreed standards for advanced level practice are required for nurses working in extended, advanced and autonomous roles, both in the NHS and in the independent and other sectors. We will work with the Council for Healthcare Regulatory Excellence and the professional regulators to ensure a consistent definition of advanced practice across the health professions. (DH 2008b, p. 20)

However, a final decision from the Privy Council to approve the opening of a new part of the NMC Register is still awaited (NMC 2006) and so there is likely to be a further period of uncertainty before the matter is settled.

Advanced nurses as policy implementers

The political processes by which policy is mediated, negotiated and modified during its formulation continue when it is implemented by individuals in the clinical setting. Policy may thus be regarded as both a statement of intent on the part of those seeking to change or control behaviour, and a negotiated outcome of the implementation process (Barrett 2004). In the past, few nurses practising in clinical settings have regarded health policy as a nursing issue (Toofany 2005), believing that public policy is of little relevance to practice (Spenceley *et al*. 2006). However, it is at this *micro-level* that practitioners and patients engage, making nurses *de facto* creators of health policy through the exercise of their professional autonomy, regardless of whether they are aware of this or not (Hanningan and Burnard 2000, Hudson and Lowe 2004). If advanced nurse practitioners are to secure the longevity of their posts and to realise the full potential of their practice, then engagement with policy on a number of levels would seem to be required. Indeed, policy activity is identified as a key element of the role in recent guidance (WISE 2006) and some of the recommendations that have been made for action in this area are examined in the following text.

First, all nurses can assess, identify and articulate for, or on behalf of, patients' broad policy factors, provide information to patients on options for impacting policy and work to effect policy change through policy advocacy organisations (Malone 2005, p. 136). Malone (2005) recommends the development of *policy literacy*, whereby nurses develop some understanding of the way policy issues have been shaped by larger social forces and how they have been addressed in the past. By understanding more about policy and acting to shape the introduction of policy, advanced nurse practitioners can work towards ensuring that the role is designed to serve patients' best interests.

Second is *policy advocacy*, which is knowledge-based action intended to improve health by influencing system-level decisions (Spenceley *et al*. 2006). This is presented as a logical extension of patient advocacy to engagement in strategies to bring about change at the level of government. Calls for nurses to increase their involvement in the policy arena have been made before (see, e.g. Hennessy 2000, ICN 2001, Lee *et al.* 2002) and can appear somewhat daunting. However, if *policy advocacy* of this type is achieved, it would be one means of ensuring that a nursing voice contributes to the process of policy development.

Third, *policy competence*, is a level of involvement that lies somewhere between policy literacy and advocacy (Longest 2004). Presented as a collection of skills that managers need if they are to be successful in leading their organisations, it can also be applied to advanced nursing practice. Policy competence requires not only a thorough understanding of policies that are relevant to the strategic management of organisations but also an understanding of the complex process through which policy is made (Longest 2004). With such understanding, advanced nurse practitioners will be well equipped to guide the development of their own roles within the organisation.

Advanced nurse practitioners need to not only be conversant with the language of health policy but also have the ability to effectively navigate health policy arenas. Health policy activity is now the single largest influence in determining the nature of nursing and heath-care provision (Whitehead 2003). Without some level of *policy competence* those in advanced nursing roles are likely to flounder.

Conclusion

The amount and pace of reform in the NHS has led some to conclude that we are all engaged in a massive experiment and that the only certainty is that at no other time in the NHS's history has its future appeared so uncertain (Hunter 2005). Within the broad sweep of this experiment, advanced nursing practice is one, albeit, crucial element. However, a number of factors have come together to create a policy environment that is conducive to the further development of the role: national government regards it as essential; a pay and career structure is being put in place to support it and the NMC is committed to adding it to the professional register as a recognised level of practice.

It is difficult to predict how things will develop from this point because the NHS has recently experienced a period of financial deficit. Estimated at about £700 million in 2005–2006, the deficit led to job losses and cutbacks (Ham 2006). Also, greater pressure on the system resulting from a combination of rising numbers of older people, increased public expectations and advances in medical technology could lead to a £6 billion funding gap in 20 years' time (Glasby 2008). Add to this the current 'credit crunch', which is going to add to the tax burden of all those in the United Kingdom, western Europe and the United States (Peston 2008), and it becomes clear that when there are such immediate and pressing concerns, advanced nursing practice may slip down the policy agenda again. However, the commitment to reform remains (Ham 2006), the importance of regulating advanced nursing practice has been identified (DH 2008b) and advanced nurse practitioners themselves may be able to affect policy more directly, particularly as it is a requirement of their roles. This is likely to be a crucial determinant of their future. The term *advanced* is recognised as reflective of a relative developmental position, where practice is progressive or is in some way ahead in terms of its development. Advanced practice within a health-care system will always be a relative and changing position, relevant to a particular socio-historical context. As such, it is in the nature of advanced practice that it will remain subject to ongoing debate (Atkins and Ersser 2000, p. 523). Advanced nurse practitioners need to be actively contributing and indeed leading that debate in order that the evidence concerning patient benefits that can accrue from their practice is available to inform the formulation of local and national policy.

 Key questions for Chapter 2

In your field of practice:
(1) Which elements of the policy environment have contributed to the development of advanced nursing practice?
(2) In what ways can nurses actively influence the policy agenda in order to establish advanced nursing roles?
(3) What skills do advanced nurse practitioners need if they are to engage more directly in the policy process?

References

6P and Peck, E. (2005) The role of organisational development in policy implementation in health care. In *Organisational Development in Health Care*, (ed. E. Peck), pp 27–42. Oxford, Radcliffe Press.

Atkins, S. and Errser, S.J. (2000) Education for advanced nursing practice: an evolving framework. *International Journal of Nursing Studies* **37** 523–33.

Barrett, S.M. (2004) Implementation studies: time for a revival? Personal reflections on 20 years of implementation studies. *Public Administration* **82** (2) 249–62.

Bate, P. and Glenn, R. (2003) Where next for policy evaluation? Insights from researching National Health Service modernisation. *Policy & Politics* **31** (2) 249–62.

Bate, P. and Glenn, R. (2006) 'Build it and they will come' – or will they? Choice, policy paradoxes and the case of NHS treatment centres. *Policy & Politics* **34** (4) 651–72.

Bergen, A. and While, A. (2005) 'Implementation deficit' and 'street level bureaucracy': policy, practice and change in the development of community nursing issues. *Health and Social Care in the Community* **13** (1) 1–10.

Bryant-Lukosius, D., DiCenso, A., Browne, G. and Pinelli, J. (2004). Advanced practice nursing roles: developing, implementation and evaluation. *Journal of Advanced Nursing* **48** (5) 519–29.

Carnwell, R., Daly, W. and Helm, R. (2001) *An Evaluation of the Developing Role of the Advanced Nurse Practitioner and its Impact upon Primary Care Practice*. Birmingham, NHS Executive.

Cookson, R. (2005) Evidence-based policy making in heath care: what it is and what it isn't. *Journal of Health Services Research & Policy* **10** (2) 118–21.

Crinson, I. (2005) The direction of health policy in New Labour's third term. *Critical Social Policy* **25** (4) 507–16.

Currie, G. and Suhomlinova, O. (2006) The impact of institutional forces upon knowledge sharing in the UK NHS: the triumph of professional power and the inconsistency of policy. *Public Administration* **84** (1) 1–30.

Daly, W.M. and Carnwell, R. (2003) Advanced nursing practitioners in primary care settings: an exploration of developing roles. *Journal of Clinical Nursing* **12** 630–42.

Daly, W.M. and Carnwell, R. (2003) Nursing roles and levels of practice: a framework for differentiating between elementary, specialist and advancing nursing practice. *Journal of Clinical Nursing* **12** (2) 158–67.

Department of Health (1997) *The New NHS Modern Dependable*. London, DH.

Department of Health (1997a) *Junior Doctors Hours: The New Deal*. London, HMSO.

Department of Health (1999) *Making a Difference: Strengthening the Nursing, Midwifery and Health Visiting Contribution to Health and Health Care*. London, DH.

Department of Health (2000) *The NHS Plan: A Plan for Investment, a Plan for Reform*. London, DH.

Department of Health (2004) *Annual Report*. London, The Stationery Office.

Department of Health (2005) *Health Reform in England: Update and Next Steps*. London, DH.

Department of Health (2005a) *Creating a Patient Led NHS: Delivering the NHS Improvement Plan*. London, DH.

Department of Health (2005b) *Agenda for Change: NHS Terms and Conditions Handbook 3617*. London, DH.

Department of Health (2006) *Our Health, Our Care, Our Say: A New Direction for Community Services*. London, DH.

Department of Health (2006a) *Modernising Nursing Careers*. London, DH.

Department of Health (2008) *Towards a Framework for Post-Registration Nursing Careers: Consultation Response Report*. London, DH.

Department of Health (2008a) *High Quality Care for All – Next Stage Review Final Report*. London, DH.

Department of Health (2008b) *A High Quality Workforce – NHS Next Stage Review*. London, DH.

Dunn, L. and Morgan, E. (1998) Creating a framework for clinical nursing practice to advance in the West Midlands Region. *Journal of Advanced Nursing* **7** 239–43.

Exworthy, M. and Peckham, S. (2006) Access, choice and travel: implications for health policy. *Social Policy & Administration* **40** (3) 267–87.

Furlong, E. and Smith, R. (2005) Advanced nursing practice: policy, education and role development. *Journal of Clinical Nursing* **14** (9) 1059–66.

Glasby, J. (2008) *'Who cares?' Policy Proposals for the Reform of Long-term Care*. Health Services Management Centre Policy Paper. Birmingham, University of Birmingham.

Greener, I. (2004) The three moments of New Labour's health policy discourse. *Policy & Politics* **32** (3) 303–16.

Greipp, M.E. (2002) Forces driving health care policy decisions. *Policy, Politics & Nursing Practice* **3** (1) 35–42.

Griffin, M. and Melby, V. (2006) Developing an advanced nurse practitioner service in emergency care: attitudes of nurses and doctors. *Journal of Advanced Nursing* **56** (3) 292–301.

Ham, C. (2004) *Health Policy in Britain*, 5th edn. Houndmills, Palgrave-Macmillan.

Ham, C. (2005) Lost in translation? Health systems in the US and the UK. *Social Policy & Administration* **39** (2) 192–209.

Ham, C. (2006) Creative destruction in the NHS. *British Medical Journal* **332** (7548) 984–5.

Hanningan, B. and Burnard, P. (2000) Nursing, politics and policy: a response to Clifford. *Nurse Education Today* **20** (7) 519–23.

Harrison, S. and Wood, B. (1999) Designing health service organization in the UK, 1968–1998: from blueprint to bright idea and 'manipulated emergence'. *Public Administration* **77** (4) 752–68.

Health Service Circular (1998) *Reducing Junior Doctors' Hours* HSC1998/240. Wetherby, National Health Service Executive.

Health and Social Care Act (2001) Available at http://www.dh.gov.uk/en.

Hennessy, D. (2000) The emerging themes. In *Health Policy and Nursing – Influence, Development and Impact*, (eds D. Hennessy and P. Spurgeon), pp 1–38. Houndmills, Macmillan Press Limited.

Hill, M. (1997) *The Policy Process in the Modern State* 3rd edn. London, Prentice Hall.

Hill, M. and Bramley, G. (1986) *Analysing Social Policy*. Oxford, Basil Blackwell.

Hogwood, B.W. and Gunn, L.A. (1984) *Policy Analysis for the Real World*. Oxford, Oxford University Press.

House of Commons (2001) *The Health and Social Care Act*. London, HMSO.

Hudson, J. and Lowe, S. (2004) *Understanding the Policy Process*. Bristol, The Policy Press.

Humphrey, C., Ehrich, K., Kelly, B., Sandall, J., Redfern, S., Morgan, M., *et al.* (2003) Human resources policies and continuity of care. *Journal of Health Organization and Management* **17** (2) 102–21.

Hunter, D.J. (2005) The National Health Service 1980–2005. *Public Money & Management* **25** (4) 209–12.

International Council of Nurses (2001) *Guidelines on Shaping Effective Health Policy*. Geneva, ICN.

Ketefian, S., Redman, R.W., Hanucharurnkul, S., Masterson, A. and Neves, E.P. (2001) The development of advanced practice roles: implications in the international nursing community. *International Nursing Review* **48** 152–63.

Kingdon, J.W. (1995) *Agendas, Alternatives and Public Policies*. 2nd edn. New York, Longman.

King's Fund (2005) *An Independent Audit of the NHS under Labour (1997–2005)*. London, King's Fund.

King's Fund (2006) *Deficits in the NHS (June Briefing)*. London, King's Fund.

Larsen, T.P., Taylor-Gooby, P. and Kananen, J. (2006) New Labour's policy style: a mix of policy approaches. *Journal of Social Policy* **35** (4) 629–49.

Lee, M.B., Tinevez, L. and Saeed, I. (2002) Linking research and practice: participation of nurses in research to influence policy. *International Nursing Review* **49** 20–6.

Lee, S. and Woodward, R. (2002) Implementing the Third Way: the delivery of public services under the Blair government. *Public Money & Management* **22** (4) 49–56.

Lindblom, C.E. (1959) The science of 'muddling through'. *Public Administration Review* **19** 78–88.

Lindblom, C.E. (1979) Still muddling, not yet through. *Public Administration Review* **39** 517–25.

Lloyd-Jones, M. (2005) Role development and effective practice in specialist and advanced practice roles in acute hospital settings: systematic review and meta-synthesis. *Journal of Advanced Nursing* **49** (2) 191–209.

Longest, B.B. (2004) An international constant: the crucial role of policy competence in the effective strategy management of health service organizations. *Health Services Management Research* **17** (2) 71–78.

Malone, R.E. (2005) Assessing the policy environment. *Policy, Politics & Nursing Practice* **6** (2) 135–43.

Manley, K. (1997) A conceptual framework for advancing practice: an action research project operationalizing an advanced practitioner/consultant nurse role. *Journal of Advanced Nursing* **6** 179–90.

Maslin-Prothero, S. and Masterson, A. (1998) Continuing care: developing a policy analysis for nursing. *Journal of Advanced Nursing* **28** (3) 548–53.

Masterson, A. (2001) Cross-boundary working: a macro political analysis of the impact on professional roles. *Journal of Clinical Nursing* **11** (3) 331–39.

McKenna, H., Richey, R., Kenney, S., Hasson, F., Sinclair, M. and Poulton, B. (2006) The introduction of innovative nursing and midwifery roles: the perspective of healthcare managers. *Journal of Advanced Nursing* **56** (5) 553–62.

Modernisation Agency (2004) *A Career Framework for the NHS* (Version 2 June 2004). London, DH.

Morrell, K. (2006) Policy as narrative: new labour's reform of the National Health Service. *Public Administration* **84** (2) 367–85.

Nursing and Midwifery Council (2005) *Mapping of the NMC Approved Competencies against the KSF. Annexe 1 of Implementation of a Framework for the Standard for Postregistration Nursing (C/05/160)*. London, NMC.

Nursing and Midwifery Council (2006) *Advanced Nursing Practice* – update 4 July 2006. http://www.nmc-uk.org/aArticle.aspx?ArticleID = 2038. Accessed 8 September 2006.

Peckham, S. (2000) Health-care policy making. In *Nursing for Public Health: Population-Based Care*, (eds P.M. Craig and G.M. Lindsay). pp 241–61. Edinburgh, Churchill Livingstone.

Peston, R. (2008) *The Day the Bill Arrived*. 29th September 2008. BBC News. http://www.bbc.co.uk/blogs/thereporters/robertpeston. Accessed 2 October 2008.

Schofield, J. (2004) A model of learned implementation. *Public Administration* **82** (2) 283–308.

Scott, C. (1998) Specialist practice: advancing the profession? *Journal of Advanced Nursing* **28** (3) 554–62.

Skills for Health (2006) *Key Elements of the Career Framework*. http://www.skillsforhealth.org.uk/careerframework/key_elements.php. Accessed 21 September 2006.

Spenceley, S.M., Reutter, L. and Allen, M.N. (2006) The road less travelled: nursing advocacy at the policy level. *Policy, Politics & Nursing Practice* **7** (3) 180–94.

Toofany, S. (2005) Nurses and health policy. *Nursing Management* **12** (3) 26–30.

United Kingdom Central Council for Nursing Midwifery and Health Visiting (1999) *A Higher Level of Practice*. London, UKCC.

Whitehead, D. (2003) The health-promoting nurse as a health policy career expert and entrepreneur. *Nurse Education Today* **23** 585–92.

Wilson-Barnett, J., Barriball, L., Jowett, S., Reynolds, H. and West, P. (1999) *Evaluation of Advancing Nursing Practice Courses in the West Midlands*. Birmingham, King's College London/NHS Executive West Midlands.

Wilson-Barnett, J., Barriball, K.L., Reynolds, H., Jowett, S. and Ryrie, I. (2000) Recognising advancing nursing practice: evidence from two observational studies. *International Journal of Nursing Studies* **37** 389–400.

WISE (2006) http://www.wise.nhs.uk/cmsWISE/Workforce+Themes/Using Task Skills Effectively/roleredesign. Accessed 21 September 2006.

WISE (2006a) National Profiles for Nursing Services. http://www.wise.nhs.uk. Accessed 15 November 2006.

Woods, L. (1998) Implementing advanced practice: identifying the factors that facilitate and inhibit the process. *Journal of Clinical Nursing* **7** 265–73.

Chapter 3

Advanced Practice in Allied Health Professions

Paula McGee and David Cole

Introduction

The programme of UK National Health Service reforms that began after the general election in 1997 was intended to reduce health inequalities by providing better access to treatment and care delivered through patient-focused services (DH 2000a). Implicit in the achievement of this vision of what the health service could become was the need for professionals to adopt new ways of working that inspired and promoted confidence based on the application of current best practice and guidance from the National Institute of Clinical Excellence (http://www.nice.org). Ten areas of practice were identified as particularly influential in bringing about the changes envisaged to provide faster access to diagnostic tests and treatment, overhaul services to reduce queues and length of hospital stay and apply a systematic approach across a range of disciplines so that patients received coherent packages of care based on actual need (Box 3.1). This was seen as particularly important for those with complex or long-term conditions who needed continuity in care from a multi-professional team (DH 2005). Promoting and maintaining health was also high on the agenda; people were to be encouraged to maintain their own health and engage in more self care activities rather than rely on professionals (DH 2000a). Partnerships with organisations, communities and individuals were regarded as a base from which health professionals could actively promote health and enable healthy people to stay well (DH 2000b).

Box 3.1   Ways of improving access to diagnostic tests and treatment

Day surgery
Managing variation in patient discharge to reduce length of stay
Managing variation in patient admissions to reduce cancellations
Avoiding unnecessary follow-up appointments
Increasing the reliability of therapeutic interventions
Providing a systematic approach to care for people with long-term
    conditions
Reducing queues
Redesigning and extending professional roles

Source: Summarised from NHS Modernisation Agency (2004) *10 High Impact Changes for Service Improvement and Delivery.* Available at http://www.ogc.gov.uk/documents.

These reforms offered many new opportunities to members of allied health professions; the field was wide open, giving freedom to professionals who were now able to creatively exploit their potential in pioneering new forms of practice and service delivery. They were to be supported in this by changes in the recruitment and education of aspiring allied health professionals and the introduction of an improved career structure linked to Agenda for Change, which encouraged experienced practitioners to continue working with patients rather than move into teaching or management; this retention of expertise in the practice setting was to be achieved through the introduction of the *therapist consultant* (DH 2000b, p. 37; 2004).

This chapter begins by outlining the introduction of this consultant's role and then describes how it has developed in two professions: physiotherapy and radiography/sonography. The chapter closes with a discussion of the similarities and differences between consultants' posts in the two professions based on a combination of McGee and Castledine's view of the concept of advanced practice and the ideas of Hamric *et al.* (2005) about the core competencies. The chapter closes with some key questions for further reflection on this subject.

The introduction of the consultant allied health professional

The term *allied health professional* spans a very wide range of activities directed, in each case, towards clearly defined roles in the care and treatment of patients (Box 3.2). These roles form a central part of the delivery of health care in both hospital and community settings, complementing the input from medicine and nursing. It was, therefore, entirely appropriate that the health service reforms should include allied health professionals in order to provide better access to care based on multi-professional working focused on patient need rather than traditional professional boundaries (DH 2000b, 2003a). Allied health professionals had the potential to act as the first point of contact with the health service and refer patients on to others as necessary. They could manage and lead teams, request diagnostic tests, treat and even prescribe within stated protocols; they could play a central role in the planning and delivery of health care (Box 3.3).

Box 3.2   Allied health professions

Art therapists	Occupational therapists
Chiropodists/podiatrists	Orthoptists
Chiropodists/podiatrists	Paramedics
Diagnostic radiographers	Physiotherapists
Dietitians	Prosthetists and orthotists
Drama therapists	Speech and language therapists
Music therapists	Therapeutic radiographers

Source: Summarised from Department of Health (2000b) *Meeting the Challenge. A Strategy for the Allied Health Professions*. London, DH.

Box 3.3   Ten key roles for allied health professionals

To provide a first, and in some cases only, point of contact with health services

To provide complete episodes of care by assessing, initiating investigations, diagnosing and treating patients within established protocols

To discharge and/or refer patients to other services, working with protocols

To educate and guide colleagues and other professionals, patients and carers

To develop new ways of working that transcend the traditional boundaries of practice in their field

To provide clinical and professional leadership

To ensure that practice is based on the best available research evidence

To promote health

To participate in planning and policy development at organisational level

To work collaboratively with other professions and services

Sources: Summarised from Department of Health (2003a) *Implementing a Scheme for Allied Health Professionals with Special Interests*. London, DH.
Department of Health (2003b) *Ten Key Roles for Allied Health Professionals*. London, DH.

While the intention was to provide more accessible, appropriate and coherently organised care for patients, the health service reforms also instigated the first systematic consideration of post-qualifying practice in allied health professions. Fulfilling the expectations outlined in the National Health Service (NHS) plan (DH 2000a) required an appraisal of the nature of practice beyond qualification and how this was likely to change in response to both the reforms and advances in medicine to determine what patients, the professions and society wanted allied health professionals to provide.

In determining a way forward it was essential to address the issue of post-qualifying education, which had so far developed in a rather haphazard manner that was 'informal, uni-disciplinary, unaccredited, and not tied into organisational requirements' (DH 2000b, p. 34). There were signs of a move towards improvements in this situation by linking the professional schools of study with higher education establishments but these had to be developed into courses leading to qualifications that carried both academic and professional weight. Better education was needed to equip practitioners with the knowledge and skills required for their new roles, especially with regard to interprofessional working, which was intended to facilitate understanding of the contributions that diverse professions can make to patient care. At the same time, the qualifications gained would be recognisable outside the respective professions, allowing practitioners to demonstrate their competence alongside those of other professionals. Post-qualifying education and a new pay structure were to pave the way for new clinical career pathways.

However, realising potential in this way was not without problems. Developing new roles, pioneering new practice, redesigning services and so on does not alter the fact that, on each working day, practitioners still have to attend to a whole range of day-to-day activities. These may be regarded as routine but remain very important to patients: accompanying patients learning to walk on artificial limbs, helping patients re-learn how to dress themselves, breast screening and toenail trimming. The problem is that performing these tasks inevitably reduces the amount of time available for expanding practice. If society, the professions and the policy makers wanted a different type of allied health professional, it was essential to find a solution for the day-to-day, routine tasks. The solution arrived in the guise of assistant practitioners who were first introduced in radiography 'to take mammograms under the supervision of a radiographer. The aim is to enable radiographers to extend their role into some of the tasks traditionally undertaken by radiologists, in turn increasing the capacity of the NHS to deliver the national breast screening service' (DH 2000b, p. 36). Assistant radiography practitioners were to receive a recognised form of training at National Vocational Qualification (NVQ) levels 2 or 3 and are now accredited as assistant practitioners in order for their qualifications and practice to be recognised within the NHS. For individuals to receive accreditation, it is necessary for them to demonstrate knowledge, skills and achievement at the relevant level as identified in the Society and College of Radiographers' Curriculum Framework of 2008 (http://www.sor.org). Assistant practitioners' roles have now been extended to other allied health professionals and training is provided at foundation degree level under the auspices of Foundation Degree Forward (http://www.fdf.ac.uk).

The introduction of assistant practitioners and better post-qualifying education were complemented by a new pay structure that dispensed with the old grading system and purported to take account of the work that individual practitioners actually did (DH 2004). Allied health professionals were free to develop new roles and services. For example, in Birmingham, a new community orthoptic/optometric service meant that children who were identified in school as needing glasses could be seen in a local clinic/health centre thus reducing both waiting time and inconvenience to parents who might otherwise have to travel. In Hinchingbrooke Healthcare, NHS trust patients could access physiotherapy without the need for referral by a doctor. This scheme improved clinical outcomes, increased access to the service and reduced waiting times. Patients sought and received treatment at an earlier stage, thus avoiding complications. In a final example, in Bournemouth, a dietician-led coeliac clinic ensured that patients were seen quickly after diagnosis to receive education about the need for a gluten-free diet. This improved patient satisfaction and reduced the number of patients needing to see the consultant gastroenterologist (DH 2003a).

Crucial to the success of many of these initiatives were the new *therapist consultants*, senior and experienced practitioners whose role was to 'provide better outcomes for patients by improving quality and services' and by strengthening 'professional leadership' (DH 2000b, p. 37). *Therapist consultants* were envisaged as having four core functions: 'expert practice; professional leadership and consultancy; education, training and development and practice and service development research and evaluation' (DH 2000b, p. 37). Therapist consultant posts were to be specific to single professions and so the core functions were to be interpreted by each allied health profession to fit its own area of expertise.

Physiotherapy

The Chartered Society of Physiotherapists (CSP) began to address the concept of specialist roles in 2001. There appears to be no definitive statement about specialist practitioners prior to this date although individuals undoubtedly developed expertise in working with people who had particular conditions. In some instances this expertise was recognised at local level through the creation of specific posts with enhanced grading but there was no national strategy and no pay scales (CSP 2001). From 2001 the CSP, with government support (DH 2000a), introduced three roles, all of which were considered to be forms of advanced practice. *Clinical specialist roles* were linked to specific fields, such as sports medicine, paediatrics, learning disabilities, trauma and orthopaedics and were intended to encompass clinical practice, clinical teaching, evaluation, practice and service development (Table 3.1). *Extended scope practitioners' roles* were those in which practice extended outside the usual scope of physiotherapy.

The CSP's descriptions of these two roles clearly drew on the works of Benner (1984) and Dreyfus and Dreyfus (1980) in terms of levels of skill acquisition. The key component of each was described as advanced clinical reasoning, which the CSP regarded as 'the thinking and decision-making processes associated with a physiotherapist's assessment and management of a patient (*and*) therefore related to the individual practitioner's exposure to learning, clinical practice and experience' (CSP 2001, p. 4). These two roles were to form stepping stones to *consultants' roles* based on a specified core of activities centred on direct and expert clinical practice (Table 3.2). Principal competencies focused on professional leadership, education,

Table 3.1   Clinical specialists in physiotherapy.

Aspect of the role	Role activities
Clinical practice	Advanced clinical knowledge, skills and reasoning; the ability to deal with complex cases; providing clinical support for colleagues
Clinical teaching	Providing in-service education across a region; acting as mentor/supervisor; participating in post-qualifying education; involvement in teaching at pre- and post-qualifying levels
Evaluation	Active participation in research and audit; the ability to critically appraise evidence and apply it to practice; publishing in peer reviewed journals
Practice and service development	Clinical supervision of colleagues; participation in clinical governance activities; active participation in professional networks providing clinical leadership

Source: Summarised from Chartered Society of Physiotherapists (2001) *Specialisms and Specialists: Guidance for Developing the Clinical Specialist Role.* Available at http://www.csp.org.uk.

Table 3.2   Consultant physiotherapy role.

Aspect of the role	Role activities
Expert clinical practice	Includes the management of a complex caseload, creating and developing evidence-based protocols for care with best practice examples, recognition as a national/international expert, responsibility for ensuring that the moral and ethical dimensions of practice are addressed, high levels of personal autonomy
Professional leadership	Incorporates effective communication, developing innovative models of practice, acting as a change agent and contributing to the development of quality care through clinical governance
Practice and service development, research and evaluation	To ensure high-quality evidence-based care, providing leadership for the development of protocols, contributing to the implementation of national policies, evaluating clinical services, identifying gaps in the evidence base and initiating research, forming partnerships with higher education settings
Education and professional development	To promote and facilitate a learning environment, providing education in a specific field of clinical expertise, enhancing links between practice, professional bodies, academic and research institutes

Source: Summarised from Chartered Society of Physiotherapists (2002) *Physiotherapist Consultant (NHS): Role, Attributes and Guidance for Establishing Posts.* Available at http://www.csp.org.uk.

practice and service development. Eligibility for consultant posts required a suitable career portfolio and preparation at Master's level (CSP 2002).

Radiography and sonography

A shortage of both radiographers and radiologists coupled with the development of new imaging technologies created an increased demand for services that provided the impetus for change in radiography. The aim was to create a better career structure that would attract and retain more recruits, providing equal pay for work of equal value (DH 2004). This culminated in the introduction of four practitioner roles: assistant, professional practitioner, advanced practitioner and consultant practitioner (Table 3.3). In this context, sonography is a form of advanced practice for which a postgraduate diploma is required. The sonographer is an autonomous practitioner who performs a wide-ranging role, defines the scope of practice of others and continuously develops the field. Not all sonographers are radiographers; midwives, nurses, obstetricians, cardiology technicians and medical physicists can also perform sonography if they have the appropriate qualifications.

To date the Society of Radiographers has not issued any position papers on the advanced or consultant roles and there seems to be a dearth of literature on this subject. However, analysis of job descriptions has highlighted commonalities that may be deemed key components. This analysis shows a move towards autonomous practice. First, advanced and consultant practitioners are able to formulate diagnoses and compile reports. In comparison, a professional practitioner possesses only limited autonomy. He or she produces images that are reported and acted upon by a radiologist or another clinician. Therefore, in the ordinary course of events, the professional practitioner does not make decisions or recommendations that affect the management of the patient, whereas advanced and consultant radiographers are able to do both.

Second, there is evidence of pioneering new practice in response to the introduction of new imaging modalities such as computerised tomography (CT) scanning, magnetic resonance (MR) imaging and medical ultrasound. Advanced and consultant radiographers have become specialist experts. They have developed new skills and are now able to offer more comprehensive care and services. For example, they are now able to perform complete examinations such as barium meals and enemas and procedures that involve injecting contrast media or radiopharmaceuticals. Previously a radiologist would be required for certain parts of these procedures; in pioneering new practice advanced and consultant radiographers are able to provide more holistic services to patients (Table 3.3).

Pioneering new skills and a more holistic approach have led to increased professional autonomy; advanced and consultant radiographers are now equipped to make diagnoses and report on medical images, thus blurring the traditional boundaries between their sphere of practice and that of other professional roles. This particular development is attributable to the introduction of ultrasound examinations. In this procedure, diagnosis is made on the spot, from a dynamic image produced while scanning. Once it was established that radiographers could act as diagnosticians

Table 3.3   Levels of practice in radiography.

Assistant practitioner	Radiographer	Advanced radiographer	Consultant radiographer
Qualifications			
Does not hold a degree in radiography	Bachelor's degree in radiography	Bachelor's degree in radiography Postgraduate degree in radiography	Bachelor's degree in radiography Postgraduate research degree in radiography
Responsibilities			
Carries out imaging procedures Assists radiographers in carrying out specialist procedures Undertakes administrative and clerical duties	Assesses the referral information Selects and performs the most appropriate X-ray examination within departmental protocols Explains the procedure to the patient and obtains his or her consent Assesses the X-ray images for diagnostic value and reports to the referring practitioner Maintains records Teaches and supervises assistant practitioners and students Participates in/undertakes clinical audit and quality assurance Evaluates and implements research as appropriate Undertakes rotation into specialist areas for further professional development	Specialises in a specific field of radiography Performs imaging techniques traditionally carried out by radiologist/other clinician Formulates diagnoses and reports to referring practitioners Manages staff and service provision Teaches and supervises professional and assistant practitioners and students Performs clinical audit and quality assurance Evaluates and implements research as appropriate and may participate in research investigations	Expert practice Provides advice and clinical leadership to radiography practitioners and the NHS trust about evidence-based changes in practice Undertakes research Coordinates specialist training

in sonography, it was only a matter of time before this became the norm in other modalities such as conventional radiography and barium studies (Table 3.3).

Third, analysis of job descriptions shows that advanced and consultant radiographers work collaboratively with members of other professions and thus require a greater understanding of their clinical roles in relation to patient care. They are thus well placed to provide leadership both within their own profession and in a multi-disciplinary context.

Fourth, they have teaching and supervisory responsibilities in relation to colleagues within their own profession: assistant practitioners, students and professional practitioners. However, their roles as expert specialists also carry teaching and supervisory responsibilities towards members of other professions who may be learning specific procedures such as sonography.

Fifth, as pioneers of new practice and autonomous practitioners, advanced and consultant radiographers are responsible for ensuring that both their practice, and that of those they teach or supervise, are based on the best available evidence. They also have roles in monitoring, evaluating and auditing practice to ensure that patients receive a high standard of care. While some evidence may be based on professional opinion, research is of paramount importance. Expert specialists have a role in ensuring that research findings are introduced into practice in an appropriate way and in participating in or leading projects. Finally, advanced and consultant practitioners have managerial roles as practice development cannot be achieved without control over personnel and resources (Table 3.3).

Sonography: an example of advanced radiography role

A majority of sonographers (over 70%) are radiographers and require a postgraduate qualification in order to practice. This qualification enables them to specialise in what is still a new imaging modality, practise autonomously, formulate diagnoses and report directly to the referring clinician. The scope of practice and the range of activities indicate that sonography can be viewed as a form of advanced practice (Table 3.4). However, it must be noted that, until 2000, the term *advanced practitioner* was not associated with radiography or sonography and was generally applied only to nurses. In 2000 a number of NHS trusts advertised for sonographers, offering a senior I radiographer pay scale plus a reporting or advanced practitioner allowance of normally £2000–4000 per annum. This led to sonographers in other trusts applying pressure on their employers for a similar allowance. As a result, the West Midlands Sonography Action Group (WMSAG) was formed in 2000 with the aim of addressing issues such as poor pay, reporting and training allowances and work-related upper limb disorders prevalent among radiographers (http://health.groups.yahoo.com/group/wmsag). Pressure from this group led more NHS trusts in the region to award reporting/advanced practitioner allowances and with some advertising for advanced practitioners rather than sonographers.

Sonography is a highly skilled, non-invasive, flexible and dynamic procedure in which real-time images of organs are visualised directly onto a screen and measured. Each person may require variations in technique and measurement because of differences in size and shape. Consequently, the sonographer must adapt his or her skills to suit the dimensions of each person's body and in order to obtain optimal visualisation.

Sonographers, therefore, have to be able to conduct detailed assessments in order to identify exactly where the site of the problem might lie. For example if a patient presents with haematuria, the appropriate ultrasound examination would be that of kidneys, ureters and urinary bladder. However, if information supplied by the patient suggests that other areas should be examined then the sonographer can extend the examination.

The sonographer is able to obtain the patient's consent for the procedure without recourse to another professional and to move beyond simply explaining the procedure to the patient towards interpreting what appears on the screen. This dynamic image

Table 3.4   A comparison of sonography with the advanced radiography role.

Advanced radiographer	Sonographer
Qualifications	
Bachelor's degree in radiography Postgraduate degree in radiography	Bachelor's degree in radiography Postgraduate degree in radiography
Responsibilities	
Specialises in a specific field of radiography Performs imaging techniques traditionally carried out by radiologist/other clinician Formulates diagnoses and reports to referring practitioners Manages staff and service provision Teaches and supervises professional and assistant practitioners and students Performs clinical audit and quality assurance Evaluates and implements research as appropriate and may participate in research investigations	Specialises in a specific field, i.e. sonography Performs imaging techniques traditionally carried out by radiologist/other clinician Performs detailed assessment of the patient, adapts skills to suit the dimensions of each person's body; makes decisions about what to include in the scan Interprets the images and formulates a diagnosis Produces a report for the referring clinician Discusses images and their implications directly with patients Develops protocols in line with technological developments and monitors their impact Ensures that equipment is fit for purpose Teaches and supervises trainee sonographers Conducts clinical audits and evaluates all aspects of practice and changes in practice including adherence to protocols, performance in measuring anatomical structures, accuracy of diagnosis and patient satisfaction Evaluates and implements research as appropriate and may participate in research investigations

is not usually recorded; the only permanent records are still images. Interpretation and diagnosis have to take place immediately and a decision made as to whether to extend the examination. For instance, if a scan of a woman's pelvis were to reveal a mass lesion then the examination may be extended in order to search for metastases in the upper abdomen (Table 3.4).

This means that the sonographer is able to discuss findings with the patient, as they occur. For example, in obstetric ultrasound, the sonographer will be able to explain the significance of what appears on the screen. In some instances, this may involve the very sensitive matter of breaking bad news to parents if there are abnormalities present. Finally, the sonographer is equipped to compile reports for referring clinicians in ways that convey the nature and significance of the images obtained and the diagnosis. This is crucial in ensuring that clinicians are correctly informed so that suitable treatment and care can be provided for the patient (Table 3.4).

In addition to these activities, the sonographer's role requires managerial skills. Newly qualified practitioners would expect to spend 80–90% of their work time in scanning but ultrasound departments generally have fewer members of staff compared to radiology departments, typically five or six. Thus all members of staff carry some managerial responsibility especially as sonographers are usually senior members of staff with at least 2 years' experience as radiographers before enrolling on an ultrasound degree programme and so should have the professional maturity and experience required. Their responsibilities include the setting and monitoring of standards. Ultrasound is a rapidly developing imaging modality. Images are becoming much clearer and of higher resolution. Technological advances such as colourflow imaging mean that a map of the blood vessels can be superimposed on the normal greyscale image. With each improvement more information is available to the operator and so protocols, which specify the organs to be examined, need to be continually updated. Sonography managers have a role in developing and monitoring protocols that reflect these advances in technology (Table 3.3).

The management role extends to ensuring that equipment is maintained and fit for purpose. There is a range of quality assurance tests that can be undertaken on ultrasound equipment to measure the image characteristics and accuracy of measurement. Clinical audit is also required to evaluate all aspects of practice and changes in practice. Typical areas for clinical audit include adherence to protocols, performance in measuring anatomical structures, accuracy of diagnosis and patient satisfaction. All sonographers will have learnt the fundamentals of research in their postgraduate ultrasound degree and there is an expectation that they will carry out research to ensure that current practice is evidence based. Finally, a majority of ultrasound departments have heavy teaching commitments because of the number and range of practitioners learning to undertake scans. These may include radiographers and midwives, junior doctors specialising in obstetrics and trainee radiologists (Table 3.4).

Are these new roles in physiotherapy and radiography/sonography advanced?

The limited literature on new roles in physiotherapy and radiography/sonography create something of a challenge in determining whether these are advanced. McGee's views (see Chapter 4) about advanced practice in nursing help to provide at least one way of approaching this topic. First is the issue of *professional maturity;* the advanced practitioner should have gained experience in a wide variety of settings with diverse client groups, hold a senior position and have obtained formal academic qualifications beyond initial degree level. This, she argues, is the foundation for autonomous practice. In physiotherapy and radiography/sonography this *professional maturity* is evident in that the roles appear to require the type of clinical knowledge, skills and reasoning that can only be developed through working with patients and postgraduate study is mandatory (CSP 2001).

Second, McGee argues that advanced practice requires the confidence and ability to *challenge the status quo*, introducing new approaches to practice – new ideas, new technologies. Inherent in this is the vision and drive to critically appraise traditional professional boundaries and the extent to which the preoccupations, priorities and concerns associated with them enable or hinder practitioners in meeting the demands of a modern health service. Advanced practice in this context requires high levels of interpersonal competence that enable the practitioner to collaborate with members of different professions and to provide leadership. These qualities appear to be implied rather than overtly stated in physiotherapy and radiography/sonography roles.

Third, McGee proposes that the advanced practitioner engages in critical practice, adopting an open minded and reflective approach to care (Brechin 2000). Critical analysis of and reflection about situations provide a basis for identifying where change is required and the form it should take. In McGee's view the advanced practitioner *pioneers innovations*, providing leadership for new ventures and ensuring that, once established, these are audited and evaluated. Both physiotherapy and radiography/sonography roles have the potential to pioneer innovations. Certainly, advanced radiography and sonography roles seem to demonstrate a move to new developments in practice that are systematically monitored (Table 3.4). Like nursing, clinical specialists and consultants in physiotherapy are clearly expected to be active in professional networks and develop care (Table 3.2).

A second way of determining whether physiotherapy and radiography/sonography roles are advanced is to examine competencies. Hamric *et al.* (2005, p. 95) argue that while nursing is a very diverse professional field, advanced nursing practice roles share a number of common elements at the centre of which is direct clinical practice. Practitioners may engage in many other activities but 'direct care expertise provides the foundation necessary' for competency in every other aspect of the role. This statement appears to apply also to physiotherapy and radiography/sonography. In both cases, specialist, extended, advanced and consultant roles carry a strong emphasis on direct engagement with patients, especially those with complex needs. Given that advanced roles in all three professions were initially intended to ensure that clinical expertise remained in patient care rather than being transferred to management or education, this emphasis on direct clinical practice is important.

Hamric *et al.* (2005) go on to identify six other core competencies that underpin direct practice: research, clinical and professional leadership, collaboration, ethical decision-making skills, acting as a consultant for others and providing expert coaching and guiding. Advanced radiography/sonography roles include elements of research, collaboration, leadership, teaching and supervision but ethical decision-making and consultation are implied rather than stated (Table 3.4). Likewise, consultant physiotherapy roles encompass consultancy, leadership, research and education but collaboration and ethics are not overtly included (CSP 2002). Thus both roles appear to fulfil some but not all of the criteria of Hamric *et al.* (2005) for advanced practice.

Nevertheless, using these criteria shows that there appears to be sufficient similarity between advanced practice in nursing and the two allied health professions considered here, indicating the possibility of some emergent consensus about the nature of advanced practice. However, the influence of theoretical ideas drawn from nursing may simply have been transferred to physiotherapy without critical evaluation of their suitability and applicability. It is possible that, in the wake of the publication of the NHS plan, some allied health professionals simply seized on whatever was available in order to launch their own developments and that more time and research are needed to determine whether the theoretical ideas developed by nursing can be applied across professional boundaries. Radiography and sonography appear to have taken a completely different approach. The combination of staff shortages, new technologies, low pay and other grievances created a catalyst for change that was effected by lobbying employers. Theoretical considerations seemed not to have featured in this and yet some of the ideas put forward by nurse theorists are discernible in sonography roles. There is an urgent need for research to determine in more detail the competencies required for advanced practice in these and other allied health professions and the theoretical ideas that underpin them.

Conclusion

This chapter has presented an account of the introduction of consultant roles in allied health professions. While health service reforms provided the impetus for change, each professional body concerned has begun to configure consultant posts in ways that are commensurate with its sphere of practice. In doing so, they appear to have drawn heavily on nursing theory about advanced practice. However, more research is needed to determine whether this is the most suitable approach and more literature is needed to stimulate debate. The following key questions are intended to promote discussion on this issue.

 Key questions for Chapter 3

In your field of practice:
(1) How might advanced competencies in physiotherapy and radiography/ sonography be explored?
(2) What might a set of pan-professional core competencies for advanced practice contain and why?
(3) To what extent might a set of pan-professional core competencies for advanced practice help or hinder patient-centred care and why?

References

Benner, P. (1984) *From Novice to Expert: Excellence and Power in Clinical Nursing Practice*. Menlo Park, California, Addison Wesley.

Brechin, A. (2000) Introducing critical practice. Chapter 2 in *Critical Practice in Health and Social Care*, (eds A. Brechin, H. Brown and M. Eby), pp 25–47. Buckingham, OUP.

Chartered Society of Physiotherapists (2001) *Specialisms and Specialists: Guidance for Developing the Clinical Specialist Role*. Available at http://www.csp.org.uk.

Chartered Society of Physiotherapists (2002) *Physiotherapist Consultant (NHS): Role, Attributes and Guidance for Establishing Posts.* Available at http://www.csp.org.uk.

Department of Health (2000a) *The NHS Plan. A Plan for Investment. A Plan for Reform.* Wetherby, DH.

Department of Health (2000b) *Meeting the Challenge. A Strategy for the Allied Health Professions.* London, DH.

Department of Health (2003a) *Implementing a Scheme for Allied Health Professionals with Special Interests.* London, DH.

Department of Health (2003b) *Ten Key Roles for Allied Health Professionals.* London, DH.

Department of Health (2004) *Agenda for Change. Final Agreement.* Available at http://www.dh.gov.uk.

Department of Health (2005) *Supporting People with Long Term Conditions: Liberating the Talents of Nurses Who Care for People with Long Term Conditions.* London, DH.

Dreyfus, S.E. and Dreyfus, H.L. (1980) *A Five Stage Model of the Mental Activities Involved in Directed Skill Acquisition.* Unpublished report supported by the Air Force Office of Scientific Research (Contract F49620-79-C-0063). Berkeley, University of California.

Hamric, A., Spross, J. and Hanson, C. (2005) *Advanced Nursing Practice. An Integrative Approach*, 3rd edn. St Louis, Elsevier Saunders.

NHS Modernisation Agency (2004) *10 High Impact Changes for Service Improvement and Delivery.* Available at http://www.ogc.gov.uk/documents.

Chapter 4

The Conceptualisation of Advanced Practice

Paula McGee

Introduction

In the previous edition of this book, McGee and Castledine presented their ideas about the nature of advanced nursing practice. In their view advanced practice was 'a state of professional maturity in which the individual demonstrates a level of integrated knowledge, skill and competence that challenges the accepted boundaries of practice and pioneers new developments in health care' (McGee and Castledine 2003, p. 24). This chapter presents an updated examination of this definition in the light of current developments in advanced nursing in the United Kingdom and changes in the roles of allied health professionals. The chapter begins with a brief overview of the context in which advanced practice has developed but then goes on to discuss the current view of advanced practice on which this book is based. This discussion examines the three core elements of McGee's ideas in more detail and then moves on to consider their application to allied health professions. The chapter closes with some key questions for further debate.

The context of the development of advanced practice

Advanced practice is an evolving concept first developed by nurses in rural areas of the United States. It subsequently attracted considerable interest in many different countries and societies in response to continued technological advances, the increased complexity of health care, structural changes in health-care delivery and changing health-care needs (Schober and Affara 2006). These four factors provided opportunities for nurses to extend their roles and develop new forms of practice particularly in primary care settings and especially with regard to the prevention and management of communicable diseases such as tuberculosis, malaria and HIV/AIDS (Schober and Affara 2006). In taking advantage of these opportunities and as the most numerous part of any health service, nurses demonstrated that, given suitable education, they had a considerable amount of untapped potential. The report of the Global Advisory Group on Nursing and Midwifery, therefore, encouraged governments to exploit this as a means of making health services more appropriate and accessible to vulnerable and marginalised groups while, at the same time, meeting escalating societal expectations and grappling with rising costs (World Health Organisation 2000).

The Global Advisory Group's vision implied that nursing could develop in response to local requirements and the social context of each society; extended, specialist, advanced and other roles could, therefore, be developed in response to specified needs. While this afforded strengths in terms of freedom to explore the most suitable local solutions to health-care needs, the development was, in the long term, hampered by a lack of agreement about the nature of advanced practice. Eventually, the International Council of Nurses defined the advanced practitioner as 'a registered nurse who has acquired the expert knowledge base, complex decision-making skills and clinical competencies for expanded practice, the characteristics of which are shaped by the context and/or country in which she/he is credentialed to practice. A master's degree is recommended for entry level' (International Council of Nurses 2002). The council went on to delineate a broad scope of practice that reflected an emphasis on professional autonomy, enhanced assessment and diagnostic skills and clinical expertise. The advanced practitioner was seen as the potential first, and in some instances, the only point of contact between the patient and the health service. The council also recommended that each country should introduce specific legal and regulatory mechanisms to ensure that the professional titles given to advanced practitioners were protected and to allow the nurses concerned to diagnose, prescribe medication and perform other activities outside the scope of current legislation (International Council of Nurses 2002, Schober and Affara 2006). Nevertheless, there is still a considerable amount of work to be done in interpreting the council's views and applying them to practice in each country.

Moreover, the professional and political debates about advanced practice are no longer confined to nursing. As nursing has demonstrated the ability to undertake advanced roles, incorporating at times the work that was previously the preserve of medicine, questions have arisen about the untapped potential of other health-care professions to do likewise (DH 2000a, b). The ensuing debates have made clear that, both in nursing and in allied health professions, there are levels of practice beyond initial qualification for which some kind of additional preparation is required. These levels of practice are needed to provide treatment and care within the increasingly complex field of health care. They are not medicine, although they may incorporate some aspects of it; rather, they are new directions that enable separate professional roles to meet modern health-care needs.

This development in allied health professions calls into question the nature of advanced practice. Nursing has clearly led the way in exploring this concept, formulating theoretical ideas and definitions that reflect its sphere of practice. Other professions such as physiotherapy have borrowed heavily from nursing discourse to determine the nature of advanced practice for their own particular fields (Chartered Society of Physiotherapists 2002). Inherent in this situation is the possibility that advanced practice contains elements that can be shared across professional boundaries.

The nature of advanced practice

The ideas with which this chapter began were based on McGee and Castledine's experience as senior nurses working as consultants in National Health Service (NHS) trusts and their research documenting certain aspects of the national development of advanced nursing practice in England (McGee and Castledine 2003). It was also strongly influenced by the United Kingdom Central Council (UKCC)'s work on higher-level practice, in which Castledine took a lead role (UKCC 2002). Recent events, such as the Nursing and Midwifery Council (NMC)'s and Royal College of Nursing (RCN)'s statements about advanced practice, have required a degree of reappraisal and the remainder of this chapter presents a current explanation of the three core elements of professional maturity, challenging *professional boundaries* and *pioneering innovations* (McGee and Castledine 2003, NMC 2005, RCN 2008) (Figure 4.1).

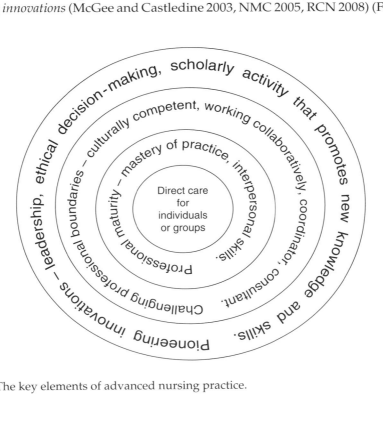

Fig. 4.1   The key elements of advanced nursing practice.

Professional maturity

Direct practice is the essential criterion for all advanced roles irrespective of the profession in which the practitioner is based (Manley 1998, Hickey and Patton 2003, Hamric 2005) (Figure 4.1). Those who do not engage in direct practice cannot be considered to be advanced practitioners. Nursing and allied health work is primarily aimed at providing treatment and care directly to patients, their relatives, carers and communities; thus, advanced status depends first and foremost on performance. Direct treatment and care can take diverse forms: working with individuals or groups, working towards crisis prevention or intervention, teaching through example, forming partnerships with patients or carers or looking after those with complex or unusual needs (Koetters 1989). A key component of this direct practice is a broad repertoire of technical and clinical knowledge and skills, acquired through practice in a wide range of settings and with diverse patient populations (Spross 2005). This repertoire and experience equip the advanced practitioner to deliver culturally competent treatment and care based on multiple strategies and interventions. Thus, advanced practice is inherently flexible as the practitioner can select the course of action that needs to be taken rather than rely on a single approach.

However, technical and clinical knowledge and skills do not, of themselves, mean that the practitioner is working at an advanced level. Direct practice requires engagement with patients as people – listen attentively to what they say and interact effectively with them, regardless of their background and circumstances. Achieving this type of engagement takes time and effort. Most importantly, it requires practitioners to work on themselves, to become aware of their personal interactional styles and how these may differ from those used by patients (Campinha-Bacote 1994, 2002). Such work on the self can be painful; attitudes and prejudices have to be consciously addressed in terms of their capacity to affect interaction and strategies devised to offset negative consequences. Individuals cannot always stop being who they are but, as professionals, they can develop personal insights and strategies that serve to enhance their interpersonal capabilities. In other words, achieving interpersonal competence is dependent on a form of emotional labour on the self (Smith 1992).

Formal education at postgraduate level is an essential part of this labour, raising consciousness, challenging perceptions and understanding while, at the same time, enhancing technical knowledge and skills. Education facilitates the integration of theoretical ideas with those gained through experience to enable the advanced practitioner to function as a mature professional whose qualifications can be readily understood by members of other disciplines and who is a master practitioner (Oberle and Allen 2001).

Challenging professional boundaries

Health professions have tended to develop in response to either the needs of under-served populations, such as those requiring physical rehabilitation, or technological advance, for example, the use of radiation. Each grew to occupy a specific niche within health services, providing treatment and care at the discretion of the patient's doctor who was regarded as having overall control and responsibility. Thus the doctor could decide to refer a patient for physiotherapy but if that therapist thought that the patient would benefit from help with speech problems, the physiotherapist could only recommend this to the doctor, who could then choose whether to act on this.

This pyramidal system that placed the doctor at the top is no longer viable. There is now no room for such autocracy, however benign it may appear to be. The complexity of modern health care means that no single profession, even medicine, can encompass all the expertise needed to treat and care for patients. Referring every decision to a single profession creates a cumbersome system that can work to patients' disadvantage, especially if they need urgent intervention. It also undermines the professionals whose expertise is either ignored or over ridden. Technological and clinical advances have not only brought changes to initial professional education in all fields but also contributed to an increase in the amount and level of post-qualifying education required. The result is highly qualified professionals with extensive expertise about which members of other professions may be ill-equipped to make decisions. One example is sonography. This is a specialist field in radiography and one which requires high levels of expertise and education, which may in time lead to the formation of a new professional group.

Policy makers reflect the need for change, seeking to place the patient at the centre of activity – to act and make choices in ways that are appropriate for the individual concerned rather comply unquestioningly with professional dictates. In this context doctors, nurses and allied health professionals may form only part of the sources of help and advice available to the patient. Consequently, within a modern health-care system, professionals have to find new ways of working together for the benefit of patients. The advanced practitioner is well placed to broker such a development. Extensive experience in diverse settings provides a sound understanding of the various professional roles that contribute to the specific care setting. Interpersonal competence provides a basis for empowering colleagues to work collaboratively as a means of achieving seamless care for patients (Figure 4.1).

Collaboration is 'a dynamic, interpersonal process in which two or more individuals make a commitment to each other to interact authentically and constructively to solve problems and learn from each other to accomplish identified goals, purposes or outcomes' (Hanson and Spross 2005a, p. 344). It may also be described as 'a dynamic, transforming process of creating a power-sharing partnership' among patients, professionals and carers in order to improve health and quality of life (Sullivan 1998, p. 19). Collaboration is dynamic because it requires the motivation to address a specific purpose to which all those concerned must contribute if success is to be achieved; it is, therefore, both problem and solution focused (Sullivan 1998). That purpose may differ but the underlying commitment is essential. For example, collaboration may be required to address a particular patient need, supervise and teach students or to introduce new technology (Keuhn 2004). No one can act alone in any of these situations because each person has knowledge, skills, expertise and experience that complement another's and which are perceived as valuable (Hanson and Spross 2005a, Sullivan 1998). Thus, the first and most essential element of collaboration is the clinical credibility of the practitioners concerned and their ability to articulate clearly what they are able to do, their strengths as well as their individual and professional limitations. This requires the professional maturity of the advanced practitioner and confidence in one's own abilities while at the same time valuing the skills and expertise of colleagues in other disciplines.

Valuing one's own and others' expertise contributes to the transformative nature of collaboration. It enables individual professionals to recognise themselves and others as equals, each able to freely put forward their contributions, discuss, cooperate and even disagree or criticise without deference. Those involved may all be advanced practitioners from different professions consulting with and referring to one another easily. Alternatively, an advanced practitioner may facilitate collaboration as a means of enabling colleagues to improve their competence (Keuhn 2004). In both examples, collaborators have to be able to engage outside their own professional spheres. To do so they have to be able to depend on each other. Trust and respect are essential so that 'they can count on satisfactory resolution of the problem even when they know as individuals that they may have approached the situation differently' (Hanson and Spross 2005a, p. 360).

Equality, trust, respect and partnership distinguish collaboration from other styles of working. Team work may incorporate some of these characteristics but teams are usually based on some form of hierarchical structure (Sullivan 1998). Collaboration is not consistent with inequality; traditional health-care hierarchies do not allow the freedom and creativity that collaboration can provide because someone can always veto whatever is proposed.

This is not to say that collaboration may not require coordination and leadership. Coordination is essential in ensuring that the contribution of each collaborator takes place at an appropriate time in the patient's overall treatment and care. Coordination is a neglected topic. A patient with bronchopneumonia will require treatment and care from several different disciplines including medicine, nursing, physiotherapy, dietetics and possibly occupational therapy. Someone has to take responsibility for ensuring that the patient has adequate rest periods and is not over-tired by too many interventions being delivered at the same time. The rhetoric of patient choice seems at times to be based on the assumption that patients can do this for themselves. A few may be able to do so but, for the majority, poor health, social circumstances or a combination of the two, make this nigh on impossible. This is particularly the case when patients have multiple diagnoses that require treatment from several separate sources. For example, an elderly patient may be receiving treatment and care for cancer while also suffering from arthritis, oral thrush, an underactive thyroid and eczema. Engagement in direct care means that the advanced practitioner is able to develop a comprehensive picture of the patient's needs and develop a clear strategy based on what the patient wants to happen and what is feasible. This may mean that the advanced practitioner has to advocate for the patient to collaborating colleagues, adopting a non-judgemental approach to helping them understand the patient's view of the situation and what it is like to be the recipient of the collaborative venture (Reinhard *et al.* 2004). It also means empowering the patient to take an active part in decision-making.

Coordination and advocacy emphasise an important aspect of collaboration: a willingness to look at new ideas without being obstructive and to reflect on and give due consideration to the views of others; to assist and cooperate with them when there are difficulties. Inevitably this will involve some conflict. Collaborators need to be able to manage conflict effectively and be willing to moderate, conciliate, arbitrate and respect people's differences in order to assist the team to continue effectively (Keuhn 2004). Working cooperatively means respecting the skills, expertise and contributions of colleagues, treating them fairly and communicating effectively while remaining accountable for one's own professional conduct (NMC 2004). The advanced practitioner has the interpersonal competence and experience to provide leadership by facilitating power-sharing. Collaborators need not rely on one person to provide leadership. Depending on the goals to be achieved, the role of leader may rotate as differing professional expertise may be required at various stages (Hanson and Spross 2005a, Sullivan 1998). However, such rotation can only be considered if the collaborators feel able to trust each other to the extent of transferring authority and power from one to another as the situation demands (Sullivan 1998).

A key consideration here is the context in which collaboration takes place. Health services tend to run along hierarchical lines with designated individuals fulfilling specific roles and functions. Responsibility and accountability are clearly defined management terms. In such contexts, collaborative working in which leadership rotates presents a challenge to the status quo. Thus while collaborative working is supported and encouraged by health policy, it may be limited by what the individual organisation will allow. Moreover, the advanced practitioner may find that professional regulation militates against true collaboration by retaining the pre-eminence of the doctor. For instance, some US states require the advanced nurse practitioner to work under the supervision of a doctor thus perpetuating a system of professional dependence (Phillips 2007). Consequently, the advanced practitioner may find that collaborative ventures have to be negotiated around such restrictions which may in turn limit success (Keuhn 2004). Dependence on medical support may militate against the development of collaborative ventures that are not valued by medicine and thus contribute to the medicalisation of advanced practice (Carroll 2002). Consequently, the advanced practitioner must have a thorough understanding of the way in which the organisation functions and why, and the ability to think and act politically (O'Grady 2005). Challenging professional boundaries, therefore, requires the advanced practitioner to be culturally competent in organisational terms, understanding thoroughly *the way we do things round here* (Jason Martin 2006). This understanding forms a basis for systems advocacy, complex negotiation in which the advanced practitioner seeks to help the organisation to reconsider its values and attitudes expressed in its policies and procedures (Reinhard *et al.* 2004).

Pioneering innovations

The advanced practitioner engages in *critical practice*, which facilitates the identification of need, opportunities for change and future possibilities (Figures 4.1 and 4.2). *Critical practice* begins with critical analysis in which the identification of need arises from engagement in direct practice with patients. Listening to patients' concerns, assessing their responses to treatment and care leads the advanced practitioner to critically analyse the effectiveness of interventions and patients' experiences. This analysis leads directly to *critical reflection*, which allows the advanced practitioner to develop two complementary but distinct ways of knowing.

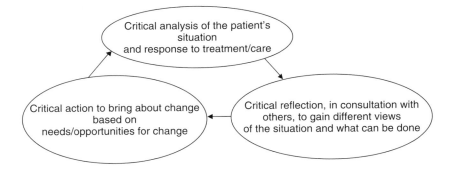

Fig. 4.2   The elements of critical practice. Summarised from Brechin (2000).

The first is theoretical knowing, *knowing that*, which is concerned with describing, explaining and predicting events. The second is practical knowing, *knowing how*, that is rooted in the performance of activities. Benner's (1984) study set out to clarify practical nursing knowledge, 'knowledge that accrues over time in the practice of an applied discipline' (Benner 1984, p. 1), and which cannot always be explained theoretically. The development of practical knowledge is based on the recognition that patients do not present their problems in the straightforward manner of textbooks; no two patients have identical needs. The development of expertise, therefore, requires more than the knowledge and skills provided by formal education. Professionals need 'an active synthesis of skill, an art of practice which goes beyond established boundaries' (Schön 1983, p. 19) and that takes into account 'the process by which we define the decision to be made, the ends to be achieved, the means which may be chosen' (Schön 1983, p. 40). To achieve this synthesis the professional draws on different types of knowledge that, in nursing, may include empirical, ethical, aesthetic and personal domains (Carper 1978). Reflection may be undertaken alone but it is more productive if others are involved. In consulting with others, the advanced practitioner is able to gather feedback from diverse sources: patients, relatives, other professionals and managers.

Critical reflection enables the advanced practitioner to clarify what is going well, what, and for whom, problems have arisen. It can facilitate the development of paradigm cases, a term used by Benner (1984) to denote situations that in some way challenge the advanced practitioners' view of the *status quo* and from which individuals learn to change their practice. Such cases serve to guide future practice by allowing practitioners to grasp situations quickly. Thus critical reflection can serve to educate colleagues and students or provide guidance for future practice situations.

Critical reflection can also serve as a basis for *critical action* in which the advanced practitioner facilitates ethical decision-making about the best course of action to be taken. This requires an understanding of theories about ethics and application of these in ways that facilitate an ethical working environment in which all concerned feel able to express their views. Such an environment 'supports and values the critical exchange of ideas and promotes collaboration' (Hamric and Reigle 2005, p. 391). Interpersonal skills are vital here in helping those involved to identify and articulate problems and clearly separate feelings from events. As with collaboration, conflict may arise because of individual values or differences of opinion about what should be done. The advanced practitioner has the skills to act as broker so that all parties can hear and try to understand each other. This allows unhelpful or resistant behaviour or positions to be brought into the open and challenged constructively so that consensus or a compromise can be reached (Hamric and Reigle 2005).

The critical action to be taken may lead the advanced practitioner to experiment with new and radical approaches to care or service provision. For example, critical analysis of and reflection about the experiences of some orthopaedic patients may show that they experience persistent pain. Complaints about the effectiveness, and the unwelcome side effects of analgesic drugs, indicate a need for new approaches to pain relief. Acupuncture is a technique that originated in traditional Chinese medicine and involves the insertion of needles into specific points on meridians in the body. There is evidence to suggest that, for some people, this provides pain relief without the side effects of medication. It may, therefore, be appropriate for advanced practitioners to gain the qualifications necessary to use acupuncture as a part of their repertoire in the management of pain (Oliver 2004, The British Medical Acupuncture Society, http://www.medical-acupuncture.co.uk.).

What is important in such a development is that there is clear justification for the course of action selected and that those concerned understand what is involved. This means that managers and senior personnel in the organisation must concern themselves with proposed new initiatives. They are responsible for ensuring that such initiatives are clearly thought out in terms of the anticipated benefits, costs and any potential difficulties. They must also ensure that members of staff concerned achieve the competence required for the performance of their new activities. Policies and procedures must be formulated to address practice standards and monitor performance. The advanced practitioner will be able to assist in this through systems advocacy and in facilitating rational debate.

People often respond emotionally to new ideas; they get carried away by enthusiasm or feel so threatened that they automatically oppose anything new. To counter this, the advanced practitioner needs to help others to think clearly by devoting an equal amount of time to each of six activities: gathering information about what is proposed, identifying the ways in which the proposal might work in the setting concerned, examining the value and benefits of what is proposed, expressing feelings, looking honestly at what may go wrong and identifying the management issues involved (De Bono 1991). In this way the proposed development can be examined from multiple perspectives; everyone has a chance to contribute but no single point of view is allowed to dominate until all the angles have been considered.

An additional strength in this approach is that it allows the advanced practitioner to ensure that new developments are firmly embedded in the organisation and that they are clearly justified in practice. Too often advanced practice developments are defined in terms of setting up nurse-led clinics or taking on prescribing roles. These activities are not, of themselves, advanced practice; in nursing, for example, specialists and other practitioners may run clinics or prescribe within their speciality but they are not advanced practitioners. However, clinic work and prescribing may become part of the advanced practitioner's repertoire if they are required as part of that practitioner's direct engagement with patients.

Finally, critical practice and rational thinking enable the advanced practitioner to identify aspects of practice that require investigation. These may range from evaluating new initiatives to leading and conducting a research team and take place at several different levels in the organisation (Box 4.1). The degree and level of involvement depends on the situation and the individual advanced practitioner's strengths. Advanced practitioners often seem to take a narrow view, believing that they should be *doing research projects* but a broader perspective shows that there are many different possibilities (Box 4.1). What matters is that the advanced practitioner has the skills to engage in scholarly activity that promotes new knowledge and skills. How this is achieved, whether it is through the self or others, is not particularly important.

Box 4.1   The advanced practitioner's involvement in research

Developing academic research skills
Facilitating the developing of critical skills that enable staff to understand and
    critique research reports
Encouraging junior colleagues to work with experienced researchers to
    investigate a particular topic
Undertaking small-scale project work that demonstrates the ability to apply
    research skills
Facilitating collaborative working as a basis for research
Evaluating treatment and care
Working as a member of a research team
Leading a research team
Working within the organisation to provide resources and support for
    research
Acting as a source of advice and support for researchers

Inherent in all this activity – *pioneering new practice, challenging professional boundaries, achieving professional maturity* – is the need for leadership (Figure 4.1). In advanced practice, leadership is a process in which leaders and followers work together to create shared goals and work collaboratively towards these. Transformational leadership raises followers' aspirations and enables them to achieve their own goals (Marriner Tomey 1993). Transformational leadership 'occurs when people interact in ways that raise each other to higher levels of motivation and morality. Leaders motivate, stimulate, share with, conciliate and satisfy their followers in an interdependent, interactive exchange' (Hanson and Spross 2005b; p. 306).

Transformational leadership is essentially a democratic process in which power is shared rather than concentrated in one individual (McGee 2005). It may occur at clinical, professional or organisational levels and is characterised by four elements: *envisioning* what is to be achieved, *enabling* followers to understand the vision and collaborate with them to achieve this, *empowering* followers to develop and achieve and *energising*, inspiring followers to achieve. The advanced practitioner uses these elements to lead others in developing and providing the best possible treatment and care for patients (Hanson and Malone 2000, Close 2003, Hanson and Spross 2005b).

Is advanced practice a generic term?

This examination of advanced practice has been inevitably drawn on nursing research and experience as these provide most of the sources available for such a discussion. However, this is not to imply that advanced practice is the sole preserve of nursing. Professional maturity would seem to be a necessary requisite for the development of roles in allied health professions. Post-qualifying education is essential in enabling practitioners to develop the academic and professional knowledge and skills needed to meet the needs of patients in a modern health service. Given that initial professional education in most allied health professions is at bachelor's degree level, it is reasonable to argue that further courses should at least lead to master's degrees. Professional experience in a wide range of settings and with differing client groups is also essential given the diverse nature of society and the importance attached to ensuring parity in access to health services.

The complexity of need that many patients present demands an approach to service provision in which members of different professions can work efficiently together. A great deal of work is required to make this a reality because there is no tradition of collaborative working. As professional maturity raises the consciousness of both nurses and allied health professions, it should liberate them from dependence on medicine but sustained effort is needed to challenge existing professional boundaries and run the risk of creating something new. What are needed first are individuals who are willing to take such risks, to leave aside tradition and explore fresh territory.

Creativity is needed to fashion new practice and research skills to determine what works best. In particular, allied health professionals must explore for themselves rather than continue to rely on nursing to lead the way. There may be much that is useful in the development of advanced nursing to date but that is no reason to avoid investigating physiotherapy or any other discipline as a separate field. It is, therefore, too early to say for certain whether advanced practice in allied health professions will have the same attributes as that in nursing but the key elements of the ideas discussed here do seem to have some potential in establishing common ground between professions.

Conclusion

This chapter has presented an examination of McGee and Castledine's ideas about the nature of advanced practice. These ideas are rooted in nursing but appear to have the potential for application in allied health fields. Research and development are needed to determine whether advanced practice is a separate issue in each profession or whether there is a generic definition that can apply to all. The following key questions are intended to promote discussion about these matters.

> **?** **Key questions for Chapter 4**
>
> In your field of practice:
> (1) How is advanced practice conceptualised in nursing and the allied health professions that normally contribute to patient care?
> (2) To what extent is collaborative practice possible?
> (3) How might the development of advanced roles be addressed and why?

References

Benner, P. (1984) *From Novice to Expert: Excellence and Power in Clinical Nursing Practice*. Menlo Park, California, Addison Wesley.

Brechin, A. (2000) Introducing critical practice. Chapter 2 in *Critical Practice in Health and Social Care*, (eds A. Brechin, H. Brown and M. Eby), pp 25–47. Buckingham, OUP.

Campinha-Bacote, J. (1994) Cultural competence in psychiatric mental health nursing. *Nursing Clinics of North America* **29** (1) 1–8.

Campinha-Bacote, J. (2002) *Readings and Resources in Transcultural Health Care and Mental Health*, 13th edn. Transcultural C.A.R.E. Associates. Available at http://www. transculturalcare.net/.

Carper, B. (1978) Fundamental patterns of knowing in nursing. *Advances in Nursing Science* **1** (1) 12–23.

Carroll, M. (2002) Advanced nursing practice. *Nursing Standard* **16** (29) 33–5.

Chartered Society of Physiotherapists (2002) *Physiotherapist Consultant (NHS): Role, Attributes and Guidance for Establishing Posts*. Available at http://www.csp.org.uk.

Close, A. (2003) Supervision and leadership in advanced practice. Chapter 6 in *Advanced Nursing Practice*, (eds P. McGee and G. Castledine), 2nd edn. pp 59–72. Oxford, Blackwell Science.

De Bono, E. (1991) *The Five-Day Course in Thinking*. London, Penguin.

Department of Health (2000a) *The NHS Plan. A Plan for Investment. A Plan for Reform*. Wetherby, DH.

Department of Health (2000b) *Meeting the Challenge. A Strategy for the Allied Health Professions*. London, DH.

Hamric, A. (2005) A definition of advanced nursing practice. Chapter 3 in *Advanced Nursing Practice. An Integrative Approach*, (eds A. Hamric, J. Spross and C. Hanson), 3rd edn. pp 85–108. St Louis, Elsevier Saunders.

Hamric, A. and Reigle, J. (2005) Ethical decision making. Chapter 11 in *Advanced Nursing Practice. An Integrative Approach*, (eds A. Hamric, J. Spross and C. Hanson), 3rd edn. pp 379–411. St Louis, Elsevier Saunders.

Hanson, C. and Malone, B. (2000) Leadership, empowerment, change agency and activism. Chapter 10 in *Advanced Nursing Practice. An Integrated Approach*, (eds A. Hamric, J. Spross and C. Hanson), 2nd edn. pp 279–314. Philadelphia, W. B. Saunders.

Hanson, C. and Spross, J. (2005a) Collaboration. Chapter 10 in *Advanced Nursing Practice. An Integrative Approach*, (eds A. Hamric, J. Spross and C. Hanson), 3rd edn. pp 341–78. St Louis, Elsevier Saunders.

Hanson, C. and Spross, J. (2005b) Clinical and professional leadership. Chapter 9 in *Advanced Nursing Practice. An Integrated Approach*, (eds A. Hamric, J. Spross and C. Hanson), 3rd edn. pp 301–29. St Louis, Elsevier Saunders.

Hickey, J.V. and Patton, C. (2003) *Advanced Nursing Practice. Changing Roles and Clinical Applications*, 3rd edn. Philadelphia, Lippincott.

International Council of Nurses (2002) Nurse Practitioner/Advanced Practice Network. *Definition of the Role*. Available at http://www.icn-apnetwork.org/.

Jason Martin, M. (2006) ''That's the way we do things around here'': an overview of organizational culture. *Electronic Journal of Academic and Special Librarianship* **7** (1). Available at http://southernlibrarianship.icaap.org/content/v07n01/martin_m01.htm. Accessed 21 April 2008.

Keuhn, A.F. (2004) The kaleidoscope of collaborative practice. Chapter 15 in *Advanced Practice Nursing*, (ed. L. Joel), pp 301–35. Philadelphia, F.A. Davis.

Koetters, T. (1989) Clinical practice and direct patient care. Chapter 5 in *The Clinical Nurse Specialist in Theory and Practice*, (eds A. Hamric and J. Spross), 2nd edn. pp 107–24. Philadelphia, W. B. Saunders.

Manley, K. (1998) A conceptual framework for advanced practice: an action research project operationalising an advanced practitioners/consultant nurse role. Chapter 8 in *Advanced Nursing Practice*, (eds G. Rolfe and P. Fulbrook), pp 118–35. Oxford, Butterworh- Heinemann.

Marriner Tomey, A. (1993) *Transformational Leadership in Nursing*. St Louis, Mosby Yearbook.

McGee, P. (2005) *Principles of Caring*. Cheltenham, Nelson Thornes.

McGee, P. and Castledine, G. (2003) *Advanced Practice*, 2nd edn. Oxford, Blackwell Science.

Nursing and Midwifery Council (2004) *The NMC Code of Professional Conduct: Standards for Conduct, Performance and Ethics. Protecting the Public through Professional Standards*. London, NMC.

Nursing and Midwifery Council (2005) *Implementation of a Framework for the Standard of Post Registration Nursing Agendum 27.1 C/05/160. December 2005*. Available at http://www.nmc-uk.org.

Oberle, K. and Allen, M. (2001) The nature of advanced nursing practice. *Nursing Outlook* **49** (3) 148–53.

O'Grady, E. (2005) Advanced practice nursing and health policy. Chapter 15 in *Advanced Practice Nursing. Emphasising Common Roles*, (ed. J. Stanley), 2nd edn. pp 374–94.

Oliver, N. (2004) The advanced practice and complementary therapies. Chapter 18 in *Advanced Practice Nursing*, (ed. L. Joel), pp 373–97. Philadelphia, F.A. Davis.

Phillips, S. J. (2007) Nineteenth annual update. *The Nurse Practitioner* **32** (1) 14–7, 19–20, 22, 24–5, 27–40, 32–42.

Reinhard, S., Grossman, J. and Piren, K. (2004) Advocacy and the advanced practice nurse. Chapter 14 in *Advanced Practice Nursing*, (ed. L. Joel), pp 280–300. Philadelphia, F.A. Davis.

Royal College of Nursing (2008) *Advanced Nurse Practitioners. An RCN Guide to the Advanced Nurse Practitioner Role, Competencies and Programme Accreditation*. London, RCN.

Schober, M. and Affara, F. (2006) *International Council of Nurses, Advanced Nursing Practice*. Oxford, Blackwell Science.

Schön, D. (1983) *The Reflective Practitioner. How Professionals Think in Action*. London, Avebury.

Smith, P. (1992) *The Emotional Labour of Nursing*. London, Macmillan.

Spross, J. (2005) Expert coaching and guiding. Chapter 6 in *Advanced Nursing Practice. An Integrative Approach*, (eds A. Hamric, J. Spross and C. Hanson), 3rd edn. pp 187–223. St Louis, Elsevier Saunders.

Sullivan, T. (1998) *Collaboration: A Health Care Imperative*. New York, McGraw Hill.

United Kingdom Central Council for Nursing, Midwifery and Health Visiting (2002) *Report of the Higher Level of Practice Pilot and Project*. London, UKCC.

World Health Organisation (2000) *Global Advisory Group on Nursing and Midwifery. Report of the 6th Meeting*. WHO. Available at http://www.who.org.

Chapter 5

Advanced Assessment and Differential Diagnosis

Paula McGee

Introduction

The ability to accurately assess a patient's problems and needs is an essential skill in all health professions. In conducting an assessment, the practitioner collects relevant information as a basis for determining the best course of action to take. What counts as relevant depends on the nature of the presenting problems and the orientation of the practitioner concerned. For example, a patient with mobility problems might be assessed by the physiotherapist for physical deficits such as reductions in movement or impairment in balance. The occupational therapist's assessment would be more concerned with daily living activities such as whether the patient could safely make a cup of tea or return to work.

Assessment is important because it lays the foundation for therapeutic decision-making and action. Consequently, initial professional education focuses attention on enabling novice practitioners to develop the knowledge and skills required to conduct assessment and on introducing them to a variety of different approaches. For example, in nursing education, considerable time is spent on learning to assess in three major domains: physical, social and psychological. Students are encouraged to examine the usefulness of a range of theoretical ideas such as Orem's (2001) theory of self care or the activities of living, which form part of Roper et al.'s (2000) model of nursing. With time and experience the novice will become competent and eventually proficient in conducting assessments using these theories as a guide but more is required if the individual wishes to become an advanced practitioner.

Advanced practice requires the development of advanced assessment skills that go well beyond what is taught during initial professional education. For example, in nursing, advanced assessment is linked to 32 competencies and the Knowledge and Skills Framework (Department of Health (DH) 2004, The Royal College of Nursing 2008). These competencies are divided into three groups: those relating specifically to health promotion, health protection and disease prevention; those specific to assessment and the management of patient illness and the remainder (which apply to both types of assessment). This chapter examines the nature of advanced assessment. It begins by explaining what advanced assessment is, how knowledge and skills differ from those learned during initial professional education. The chapter then progresses to a discussion of the different types of advanced assessment highlighting the different data sets that may be generated by each one. The limitations of advanced assessment are explored with reference to the organisational, policy and professional issues with which the advanced practitioner may have to contend. Finally, the chapter explains how a differential diagnosis is made and presents a discussion of the various factors that may influence. The chapter closes with some key questions for further debate.

The nature of advanced assessment

Advanced assessment is the detailed, systematic collection of relevant information about the patient's problems and health status. It is underpinned by a high level of specialised knowledge and skill and extensive experience that enable the advanced practitioner to focus 'on the accurate region of the problem without wasteful consideration of a large range of unfruitful, alternative diagnoses and solutions' (Benner 1984; p. 32, Zukav 1991, Jasper 1994). Thus the advanced practitioner can get right to the heart of a problem much faster and with a greater degree of success than others who are less experienced.

The central feature of advanced assessment is the meeting between two people, the advanced practitioner and the patient, to address a specific health problem with a view to determining what action, if any, should be taken (Peplau 1952). This meeting lays the foundation of the therapeutic relationship and success depends, in the first instance, on the interpersonal competence of the professional who is able to engage directly with the patient as a person (RCN 2008). In this situation, the ability to present oneself, to be there for and give full attention to another individual is essential. The advanced practitioner is able to relieve feelings of vulnerability and facilitate comfort and dignity, inspiring trust and confidence that, even if little can be done to help, will ensure that the situation will not be made worse by a lack of care (Benner 1984, Benner and Wrubel 1989, Benner *et al.* 1996, McGee 2000, RCN 2008). There is no doubt that patients value interpersonal skill in health professionals – being addressed correctly and with courtesy, knowing that someone will come when called because they promised to do so, understanding what is happening because someone has taken the trouble to explain all help to inspire trust and confidence (McGee 2000). The advanced practitioner works in ways that help patients feel in control, especially at their most vulnerable, and empowers them to make their own decisions, whenever this is possible (RCN 2008).

Patients welcome practitioners who communicate and show concern in ways that are culturally acceptable, who provide help rather than leaving them to struggle alone. In patients' minds, these factors far outweigh technical skill and clinical ability, although they too are important; no one wants to receive botched, incompetent treatment or care (McGee 2000). What is, perhaps, not appreciated is that, in advanced practice, the technical and clinical performance is so well honed that it appears effortless; it is thus less obvious to patients. Benner *et al.* (1996) argued that this expert level of performance requires a range of subtle skills that can only be demonstrated rather than described. Such skills appear deceptively simple because they are an integral part of the expert repertoire and represent a way of being with patients that takes account of emotional and physical responses and the needs of each person. Consequently, regardless of whether the meeting between the patient and advanced practitioner is a short and single event or the beginning of a series of encounters to address a more complex or ongoing problem, the level of skill and performance required remains high.

Types of advanced assessment

In preparing to undertake an advanced assessment, the practitioner must first decide on the most appropriate form this should take: *complete health profile, emergency* or *follow-up*. The *complete health profile* is based on an expanded concept of health as a dynamic state in which the individual constantly adapts and changes to challenges; it is, therefore, far more than the absence of disease or illness (Roy and Andrews 1999). The individuality of each person means that everyone will respond to challenges in a unique way; some will become ill while others will not. Health is now viewed as a personal experience rather than a single uniform state. Life for those with long-term conditions can be seen as *'healthy for them'* but punctuated by intermittent exacerbations of an underlying problem rather than a continuous unhealthy state. Individuals can describe themselves as *'well for me'* in situations that another might regard as *'very sick for me'*.

The *complete health profile* involves a comprehensive appraisal of the individual's health status, with reference to their age and development, based on a holistic approach to the systematic collection of information. This includes consideration of current, long-term and past health problems and how the patient responded to treatment and care (Rhoads 2006) (Table 5.1). It is important to ascertain what the patient believes to have been most helpful in managing current and previous health problems. There are now so many different sources of help and advice available that patients are likely to use a combination of several different types. For example, a patient who complains of back pain may wish to obtain analgesia that is only available on prescription in order to help him cope with a course of osteopathic treatment which, past experience has led him to believe, relieves the problem. Similarly, a patient with persistent eczema may use a combination of herbal remedies from traditional Chinese medicine but wish to combine these with something that conventional medicine has to offer. Patients are

Table 5.1   The complete advanced assessment.

Assessment focus	Factors to identify
Name, address and personal contact details and general practitioner	Accuracy of information
Age	Factors associated with development, maturation and aging
Next of kin/emergency contact details	Preferences about releasing information to next of kin or anyone else Any special arrangements such as individual's availability
Occupation	Current and previous work roles If retired, length of time since employment
History of current health problems	Signs and symptoms Pain Duration Remedies used so far such as over-the-counter medications, rest, ice packs
Long-term health problems	Diabetes, epilepsy, ulcerative colitis etc.
Disability	Sensory Physical Learning disability Hidden disabilities such as autism or Asperger's syndrome
Current medication	Prescribed and over-the-counter medications Use of any over-the-counter medication Medications from other sources such as the internet, complementary or other practitioners
Complementary and alternative therapies	Therapies include homeopathy, osteopathy, chiropractic for which formal academic training and qualifications are required Therapies include shamanism and faith healing, which lack formal academic training and qualifications Complementary therapies are used in addition to conventional treatment and care. Alternative therapies are used instead of conventional treatment and care
Other systems of treatment and care	Traditional Chinese medicine, Ayurvedic therapies and others
Past physical medical history	Serious illnesses Repeated illness such as tonsillitis in childhood Operations Blood transfusions Allergies

Contd.

Table 5.1 *Contd.*

Assessment focus	Factors to identify
	Drug interactions Injuries/accidents Exposure to occupational hazards such as asbestos, noise or toxic chemicals
Communicable diseases	Diseases associated with childhood, e.g. measles, mumps etc. Occupation in terms of exposure to communicable diseases Travel history especially in developing countries Possible contact with communicable diseases abroad Immunisation and vaccination history Risk of infecting others
Recreational activities	Alcohol Use of legal and illegal drugs Exercise Hobbies and interests
Mental health	History of depression, anxiety, panic attacks, excessive stress Previous diagnoses of mental health disorders such as schizophrenia Substance abuse History of violence History of voluntary or mandatory admissions to hospital Current mental health support such as regular therapy, counselling History of bereavement
Personal relationships and living arrangements	Living alone/with others Significant relationships Dependants Type of housing Health of family members – parents, children, partners and other relevant individuals
Sexuality	Treatment for developmental problems such as undescended testes History of any infections Menstrual cycle Fertility issues/treatment Pregnancies Miscarriages Abortions Menopausal symptoms Sexual preferences Transgender status History of sexual violence such as rape

also likely to use the internet and buy medication that they believe will help. Finding out which sources of help the patient has accessed can prevent further complications that may arise, for example, by prescribing medication that will interact negatively with substances that the patient is already taking (Table 5.1).

It is also important to ascertain whether the patient may have been in contact with any communicable diseases. Rough sleeping, living or travelling in places with poor standards of hygiene and working in certain occupations may expose individuals to an increased risk which, in some instances, may have implications for public health (Jarvis 2000, Rhoads 2006). Recreational activities are also relevant. An individual may be employed in a low-risk occupation but engage in hobbies or activities that pose serious threats to health. It is essential to assess the patient's mental well-being so that, if necessary, referral can be made to more specialised sources of help as quickly as possible (Table 5.1). Finally, the physical part of the assessment involves the systematic collection of data about each body system (Box 5.1). Starting at the head and working downwards towards the feet allows the advanced practitioner to begin with the least intrusive aspects of assessment and gradually progress towards those about which the patient may feel reticent (Jarvis 2000, Rhoads 2006).

Box 5.1   The complete advanced assessment – physical examination

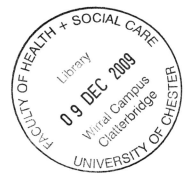

General appearance
Eyes
Ears
Nose and sinuses
Mouth, throat and teeth
Skin and hair
Neurological system
Respiratory system and smoking
Cardiovascular system
Gastrointestinal system, diet, weight and height
Urinary system
Musculoskeletal system and mobility
Reproductive system
Endocrine system
Haematological factors
Sleep and rest

The *emergency advanced assessment* is quite different in that it focuses only on the patient's immediate problems. The advanced practitioner must, therefore, be able to prioritise accurately what is important. For example, during an acute exacerbation of asthma, only information that is directly relevant to the emergency should be considered and the advanced practitioner should be able to collect this rapidly

Table 5.2   Emergency advanced assessment of an adult patient with an acute exacerbation of asthma.

Parameter	Observations	Concurrent activity
Breathing	Respiratory rate, breathlessness, wheezing, use of auxiliary muscles of respiration, signs of panic, signs of fatigue that may lead to respiratory arrest	Attempt at peak flow measurement Pulse oximetry Administration of nebulised salbutamol 2.5 mg Call for resuscitation team if respiratory arrest seems imminent
Communication	Patient unable to speak more than a few words	Finding out from those accompanying the patient about • regular medication • when the acute exacerbation began • known allergies
Maintaining body temperature	Shivering, warm flushed appearance may indicate infection	Record body temperature Consider need for broad spectrum antibiotics

while, at the same time, instigating the necessary treatment (Estes 1998, Jarvis 2000) (Table 5.2).

The *follow-up advanced assessment* may be used to review the progress of the patient once the emergency situation has subsided. Alternatively, a *follow-up advanced assessment* may be arranged to examine a particular health issue in more detail. For example, previous assessment may have shown that the patient is overweight; a *follow-up advanced assessment* may be arranged to investigate this in more detail. In this instance it will involve some sensitive questioning about dietary habits as well as measurement of height, weight and body mass index score. Signs of contributing factors, such as hypothyroidism, must also be considered. The therapeutic relationship established by the advanced practitioner will provide encouragement, dietary advice and regular monitoring to support a programme of sustained weight reduction. Most important in this type of advanced assessment is the need to assess whether the practitioner's view of the problem is shared by the patients and the extent to which they feel able to address it. For example, in dealing with patients identified as being overweight, the advanced practitioner must first seek to clarify whether patients perceive themselves in the same light. Following on from this is the degree to which patients believe that negative consequences might arise from being overweight and whether these consequences may directly affect them. The benefits of and effort required in taking action versus the possibility of doing nothing must then be weighed. In other words individuals do a form of risk assessment based on what they know about being overweight and whether they can handle change (Kleinman 1988, Ogden 2001).

Conducting an advanced assessment

Complete health profiles and *follow-up advanced assessments* should always be conducted in a private place where the patient and practitioner cannot be overheard, especially if sensitive issues are to be discussed. In emergency situations this may not always be possible but the advanced practitioner should take every reasonable precaution to ensure privacy and avoid settings in which there can be breaches of confidentiality.

As in any other encounter with patients, advanced practitioners should first introduce themselves to patients, explain who they are and ask permission to conduct the assessment. At this stage it is useful to make clear that this will involve taking notes to provide a record of the assessment as a basis for future treatment and care (Rhoads 2006). Sensory deficits that may affect communication are also noted and, if necessary, arrangements are made to accommodate those with special needs. Cultural norms should also be observed. To clarify this point, while the advanced practitioner will avoid unnecessarily exposing patients during physical examination, members of some cultural groups may have stronger views than others about what is acceptable. For example, McGee (2000) found that members of an indigenous white culture in England placed a high value on modesty. They took care to remain covered as much as possible, even within the context of close personal relationships and wanted health professionals of the same gender whenever physical examination was necessary. Furthermore, while many Western cultures emphasise individual responsibility in all aspects of life this is not universally the case. In the West the individual is regarded as capable of taking responsibility for the self and making decisions and is therefore more likely to wish to be assessed alone. Cultures that emphasise group or family responsibility prefer a collective, shared approach to decision-making and the care of group/family members. Thus, family members may expect to be included in the assessment (Paniagua 1998, Helman 2000).

During the assessment, information is gathered using a mixture of observation, physical measurements and semi-structured interviewing skills to determine the nature and severity of the situation. What this means is that the advanced practitioner enables the patients to tell their story while listening carefully to what is said and observing for any supportive or contradictory non-verbal signals. At the same time the advanced practitioner makes systematic observations and measurements. It sounds quite simple but patients rarely tell their stories in a straightforward fashion (Schön 1983). They may begin by recounting something well away from the main problem to see how the practitioner will react: *I fainted in the supermarket yesterday. I had stomach ache all day*. Eventually it will emerge that this patient has diarrhoea but feels unable to broach the matter straightaway. Alternatively, patients may present a very compressed version of their story, assuming that the practitioner will understand: *I still have the diarrhoea but I'm OK really*. Careful questioning might reveal bouts of severe diarrhoea and incontinence, which the patient is struggling to manage. The point here is that it is easy to be misled into believing that the patient is coping when this is not the case (McGee 2000).

Stories have three main elements: *orientation, complication and evaluation*. The *orientation* element sets the scene for events, the circumstances in which the problem arose. In the *complication* the patient narrates what actually happens and the evaluation provides an account of the outcome (Livo and Rietz 1986, Bell 1988). In conducting advanced assessments, practitioners must pay close attention to piecing the story together and use their critical reflective skills to marry this with the observations and measurements obtained to create a comprehensive picture of the patient's problems.

Limitations of advanced assessment

Advanced practitioners have to work within the constraints of the setting in which they are employed. This means that they may have to meet certain targets. For example, an advanced practitioner, working in primary care, who has specialised in asthma management, may be charged specifically with assessing the inhaler technique of every patient considered to have poor asthma control. This requirement may mean that a certain number of patients have to be assessed during the course of each week and it may be considered a limitation if it curtails potential engagement in other forms of direct care that helps those with asthma to improve their health.

A second set of constraints may be imposed by the wider health-care system, which imposes restrictions that appear to have no rational basis. For example, at the time of writing, suitably prepared advanced nurse practitioners working in primary care may, following advanced assessment, prescribe a wide range of medications. However, if their assessments show that a patient is unfit to work, advanced practitioners must ask a doctor to sign a certificate to that effect so that the patient can receive sickness benefits; this rule does not apply in secondary care settings. Such arbitrary restrictions reinforce a dependency on medicine, which undermines advanced practitioners and conveys to patients that doctors are still pre-eminent in deciding what is best.

Finally, advanced practitioners must be aware of their limitations and seek to refer patients to other sources of help as appropriate. This means that members of other professions must be willing to accept such referrals and that organisational processes must allow them to do so. Regrettably, the current situation seems to militate against this. Professionals who do not understand developments in advanced practice, who are reluctant to accept change, insist that they will only receive referrals from a doctor. Thus they seek to hide behind tradition rather than confront their own insecurities. While this is, to some extent, understandable, it limits the advanced practitioner's role in assessing a patient. It may also serve to deflect advanced practitioners away from direct care, where they are most needed, into spending time and energy in educating colleagues and persuading them to change.

Formulating a differential diagnosis

The systematic collection of objective data based on measurement coupled with subjective information gleaned through listening to and observing the patient leads the advanced practitioner to the first outcome of advanced assessment: a list of problems and an action plan that sets out what to do next in formulating a diagnosis (Rhoads 2006). Further objective information may be needed in which case the advanced practitioner can request laboratory tests, X-rays, ultrasound or a specialist's opinion about particular signs and symptoms. The advanced practitioner will then begin to cluster findings together and progress towards analysis and interpretation. In other words the advanced practitioner will engage in diagnostic reasoning, which is 'a scientific process in which the practitioner reviews the cause of the patient's symptoms and signs based on previous knowledge, gathers relevant information, selects necessary tests and recommends therapy' (Dains *et al.* 2003, p. 2).

Formulating an accurate diagnosis is dependent on a high-quality assessment, which provides sufficient relevant information with respect to four criteria. The diagnosis should be *credible*, providing an explanation of what has happened that reflects the objective and subjective information gained from the patient. It should be *adequate* in that it accounts for all the signs and symptoms that deviate from what is normal for the patient. This account should be *parsimonious* in that it provides the simplest explanation based on the information obtained in assessment. Finally, it should reflect the elimination of other possibilities through the synthesis of information from the patient with what is known about specific conditions in order to identify the most important features and emergent patterns (Dains *et al.* 2003) (Figure 5.1, Table 5.3).

Achieving these four criteria sounds very straightforward but, in reality, formulating a diagnosis requires complex decision-making that, at each stage, presents the advanced practitioner with a range of possibilities from which to choose. Much depends on the ability of the professional to identify and interpret the significance of signs and symptoms (Eddy 1988). Advanced practitioners are individuals and there will inevitably be some variation in response to similar information. Just as each patient presents health problems in a unique way, the professional will also bring a particular set of knowledge and skills to the consultation. Collecting information highlights the vagaries of the boundaries between what is considered normal and abnormal (Eddy 1988). If health is defined in terms of the individual's experience, ascertaining what is normal for that person can be very difficult indeed.

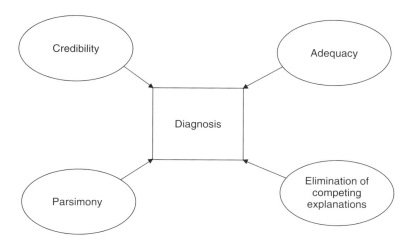

Fig. 5.1   Elements of a diagnosis.

Table 5.3 Examples of differential diagnoses.

Presenting symptoms	Competing explanations may include	Associated symptoms and signs
Sore throat	Tonsillitis	Enlarged tonsils, raised temperature, difficulty in swallowing
	Allergic reaction to substance swallowed/inhaled	Difficulty in breathing Redness and swelling in throat
	Oral thrush	Red, sore mouth with white cheesy patches on the tongue Recent course of antibiotics or chemotherapy
	Bronchitis	History of a cold Raised temperature Difficulty in breathing Productive cough with thick green sputum Chest sounds: auscultation normal with prolonged expiration, possible wheeze and crackles over affected areas, percussion resonant
	Sexually transmitted infection	History of oral sexual activity Throat swab positive for gonorrhoea
	Glandular fever	Raised temperature Headache Persistent fatigue Enlarged lymph nodes in neck Spleen may be palpable
Diarrhoea	Food poisoning	Abrupt onset Limited duration – 1 or 2 days
	Viral gastroenteritis	Raised temperature Abdominal pain and cramps Nausea and vomiting Abrupt onset Stool samples reveal causative organism Increased bowel sounds
	Ulcerative colitis	Frequent and severe bouts of diarrhoea with blood Abdominal cramps and tenderness relieved by defaecation Most common in young adults Family history
	Coeliac disease	Diarrhoea with pale fatty stools Signs of malnutrition Signs of anaemia Delayed physical development in children Lethargy Abdominal pain
	Faecal impaction	Hard faeces in rectum

Behaviour and mental health assessment help to illustrate this point. It may be normal for someone with agoraphobia to experience high anxiety if asked to go outside but abnormal when the same symptoms occur on trying to leave the bedroom. Similarly, hearing voices may be accepted as a normal part of everyday life until they begin to make statements that drive the individual to behave violently.

Formulating a diagnosis also depends on knowing how disease and illness are defined within a particular society. Western societies have allowed medicine to dominate this particular subject; disease has become a pathological abnormality arising from alterations in biological structures and function. Making a diagnosis is about interpretation of signs and symptoms: the approach by the patient to request for that interpretation (Kleinman 1988). That interpretation is itself ruled by what Western medicine has legitimated as disease; other societies and systems of medicine may put forward quite different explanations of what has happened to the patient. For example, in traditional Chinese medicine, health is conceptualised as harmony both within the self and between the self and the external environment, both social and physical (Chen 2001). In this context, disease is a result of imbalance between opposing but complementary forces, *yin* (feminine) and *yang* (masculine); in Hispanic tradition this is conceptualised as *frio* (yin) and *caliente* (yang) (Echols 1998, Chen 2001). Treatment is thus aimed as restoring harmony rather than just curing the particular ailment. Certain illnesses and conditions are described as *culture bound or folk illnesses* because they are recognised only within a particular cultural setting where they are invested with 'symbolic meanings – moral, social or psychological'; for example, the English notion of *catching a chill* (Helman 2000, p. 87). The point here is that disease and illness have to be linked to an accepted diagnostic category that permits the patient's access to treatment and care. In Western health-care systems diagnostic categories are formulated in a specific way that may or may not be meaningful to the patient.

The ability to diagnose thus involves the advanced practitioner living with a great deal of uncertainty. Medical practitioners have tended to cope with this, when dealing with patients, by engaging in a delicate balancing act between the limitations of current professional knowledge, individual weaknesses in the mastery of that knowledge and the individuality of patients (Katz 1988). It has yet to be determined whether advanced practitioners will do the same. What matters in the meantime is safe practice; even if they cannot assist patients in solving their health problems, advanced practitioners should, at the very least, do no harm.

There is limited research to date but a recent study in a neonatal unit suggests that advanced assessment by advanced nurse practitioners compares well with those of doctors. The study set out to establish whether the quality of care and clinical outcomes for premature babies, in a specialist neonatal unit, were affected by the type of practitioner responsible for their assessment and treatment during the first 6–12 hours after admission. The medical and nursing records of 61 babies were examined with reference to specific data such as Apgar score, gestation, blood pressure, temperature and blood sugar. The reviewer was a neonatologist, based in a different National Health Service (NHS) trust, who received no information regarding the identity or profession of those who had written the records. Findings showed no statistical differences between the standard of assessment and quality of care provided by neonatal nurse practitioners and medical staff with regard to gestation, Apgar scores, intubation and other procedures, although there were some slight differences with regard to physiological data (Woods 2006).

Conclusion

It is evident from this chapter that advanced health assessment is not a single entity. Rather it is an umbrella term encompassing several different activities: obtaining a *complete health profile, emergency advanced assessment* and *follow-up advanced assessment*. Undertaking an assessment enables the advanced practitioner to gain detailed insight into the patient's health problems and form a therapeutic relationship of trust. From this vantage point the professional may begin to formulate a differential diagnosis and draw up a plan of action for treatment and care. None of this is either easy or straightforward. Assessing and diagnosing require the ability to cope with multiple options and uncertainty, to select what seems to be the most appropriate explanation while recognising that it could be wrong because the essence of each diagnostic event is an individual practitioner's professional judgement, a subjective opinion based on a mixture of various types of information gained from the patient. A different practitioner might or might not share exactly the same view. Furthermore, advanced practitioners, as new phenomena in the field of diagnostics, have to contend not only with uncertainty and their own limitations but also with organisational and professional processes that have not kept pace evenly with developments in nursing or allied health professions. What all this points to is the need not only for a great deal more work to be done in determining the effectiveness of advanced assessment but also in clarifying the advanced practitioners' role and status within the health service.

 Key questions for Chapter 5

In your field of practice:
(1)   How might the complete health profile, emergency and follow-up advanced assessments be conducted and why?
(2)   What limitations can you identify with regard to assessing and diagnosing patients' health problems?
(3)   What factors might help you cope with uncertainty and why?

References

Bell, S. (1988) Becoming a political woman: the reconstruction and interpretation of experience through stories. Chapter 3 in *Gender and Discourse: the Power of Talk*, (eds A.D. Todd and S. Fisher), pp 97–124. Norwood, New Jersey, Ablex Publishing Corporation.
Benner, P. (1984) *From Novice to Expert: Excellence and Power in Clinical Nursing Practice*. Menlo Park, California, Addison Wesley.

Benner, P., Tanner, C. and Chesla, C. (1996) *Expertise in Nursing Practice. Caring, Clinical Judgement and Ethics*. New York, Springer.

Benner, P. and Wrubel, J. (1989) *The Primacy of Caring. Stress and Coping in Health and Illness*. Menlo Park, California, Addison-Wesley.

Chen, Y. (2001) Chinese values, health and nursing. *Journal of Advanced Nursing* **36** 270–73.

Dains, J., Ciofu Baumann, L. and Scheibel, P. (2003) *Advanced Health Assessment and Clinical Diagnosis in Primary Care*. 2nd edn. St Louis, Mosby.

Department of Health (2004) *The NHS Knowledge and Skills Framework and the Development Review Process*. Available at http://www.dh.gov.uk.

Echols, J. (1998) Cultural assessment. Chapter 5 in *Health Assessment and Physical Examination*, (ed. M.E.Z. Estes), pp 101–27. New York, Delmar Publishers.

Eddy, D.M. (1988) Variations in physician practice: the role of uncertainty. Chapter 1 in *Professional Judgment. A Reader in Clinical Decision Making*, pp 45–59. Cambridge, Cambridge University Press.

Estes, M.E.Z. (1998) *Health Assessment and Physical Examination*. New York, Delmar Publishers.

Helman, C. (2000) *Culture, Health and Illness*, 4th edn. Oxford, Butterworth Heinemann.

Jarvis, C. (2000) *Physical Examination and Health Assessment*, 3rd edn. Philadelphia, W. B. Saunders Co.

Jasper, M. (1994) Expert: a discussion of the implications of the concept as used in nursing. *Journal of Advanced Nursing* **20** 769–76.

Katz, J. (1988) Why doctors don't disclose uncertainty. Chapter 30 in *Professional Judgment. A Reader in Clinical Decision Making*, pp 544–65. Cambridge, Cambridge University Press.

Kleinman, A. (1988) *The Illness Narratives. Suffering, Healing and the Human Condition*. New York, Basic Books.

Livo, N. and Rietz, S. (1986) *Storytelling. Process and Practice*. Littleton, Colorado, Libraries Unlimited Inc.

McGee, P. (2000) *Culturally Sensitive Nursing: A Critique*. Unpublished PhD thesis. Birmingham, United Kingdom, University of Central England.

Ogden, J. (2001) Health psychology. Chapter 3 in *Health Studies. An Introduction*, (eds J. Naidoo and J. Wills), pp 69–100. Basingtoke, Palgrave.

Orem, D. (2001) *Nursing, Concepts of Practice*, 6th edn. St Louis, Mosby.

Paniagua, F. (1998) *Assessing and Treating Culturally Diverse Clients. A Practical Guide*, 2nd edn. London, Sage.

Peplau, H. (1952) *Interpersonal Relations in Nursing*. New York, G.P. Putnam.

Rhoads, J. (2006) *Advanced Health Assessment and Diagnostic Reasoning*. Philadelphia, Lippincott, Williams & Wilkins.

Roper, N., Logan, W. and Tierney, A. (2000) *The Roper–Logan–Tierney Model of Nursing: Based on Activities of Living*. Edinburgh, Churchill Livingstone.

Roy, C. and Andrews, M. (1999) *The Roy Adaptation Model*. Stamford, Connecticut, Appleton and Lange.

The Royal College of Nursing (2008) *Advanced Nurse Practitioners. An RCN Guide to the Advanced Nurse Practitioner Role, Competencies and Programme Accreditation*. London, RCN.

Schön, D. (1983) *The Reflective Practitioner. How Professionals Think in Action*. London, Avebury.

Woods, L. (2006) Evaluating the clinical effectiveness of neonatal nurse practitioners: an exploratory study. *Journal of Clinical Nursing* **15** (1) 35–44.

Zukav, G. (1991) *The Dancing Wu Li Masters. An Overview of the New Physics*. London, Rider and Co.

Chapter 6

Prescribing and Advanced Practice

Sue Shortland and Katharine Hardware

Introduction

This chapter presents an overview of the prescribing of medicines by non-medical prescribers in the United Kingdom. *Non-medical prescribers* is a term used to refer to nurses, pharmacists and members of allied health professions who are qualified to prescribe medication and medical products for patients. Many, but not all, of these professionals will be advanced practitioners. This chapter examines aspects of prescribing practice for these professionals. It begins by outlining recent events that have led to the development of their roles and responsibilities and some of the legal issues involved. The chapter then moves on to explain the process of becoming a non-medical prescriber, who may prescribe what, for whom and the circumstances in which they may do so. This is followed by the principles of good prescribing and the importance of clinical governance. The chapter closes by briefly considering the future for non-medical prescribing both in the United Kingdom and elsewhere. Any discussion about non-medical prescribing requires the use of terminology with

Table 6.1 Prescribing and advanced practice – a glossary of terms.

Medical prescriber	Doctor or dentist
Non-medical prescriber	Suitably qualified nurse, pharmacist or allied health professional
Independent prescriber	A practitioner who is licensed to prescribe any licensed medicine for any condition that he or she is competent to treat
Supplementary prescriber	A practitioner qualified to prescribe a limited list of medicines voluntarily agreed with a doctor or dentist and within the context of an agreed patient-specific clinical management plan
General sales list medicines	Medicines that can be sold or supplied through general retail outlets including pharmacies
Prescription only medicines	Medicines that are available only through a prescription from a supplementary or independent prescriber
Pharmacy medicines	Medicines that can be sold or supplied through registered pharmacies under the personal supervision of a pharmacist
Misuse of drugs regulations	Regulations that cover the prescription, storage and dispensing of medicines. Within these regulations, medicines are classified in groups called schedules according to the risks involved in their use
Patient group directions	A written instruction that allows the supply or administration of a licensed medicine to patients, in an identified clinical situation, such as coronary care. Patient group directions do not require individual prescriptions for each patient

Source: Summarised from National Prescribing Centre 2004 *Glossary of Prescribing Terms*. Liverpool, NPC.

which some readers may be unfamiliar; the key terms are, therefore, explained in Table 6.1.

Recent developments in non-medical prescribing*

Non-medical prescribing has been debated in the United Kingdom for nearly 20 years and began to become a reality when, in 1994, pilot sites were established to explore the possibility of allowing some nurses to prescribe from a very limited formulary. These sites demonstrated that nurses were better prescribers of wound care products and that allowing them to prescribe was more convenient for patients (Luker *et al.* 1997). Recent health service reforms aimed at improving access to services, treatment

---

*A detailed history of nurse prescribing was included in the second edition of this book. Please see Matthews, P. (2003) Nurse prescribing and advanced practice. Chapter 14 in *Advanced Nursing Practice*, (eds P. McGee and G. Castledine), pp 169–83. Oxford, Blackwell Publishing.

and care have raised the profile of non-medical prescribing and have brought major changes. The National Health Service (NHS) Plan (DH 2000a) proposed a substantial increase in the numbers of nurses able to supply medicines: 10 000 nurses were to be prepared to become prescribers by 2004. The first independent prescribing courses were launched in 2002 and, in 2006, the formulary was expanded to include all general sales list medicines, pharmacy medicines and about 240 prescription only medicines (DH 2006) (Table 6.1). Although this was a great move forward, nurses were still limited in their ability to provide complete episodes of care. Consequently, following further consultation with the MHRA (2005), it was recommended that suitably qualified nurses and pharmacists would be able to prescribe any licensed medicine, excluding some controlled medicines, for any medical condition, within their competence. In May 2006 these new regulations came into effect and have had a huge impact on the prescribing practice of independent prescribers (DH 2006, Table 6.1). This has been particularly beneficial for advanced practitioners who were previously frustrated at being unable to complete episodes of care for their patients. Despite such progress there is still a great deal of work to be done. Non-medical prescribing is plagued with misunderstanding and a degree of confusion amongst health professionals, let alone the general public. Furthermore, although it has been estimated that around 8000 nurses have qualified as independent and supplementary prescribers, very few working in the community have written prescriptions (Avery and James 2007, National Health Information Centre Prescribing Support Unit 2007). Other non-medical prescribers may show a similar trend.

Preparation for prescribing

There are currently four routes to becoming a non-medical prescriber:

1. Bachelor's degree level courses for nurses, midwives and pharmacists wishing to become independent and supplementary prescribers
2. Master's degree level courses for nurses and midwives wishing to become independent and supplementary prescribers
3. Bachelor's degree level courses for allied health professionals, including pharmacists, wishing to become supplementary prescribers
4. Separate courses for community nurse practitioners: district nurses, health visitors and school nurses

Community nurses are only allowed to prescribe from a limited formulary, which contains 13 prescription only medicines, some pharmacy medicines and general sales list medicines plus a list of dressings and appliances (British National Formulary and the Royal Pharmaceutical Society of Great Britain 2006). The separate courses for community nurses may be undertaken either as part of a specialist practitioner programme or as stand-alone modules for those who do not hold a specialist practitioner qualification.

   All prescribing courses for nurses and pharmacists must be validated by the Nursing and Midwifery Council or the Royal Pharmaceutical Society of Great Britain (NMC 2006, RPSGB 2006) and students must meet all requirements of these two bodies and the Department of Health. To be accepted on a course for independent and supplementary prescribing, nurses must be registered with the Nursing and Midwifery Council, have recent (within 3 years) Criminal Records Bureau clearance and 3 years' experience as a practising nurse, midwife or specialist community public health nurse. Of these 3 years, the year prior to application must have been in the field in which they intend to prescribe. Additionally, nurses have to be sponsored and supported by their employers. Many educational institutions also stipulate that the nurse should have undertaken post-qualifying courses in history taking and health assessment but there is a wide variation across the country regarding this. Allied health professionals must comply with the requirements of the Health Professions Council (HPC 2001) and the Department of Health (2003). These requirements reflect those for nurses and midwives and pharmacists.

Who may prescribe what?

Nurses

Nurses who have undertaken appropriate preparation are allowed to become independent and supplementary prescribers. This means that they are licensed to prescribe any medicine in the formulary with the exception of some controlled medicines and unlicensed medicines.

Allied health professionals

Allied health professionals, such as podiatrists/chiropodists, physiotherapists, radiographers and optometrists, are not allowed to become independent prescribers. However, they may become supplementary prescribers, which means that they are not allowed to diagnose but may plan and prescribe current and future treatments in conjunction with an independent prescriber who may be a doctor, dentist or a nurse (DH 2004). The cornerstone of the working arrangement between the supplementary and independent prescribers in this situation is a clinical management plan (DH 2007a). A clinical management plan is a formal, legal document developed by the independent and supplementary prescribers for an individual patient. The plan includes the names of the two prescribers and the patient, and details of any allergies or sensitivities to medication. The patient's condition and the aim of treatment are clearly set out. This information is followed by a list of the medication and dosage that the supplementary prescriber may prescribe and in what circumstances. The criteria for referral back to the independent prescriber must also be clearly stated. The plan should also include details of how the patient will be monitored and the procedure to be followed if that person has an adverse reaction to any of the medication prescribed. Both prescribers must sign and date the plan. Templates for clinical management plans can be found at http://www.cmponline.info

Many advanced nurse practitioners ask why they have to qualify as supplementary and independent prescribers. There are several reasons for this. First, the Nursing and Midwifery Council (NMC 2006) states that all registrants must undertake both elements of the programme. Second, there are still some medicines that cannot be independently prescribed by nurses: some controlled and unlicensed medicines (DH 2006). Third, supplementary prescribing is more appropriate when dealing with unlicensed medicines as the situation in which they are to be used will require working with medical or dental practitioners who are independent prescribers and a clinical management plan. Finally, there may be occasions when an independent prescriber may choose to act as a supplementary prescriber. An example might be new or inexperienced prescribers who needed the safety net of a clinical management plan until they develop their expertise. Thus, supplementary prescribing can be used as a means of developing competency or as a vehicle for evaluating the safety, efficacy and acceptability of non-medical prescribing (Jones and Jones 2006).

Controlled medicines

The use of controlled medicines for medicinal purposes only is allowed under the Misuse of Medicines Regulations 2001. This act was amended in 2005 to allow supplementary prescribers, in conjunction with a clinical management plan, to prescribe all controlled medicines except schedule 1 medicines, which are those not intended for medicinal use*. Non-medical prescribers can issue private prescriptions except for controlled medicines and supplementary prescribers can issue private prescriptions under a clinical management plan (DH 2003). Blood is not considered a medicine and therefore cannot be prescribed by non-medical prescribers (DH 2007b). However, products derived from blood, such as blood clotting factors, antibodies and albumin may be prescribed under a supplementary prescribing arrangement (DH 2006, NMC 2006).

Patient group directions

Patient group directions are written instructions that allow the supply or administration of a licensed medicine in an identified clinical situation for a specified group of patients without individual prescriptions being written (NPC 2004). A patient group direction is drawn up locally by doctors, pharmacists and other health professionals and must meet minimum legal criteria (DH 2000b). An individual patient group direction must be signed by a doctor and a pharmacist and a representative of the NHS trust. Professionals using patient group directions do not have to become prescribers or obtain any specific qualification but their employers must assess them to ensure that they are fully competent, qualified and trained.

Emergency situations

Exemptions provided by Article 7 of the Prescription Only Medicines (Human Use) Order 1997 mean that patient group directions are not required for the following countermeasures when given by anyone in an emergency, to save life: atropine sulphate

---

*See Statutory Instrument No. 2005 No. 271 Dangerous drugs The Misuse of Drugs (Amendment) Regulations 2005. Available at http://www.opsi.gov.uk.

injection, dicobalt edetate injection, glucose injection and pralidoxime chloride injection. More recently, patient group directions have been developed to enable medicines to be given *en masse* in the event of chemical or biological warfare (DH 2008).

The principles of safe prescribing

Good non-medical prescribing practice is based on seven principles outlined by the National Prescribing Centre (NPC 1999). These principles begin with a *holistic assessment* and diagnosis of the patient's problem. This assessment should follow a structured model and take into account the patient's past medical history, current health, any allergies and a full medication history. The patient is at the heart of prescribing and once a diagnosis has been confirmed the non-medical prescriber must *consider the most appropriate strategy*; issuing a prescription may not always be in the patient's best interests. Many significant factors need to be considered to aid the prescriber make the decision as to whether medication is the best course of action to take.

Once the decision to prescribe medication has been made, the non-medical prescriber must *select the most appropriate product*. Decisions about choice of medication should be based on consideration of what is most suitable for the individual, the effectiveness and the cost of the medicines available. To explain this further, a patient may be planning to become pregnant; some medicines may not be suitable for the very young or the elderly. A patient may have a history of adverse reactions to particular medicines. Some medicines are safe and effective when used singly but cannot be used in combination with others because of the risk of unwanted side effects. This is a particularly problematic issue where patients have more than one clinical condition requiring treatment; in this context, decisions about medication involve balancing the demands of different conditions and trying to avoid prescribing too many medicines at the same time. The cost of medicines is an important issue; depending on the circumstances it may be wiser to begin treatment with a less expensive medicine and progress to more expensive alternatives if the patient's problems continue. Furthermore, in the United Kingdom, some medicines such as paracetamol are available in High Street pharmacies and supermarkets at a lower price than if they are prescribed. In these circumstances the non-medical prescriber may advise the patient on the cheaper alternative.

Prescribing a medicine requires far more than completing a form. The non-medical prescriber must *negotiate with the patient* about what the prescription is for, what the medicine will do, the potential side effects, how long to take the medication for and who to contact in the case of an adverse reaction. What is important here is individual choice; the patient is asked to agree to make a decision, about whether to accept the medication, based on appropriate and understandable information. In some instances, negotiating with a patient may require further action. Taking medication may have to be incorporated into a particular individual's lifestyle to ensure maximum effect; one example is the introduction of insulin injections to someone newly diagnosed with type 1 diabetes. Other considerations may apply where a patient has a notifiable disease such as tuberculosis in which regularly taking medicines is linked to ensuring the health of others.

Once the patient has agreed to take the medication, the name of the medicine, the dose and the date should be *entered in the patient's records*. Assuming that the patient has agreed to take the medication as prescribed, it may be appropriate to *arrange a review* particularly where the patient has a long-term condition or complex health issues. Even in seemingly straightforward situations such as the treatment of a chest infection in an otherwise healthy person, a review may be advisable to check that the medication prescribed has actually worked. Feeling better may not always reflect a complete recovery and further treatment may still be needed.

Finally, the non-medical prescriber has a range of legal and professional responsibilities, which require *reflection on practice* to ensure safety. This means that non-medical prescribers can only prescribe within their area of competence and must keep up to date with the latest developments to ensure that their prescribing practice is based on the best available evidence. Like medical prescribers, non-medical prescribers are likely to attract the attention of pharmaceutical marketing departments. A critical, questioning approach to such attention is essential in maintaining both the independent integrity of non-medical prescribers and the safety of their practice. In addition, non-medical prescribers must ensure that their practice is consistent with the law and workplace policies (NPC 1999, Beckwith and Franklin 2007).

Safety and clinical governance

Clinical governance is a system in which health-care organisations strive continuously to improve the quality of health care and safeguard standards by creating an environment in which high-quality clinical care can flourish (NHSE 1998). Quality issues and standards apply to non-medical prescribing and responsibility is shared between the individual practitioner and the health-care organisation. Individual prescribers are accountable for their own prescribing practice and should adhere to the principles of good prescribing and their professional codes (NPC 1999, NMC 2008). Alongside these individual responsibilities are those of the employing organisation, which has a duty to ensure that prescribers are suitably trained and that prescribing practice is audited and monitored regularly. Moreover, the organisation must ensure that appropriate indemnity insurance is in place for all prescribers. Even with the best standards of prescribing practice in place, mistakes can and do happen. Patients do not always present their symptoms in an expected way; individuals may experience the same illness quite differently (Schön 1983, 1987). Consequently, in formulating a diagnosis, the professional is faced with a range of options on which to base a decision and may, occasionally, select the wrong one. In addition, even where the diagnosis is correctly selected, patients may have adverse reactions to treatment, sometimes with serious results. Indemnity insurance against non-negligent harm is, therefore, essential for all prescribers.

Safety and clinical governance present a number of opportunities and challenges for the advanced practitioner. As a prescriber working directly with patients, the advanced practitioner is able to identify the extent to which prescribing practice is safe and appropriate for patients' needs. Direct contact with patients will facilitate monitoring the wanted side effects of medication and patients' preferences in the management of their conditions. The emphasis is on safe prescribing and concordance with treatment (NPC 1999). Where changes are needed, the leadership and interpersonal skills of the advanced practitioner can be used to promote constructive dialogue between the different professionals involved in prescribing and interprofessional working. The research skills of the advanced practitioner can be used to monitor and audit prescribing practice; these skills can also contribute towards the investigation of specific problems. The key point of clinical governance is to ensure that all parties collaborate to create a working environment in which practice is based on the best available evidence and in which mistakes can be examined to prevent recurrence. This means, from the advanced practitioner's perspective, fostering a no-blame culture in which individuals can be honest about their mistakes and supported in their efforts to improve (NHSE 1998). In this context, advanced practitioners may draw on their coaching and guiding skills to enable prescribers to adopt new or safer ways of working.

The future of non-medical prescribing

Non-medical prescribing has the potential to improve the lives of patients by enabling advanced practitioners and other health professionals to provide complete episodes of care. Patients only have to recount their signs and symptoms once; the increased number of prescribers means that access to health care is improved and that patients have more choice. In some instances, a single episode may be all that is needed to solve a particular patient's health problem. Even when a follow-up session is required, there is the potential for greater continuity in care and better relationships between patients and professionals. From the advanced practitioner's perspective, independent prescribing is consistent with the scope of expert practice. The expert practitioner is able to hone in very quickly on the most important aspects of a patient's situation and take appropriate action. This is particularly important in emergency situations and when working with patients who have complex needs. The advanced practitioner has the skills required to promote safe and effective prescribing both at an individual level and across the health-care organisation as a whole.

However, there is still a great deal to be done in developing non-medical prescribing and promoting acceptance of it among patients and professionals. Those who express concern should not be brushed aside or derided as reactionaries. There has been considerable debate about the adequacy of the training of nurse prescribers and the risks to patient safety (see, e.g. Avery and Pringle 2005). Questions have been raised about nurse prescribers' lack of knowledge about pharmacology (Strickland-Hodge 2008) and the adequacy of stand-alone modules to adequately prepare nurses to become prescribers (Avery and James 2007). Early evaluations demonstrate that nurses are cautious and safe in their prescribing practice but need to integrate this with comprehensive accurate assessment and diagnostic skills (Latter 2008). This can be challenging because prescribing courses tend to be generic. More work is needed in helping prescribers to apply their learning within their specialities. Advanced practitioners have the skills required to facilitate the investigation of the many current concerns about non-medical prescribing, to promote dialogue between the various different points of view. Skills in communication, leadership and ethical reasoning can be harnessed to create working environments in which individuals feel able to express their opinions and be listened to with respect and enabled to participate in bringing about change.

Internationally, non-medical prescribing raises other possibilities for the advanced practitioner. For example, there are wide variations in the development and practice of nurse prescribing. In Australia, progress has been hampered because the health insurance situation means that if a nurse prescribes a medication it will cost the patient much more than if a doctor prescribes it (Dragon 2008). In the United States there are variations across the country as to what and when nurses can prescribe (Phillips 2008). In New Zealand preparation for nurse prescribing has to be integrated into a programme at master's degree level (Spence and Anderson 2007). Other non-medical prescribing roles also differ in terms of what the law in each country will allow. Advanced practitioners have the skills to involve themselves in addressing these issues both at national and international levels, for instance, by participating in the development of international professional guidelines such as those issued by the International Council of Nurses about advanced nursing practice (ICN 2008).

Conclusion

The extent to which non-medical prescribing develops in the United Kingdom will largely depend on NHS trusts and doctors having confidence in the safety and effectiveness of prescribers and their value in meeting patients' needs (Avery and James 2007). As independent and supplementary prescribers, advanced practitioners can do a great deal to promote confidence by demonstrating their competence in safe and effective prescribing practice. They are also well placed to identify the needs of patients and enable health-care organisations to bring about change.

 Key questions for Chapter 6

In your field of practice:

(1)   What are the opportunities for trained non-medical prescribers to utilise their skills in developing new or existing services?

(2)   How should non-medical prescribers be empowered to prescribe within their competence?

(3)   How should health-care organisations audit prescribing practices to ensure patient care is safe?

References

Avery, A.J. and James, V. (2007) Developing nurse prescribing in the UK. *British Medical Journal* **335** 316.

Avery, A.J. and Pringle, M. (2005) Extended prescribing by UK nurses and pharmacists. *British Medical Journal* **331** 1154–5.

Beckwith, S. and Franklin, P. (2007) *Oxford Handbook of Nurse Prescribing*. Oxford, Oxford University Press.

British National Formulary and the Royal Pharmaceutical Society of Great Britain (2006) *The Nurse Prescriber's Formulary for Community Practitioners*. London, BNF and RPSGB.

Department of Health (2000a) *The NHS Plan: A Plan for Investment, A Plan for Reform*. Wetherby, DH.

Department of Health (2000b) *Patient Group Directions (England only) Health Service Circular 2000/026*. Available at http://www.dh.gov.uk.

Department of Health (2003) *Supplementary Prescribing by Nurses and Pharmacists within the NHS in England*. London, DH.

Department of Health (2004) *Outline Curriculum for Training Programmes to Prepare Allied Health Professionals as Supplementary Prescribers*. London, DH.

Department of Health (2006) *Improving Patients Access to Medicines: A Guide to Implementing Nurse and Pharmacist Independent Prescribing within the NHS in England*. London, DH.

Department of Health (2007a) *Clinical Management Plans*. London, DH.

Department of Health (2007b) Nurse Prescribing FAQ. Available at http://www.dh.gov.uk/en/Healthcare/Medicinespharmacyandindustry/prescriptions. Accessed 02 October 2008.

Department of Health (2008) *Patient Group Directions*. Available at http://www.dh.gov.uk/en/Managingyourorganisation/Emergencyplanning/DH_4069610. Accessed 26 November 2008.

Dragon, N. (2008) A new prescription needed for nurse practitioners. *Australian Nursing Journal* **16** (3) 20–3.

Health Professions Council (2001) *Register of Approved Courses – Supplementary Prescribing*. London, HPC.

International Council of Nurses (2008) *The Scope of Practice, Standards and Competencies of the Advanced Practice Nurse*. Geneva, ICN.

Jones, M. and Jones, A. (2006) Prescribing ways of working. Non-medical prescribing is ushering in new opportunities. *Mental Health Practice* **9** (6) 20–2.

Latter, S. (2008) Safety and quality in independent prescribing: an evidence review. *Nurse Prescribing* **6** (2) 59–66.

Luker, K., Austin, L., Hogg, C., Ferguson, B. and Smith, K. (1997) Nurse prescribing: the views of nurses and other health care professionals. *British Journal of Community Nursing* **2** (2) 69–74.

Medicines Healthcare Products Regulatory Agency (2005) *Consultation on Proposals to Introduce Independent Prescribing by Pharmacists*. London, MHRA.

National Health Service Executive (1998) *Clinical Governance. Quality in the NHS*. London, DH.

National Health Service Information Centre Prescribing Support Unit (2007) *Prescribing Monitoring Report. Quarter 1, Leeds*. Available at http://www.ic.nhs.uk. Accessed 26 November 2008.

National Prescribing Centre (1999) Signposts for Prescribing Nurses – General Principles of Good Prescribing. *Prescribing Nurse Bulletin*. Liverpool, NPC. Available at http://www.npc.co.uk.

National Prescribing Centre (2004) *Patient Group Directions. A Practical Guide and Framework of Competencies for All Professionals Using Patient Group Directions. Incorporating an Overview of Existing Mechanisms for the Supply and Prescribing of Medicines*. Liverpool, NPC.

Nursing and Midwifery Council (2006) *Standards for Proficiency of Nurse and Midwife Prescribers*. London, NMC.

Nursing and Midwifery Council (2008) *The Code. Standards of Conduct, Performance and Ethics for Nurses and Midwives*. London, NMC.

Phillips, S.J. (2008) Legislative update. Twentieth anniversary. *The Nurse Practitioner* **33** (1) 10–34.

Royal Pharmaceutical Society of Great Britain (2006) *Curriculum for the Education and Training of Pharmacist Supplementary Prescribers to Become Independent Prescribers.* London, RPSBG. Available at http://www.rspgb.org. Accessed 25 November 2008.

Schön, D. (1983) *The Reflective Practitioner. How Professionals Think in Action.* London, Avebury.

Schön, D. (1987) *Educating the Reflective Practitioner.* San Francisco, Josey-Bass Publishers.

Spence, D. and Anderson, M. (2007) Implementing a prescribing practicum within a master's degree in advanced nursing practice. *Nursing Praxis in New Zealand* **23** (2) 27–42.

Strickland-Hodge, B. (2008) Nurse prescribing the elephant in the room? *Quality in Primary Care* **16** 103–107.

Chapter 7
Advanced Practice in Dietetics

Linda Hindle

Introduction

This chapter draws on the writer's experience as head of a dietetic service in establishing a consultant post within an National Health Service (NHS) trust and working in that role as a specialist in the management of obesity. Dietetics is a relatively small profession. The number of consultant roles has only recently broken into double figures and there are few publications about this aspect of practice. This chapter begins by explaining why consultant dietitians were needed in relation to the professional career structure and patient care. The role of a consultant dietitian is then outlined using the example of the author's post in the management of obesity. Finally, the process of developing a consultant role within a department is discussed; alongside this are a number of examples of current posts in different parts of the United Kingdom demonstrating how posts have developed to meet local needs. The chapter closes by considering the future for consultant roles in dietetics.

Reasons for the development of consultant roles in dietetics

Consultant posts for allied health professionals (AHPs) consultant posts were introduced by the UK Department of Health at the beginning of the twenty-first century (DH 2000a). The intention was to provide a new career opportunity to help retain experienced AHPs and recognise their clinical contribution to patient care, strengthen professional leadership and provide better outcomes for patients by improving quality and services (DH 2000a). This was a radical step because, at that time, career progression was very limited for dietitians who wanted to maintain a clinical focus. Those who wished to progress beyond the lowest grades of dietetic practice found that the only way to do this was to move into a post with management responsibility. This resulted in the loss of expert clinicians and many dietitians eventually moved out of the dietetic profession altogether to take up general management positions (Campbell and Gavaghan 2005).

Prior to the 1990s, senior I posts represented the highest clinical grade possible and allowed dietitians to specialise in a discrete area of dietetics. Thus dietitians with no desire or aptitude for management could potentially spend 95% of their careers in positions with no potential for progression; this is assuming that they worked for 40 years and reached a senior I post within 2 years, which was commonplace. Many became extremely specialised and respected within their fields; they developed clinical, education and research skills yet were not able to receive the recognition or remuneration they deserved. The development of clinical specialist roles in the early 1990s and consultant roles in 2004 meant that dietitians could, for the first time, develop clinical careers to the same levels as those who had taken a management route (Whitley Council 2007). Following the introduction of Agenda for Change, which came into full effect in 2006 (DH 2004), dietitians now begin their careers at band 5; senior I posts are now at band 6 or 7. Specialist and consultant posts are now at band 7 or 8b, respectively (DH 2004).

The consultant role

The role of consultant dietitians is based on the same four key functions as other non-medical consultant posts (DH 1998, 2001). While these functions are identified separately, they inevitably overlap. First, there is a strong emphasis on clinical practice with 4% of working time of current UK consultant dietitians spent in this way (BDA 2007). Second, education, training and professional development are considered an important part of the role, accounting for approximately 27% of activity. Both the first and second aspects of the role are linked, not only to each other, but also to the third element, the provision of professional leadership. This accounts for about 18% of the role with the final element, service development, research and evaluation making up the remainder. The British Dietetic Association also has a view on the role of consultants stating that post holders must be clinical experts able to expand practice and improve patient care (BDA 2007).

Working as a consultant in obesity management

Role development

The primary role of the consultant dietitian in obesity management is to provide clinical leadership. This role requires engagement with key stakeholders in primary and secondary care plus those in other agencies to work within available resources in developing clinical pathways that effectively manage and help prevent obesity. This includes working with multiple agencies to promote change and highlight obesity management or prevention as a priority for action. The role was established by a primary care NHS trust to address the needs of the local population, at a point when there was significant political, media and public interest in the rising prevalence of obesity. As a result of the obesity epidemic, a public service agreement target was established to halt the year-on-year rise in obesity in under-11-year-olds by 2010 (HM Treasury 2004). This target was the joint responsibility of the Department of Health, the Department of Education and the Department of Culture, Media and Sport.

Birmingham City Council's Health Overview and Scrutiny Committee undertook a review of childhood obesity in 2003/2004, which reported on the lack of progress locally (Birmingham City Council 2004). The report noted the lack of a coherent, city-wide approach that incorporated inter-agency working. Services were not well developed or easy to access and there was poor surveillance and monitoring of the prevalence of childhood obesity. The report stated that schools should be seen as an essential part of any solution to tackle obesity but noted that they were also part of the problem. It concluded that the prevalence of food poverty, the ability to obtain healthy, affordable food, cannot be underestimated. Food poverty may be due to a range of factors that include lack of local shops or difficulty in accessing them, lack of knowledge about healthy eating or cooking. People on low incomes have the lowest intake of fruit and vegetables and are far more likely to suffer from dietary-related diseases such as cancer, diabetes, obesity and coronary heart disease (Watson 2002).

The initial intention was to establish a strategic framework for the prevention and treatment of obesity and to develop a care pathway. Consequently the consultant role was at first divided between providing professional leadership, in terms of creating and maintaining enthusiasm for the development of the strategy and care pathway, consultancy, that is to say advising on strategic development and service developments. By the end of the second year, the care pathway and strategic framework had been developed and agreed, and so emphasis was redirected towards establishing services, training and clinical practice. By the end of the third year, it is anticipated that there will be an increased emphasis on evaluation, research and education (Table 7.1).

Clinical practice

Expert clinical practice is difficult to define although it has been discussed in the literature (Benner 1984, Benner and Tanner 1987, Castledine 1996, Manley 1997, McEvoy and Johnson 2005). It is a combination of theoretical and experiential knowledge and skills that enable practitioners to undertake a holistic assessment, after

Table 7.1   The approximate proportion of time spent by a consultant dietitian in obesity in the four defined functions of a consultant during the first 3 years in post.

Functions of a consultant	Year 1 (%)	Year 2 (%)	Year 3 (%)
Expert clinical practice	15	25	30
Professional leadership and consultancy	40	25	20
Education, training and professional development	15	25	20
Service development, research and evaluation	30	25	30

which they can speedily identify and address the individual's particular problems. These problems often reflect a complex array of needs for which there may be no defined treatment protocol. Many of the patients referred to the consultant dietitian in obesity management have endured a constant and losing battle to manage their weight. They may have been supported by health professionals and private practitioners without success and are often referred to the specialist weight management clinic as a last resort before considering bariatric surgery.

The clinic was established by the consultant dietitian and is staffed by a multi-professional team that includes a general practitioner (GP) with a special interest in weight management and a consultant in psychology (Table 7.2). This clinic is currently restricted to seeing those patients who are morbidly obese, that is to say, those with a body mass index (BMI) greater than 40 kg/m^2. BMI is a mathematical relationship between height and weight used to define obesity. The normal range is 20–25 with any score over 30 classed as obese (WHO 1995). Patients with conditions such as diabetes, cardiovascular disease and sleep apnoea and a BMI greater than 35 kg/m^2 are also eligible to attend the clinic.

Evidence indicates that a multi-professional approach to weight management will result in the best outcomes (HDA 2004). This approach has been recommended as part of the 2006 NICE (National Institute for Health and Clinical Excellence) guidance on the prevention and treatment of obesity (NICE 2006). Yet until recently obese patients were referred only for dietetic advice from specialist dietitians trained in the application of cognitive behavioural therapy approach. Paradoxically, developing a specialist service has reduced the cognitive therapy elements of dietetic practice as this is covered in detail by the psychotherapist. However, this has created opportunities for the consultant dietitian to concentrate on the specifics of diet therapy. Nevertheless, a grasp of cognitive behavioural therapy remains essential for work with this group of patients.

Professional leadership

Leadership comes not only from being in a position of responsibility but also from the individual's ability to articulate a vision and inspire others to contribute to it

Table 7.2   The roles of the health-care professional within the obesity clinic.

General practitioner (GP) with a special interest in weight management	Consultant dietitian	Consultant in cognitive behavioural psychology
The initial assessment of all patients is by a physician. The aims of the initial consultation are to assess the following: (1) Possible medical causes for obesity, e.g. hypothyroidism, Cushing's syndrome (2) The type of obesity, i.e. central or lower-body (3) The impact of obesity on existing co-morbidity, including mental health (4) Relevant medical history (5) Patients' understanding of obesity and its causes (6) Patients' aims and expectations (7) Patients' motivation to lose weight including details of previous attempts to lose weight and reasons for failure	All patients will be assessed by a dietician at their initial visit. The initial patient assessment will include the following: (1) Weight history (as child and adult) (2) Dieting history (previous regimes tried) (3) Dieting successes – why did this approach work well? (4) Family history (5) Disordered eating (6) Motivation and confidence (7) Nutritional knowledge (8) Current activity/exercise levels (9) Current nutritional intake (10) Body mass index and energy requirements	Mental health issues may often be associated with obesity, particularly anxiety and depression. It is therefore important to recognise and treat these appropriately if patients are to effectively tackle their obesity Psychological factors and complex relationships with food may also be an issue for some patients with obesity. Assessment and counselling will be provided for these patients by the cognitive behavioural psychologist either in group or individual sessions
Following this assessment, the physician will discuss some or all of the following depending on the individual patient: (1) The likely cause of obesity (2) The impact of the type of obesity *per se* and its impact on existing co-morbidity (3) Any misconceptions about obesity (4) Patients' aims and expectations and their motivation to lose weight	Once the initial assessment is complete, the dietitian will discuss the following issues with each patient. The level will depend on what has been covered by the physician: (1) Benefits of weight loss (2) Motivation for behaviour change (using decisional balance – look at pros/cons)	If the cognitive behavioural psychologist feels that there are any major mental health issues that need to be resolved before patients enter a weight reduction programme, the referring GP will be asked to arrange for the patient to be reviewed by a psychiatrist

Contd.

Table 7.2   *Contd.*

General practitioner (GP) with a special interest in weight management	Consultant dietitian	Consultant in cognitive behavioural psychology
(5) A management strategy to achieve goals with particular emphasis on the following: • long-term nature of such a strategy • need for and impact of good dietary habits and regular exercise (6) Role of drug therapy (7) Help from other members of the multi-disciplinary team Referral to appropriate members of the multi-disciplinary team and request referring GP to prescribe medication if appropriate	(3) A suitable healthy eating plan and set targets for weight loss including 5% weight loss at 6 months and 10% at 12 months The following may be used to help achieve target weight loss: • prescribed energy deficit (600 kcal deficit) • low fat and anti-obesity agent • change programme • very low calorie diet (VLCD) • Protein sparing modified fast (4) Advice on: • energy balance • active living • reading nutritional labels • shopping and cooking tips • healthy choices when eating out • maintaining weight loss and preventing relapses (5) Individual follow-up appointments and attendance at group sessions as appropriate in order to: • provide support to help patient make changes to achieve and maintain goals • discuss any concerns that the patient has • clarify any misconceptions regarding diet • aid the patient in overcoming barriers to changes in lifestyle	

(Marriner Tomey 1993). A consultant role brings with it the expectation of leadership based on professional skills and knowledge not only about the discipline but also about service development, quality improvements, managing change and working across organisational boundaries. In addition, consultants must be self aware, personally resilient, with excellent interpersonal and communication skills and the ability to be creative and visionary (Campbell and Gavaghan 2005). A consultant exhibiting such attributes will become a focal point for the organisation providing and advice and support on a range of issues from clinical practice to strategic development (DH 1999, 2000b) (Box 7.1).

Box 7.1   Examples of professional leadership and consultancy within the consultant dietitian's role

- Representing dietetics and the primary care trust of groups such as the City Council Children and Young People's Nutrition Task Force and the Regional Obesity Task Force, both of which are multi-agency groups attempting to reduce the prevalence of obesity.
- Chairing the Obesity Strategy Group and the Implementation Group. These multi-professional groups work across organisational boundaries. Consequently, it has been essential to maintain excellent communication and take on board a wide range of views while reaching conclusions that address all parties' needs and, more importantly, the issue of obesity.
- Liaising with commissioners to make recommendations for commissioning in relation to obesity.
- Participating in the contract awarding process for the provision of training for other professional groups. This has included developing a service specification and assessing tenders against this.
- Working with other professional groups such as school nurses and health visitors to define and develop their roles in relation to obesity.
- Making recommendations to the Professional Executive Committee and the Board of the NHS trust regarding the approach taken towards the prevention and management of obesity.
- Leading a cross-city dietetic support group for obesity with the aim of ensuring a consistent dietetic approach and supporting evidence-based practice.
- Initiating and overseeing service redesign within the dietetic service.

Education, training and professional development

Many of the elements of a consultant's role overlap. This was demonstrated using the obesity service redesign within the dietetic service. This involved professional leadership from the perspective of creating the vision and engaging the service to change. It incorporated professional development as members of the team reviewed their roles in the management of obesity and considered where the dietetic role should fit in relation to other service providers. This resulted in focusing and developing the role of the dietitian to provide input to those with severe obesity and complex or multiple diagnoses plus developing the role of dietetic assistants to provide weight management advice for those with a BMI below 30 and without multiple diagnoses. Training was provided to support dietetic assistants to undertake their new role. There was also a service development component as new specialist level services were created. Evaluation of the whole redesign is ongoing and this process has created opportunities for research in terms of approaches to weight maintenance, assessing the effectiveness of specialist services in primary care and the role of dietetic assistants in the management of obesity. Figure 7.1 shows the relationship between the various components of the consultant role during a service redesign.

Education, training and professional development are the keys to change management programmes. The dietetic consultant will be involved in the development of education and training packages for a range of professional groups and the delivery of presentations at strategic, professional, academic and community levels. Education, training and professional development may come from participation in working groups, professional organisations, special interest groups, publication mentorship and supervision as well as traditional approaches (HPC 2006).

Service development, research and evaluation

The consultant role inevitably involves service development. Audit, evaluation and research are essential if service providers and practitioners are to engage 'the

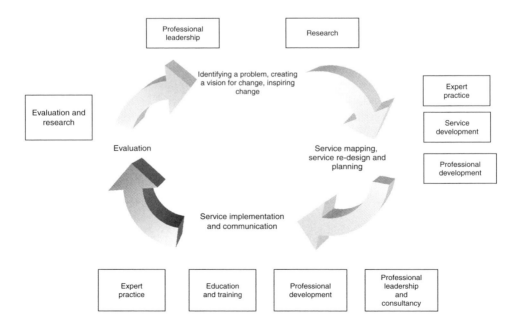

Fig. 7.1 Relationship between components of a consultant post in the redesign of services.

conscientious, explicit and judicious use of current best evidence in making decisions about the care of individual patients' (Sackett *et al.* 1996, p. 71). In today's rapidly changing health service, where departments and staff are attempting to meet frequent and challenging targets, there is a risk of moving from one initiative to the next without fully completing and evaluating each piece of work. The workplace requires a compromise between what is ideal from an evidence-based perspective – professional, legal and ethical – and what is practical within the resources available and acceptable to the users of the services. Consultant dietitians, in fulfilling the elements of the post, may provide support to others undertaking research and evaluation as well as conducting research in their own right. Some consultant posts are located in research-focused environments, such as teaching hospitals, and, therefore, post holders may undertake research as part of a wider team. Working at the cutting edge of a particular field creates opportunities to identify questions that require further investigation. While consultant dietitians will not have the time or resources to address all of these, their views and expertise will be sought from colleagues and students and, consequently, they are in a position to influence research undertaken by others.

Setting up a consultant post

Consultant posts are usually developed in response to local needs and so will vary from one place to another. The creation of consultant posts requires the approval of the relevant health authority committee responsible for ensuring that patients will benefit and how they will do so. The committee is also responsible for ensuring that adequate and appropriate resources are in place, relevant stakeholders have been involved and that the post fits the local workforce strategy; in other words, that the evidence required from NHS bodies with regard to appointing consultants has been met (DH 1999, 2001). In order to present a case for a consultant post it is useful to consider certain principles (Box 7.2). Following these will ensure that the evidence of need for the post has been justified, that the development of the post has been clearly thought through, that funding is in place and that support from stakeholders has been obtained. This will not only meet the requirements for the post to be approved but also create a positive environment for the new post holder.

Box 7.2   Guidelines for the development of a consultant post

Determine the field in which you want to establish a consultant's post, e.g. rehabilitation, oncology, obesity, paediatrics, gastroenterology, mental health, diabetes, public health.

Discuss your proposals with all key stakeholders within the local health economy.

Identify a source of funding for the post. This will usually come from a trust or consortia of trusts, e.g. a group of primary care trusts, which has identified the need to establish such a position.

Submit the proposal to the appropriate body for approval. There will usually be a given format for doing this and you will need to provide the following information:

- Outline the service benefits of establishing the post and the speciality involved.
- Draft a job description, person specification and job plan.
- Provisionally assess the salary. Consultant posts have been graded 8a–8d.
- Clarify where the post will fit within an organisation. Consultant posts are usually accountable to a Director.
- Set a timetable for the appointment process.

Examples of dietetic consultant roles

Box 7.3 presents seven examples of consultant posts in dietetics. Each has been developed in response to specific local needs and, consequently, they appear quite different. However, certain commonalities can be seen. All include elements of the four strands of consultant roles: expert clinical practice, professional leadership and consultancy, education and professional development, research and evaluation. The emphasis on each of these strands varies from post to post. Those with a public health perspective tend to have a greater emphasis on strategic service development whereas acute clinical posts have a specific focus on clinical practice and the development of protocols and guidelines. Some of the posts in hospital settings have been established to relieve work that would previously have been done by medical practitioners. Most consultant dietitians are actively involved in groups working at national level, for example, the British Dietetic Association. This enables them to provide professional leadership on a wider stage. Interestingly, a majority of consultant dietitians have previously been heads of dietetic services.

Box 7.3   Current examples of dietetic consultant roles

Role of the consultant dietitian in diabetes care

The funding for this post was identified as a means of relieving the work of medical consultants and as a means of acknowledging the unique expertise of dietitians. This expertise includes providing clinical services to patients traditionally referred to a medical consultant and leading on projects and research with regard to structured education programmes for people with diabetes in line with the National Service Framework for Diabetes (DH 2003b, 2005).

The role encompasses local and national work within the field of diabetes. The consultant is responsible for the quality and training of dietitians working in the NHS trust. Along with other medical and non-medical consultants, the consultant dietitian reviews evidence and develops guidelines and protocols in relation to patient care in order to promote evidence-based practice. The consultant dietitian is the lead clinician for a geographically defined multi-disciplinary team within the trust and, within this role, strategically develops the service to patients and practices, provides advice at national level to dietetic and multi-professional working groups and is involved in local delivery and national development of the Diabetes Education and Self Management for Ongoing and Newly Diagnosed (DESMOND) project. Future areas of work will include developing a local obesity strategy and programmes for people with impaired glucose tolerance.

Role of the consultant dietitian in a specialist hospital for cancer care

The post was established in 2004 in a large comprehensive cancer centre. The role of consultant dietitian involves responsibility for ensuring nutrition is considered at a strategic level in the development of catering and nutrition policies within the trust, developing advanced practice roles and the development of patient-focused care pathways for particular groups of patients who require a significant amount of nutritional support as part of their package of care. The role extends outside the hospital to the cancer network. The post holder is able to influence national recommendations through, for example, the National Institute for Clinical Excellence and the British Dietetic Association Oncology Group. One of the key roles is education, primarily through The Royal Marsden School of Cancer Nursing and Rehabilitation, where courses are available for AHPs and nurses, and promoting research within the rehabilitation department.

The consultant dietitian has completed her PhD on diet and body weight in patients with breast cancer and lymphoedema. She is currently a member of a number of national groups including the advisory board for the charity Cancer-BACUP; she is chair of the BDA Oncology Group. In addition to advising patients she has published a cookery book aimed at healthy eating for cancer prevention. This is a move away from advising cancer patients to give evidence-based advice to the general public on eating for cancer prevention for the general public.

Reference: Shaw, C. (2005) *Cancer: The Power of Food – Food, Facts and Recipes from the Royal Marsden Hospital*. London, Hamlyn.

Role of the consultant dietitian in nutrition

This consultant dietitian post is based in the Channel Islands. With a small island population and limited dietetic resources, the post is more general and wide-ranging than other consultant dietitian roles. The service priority remains the provision of strong leadership across diverse clinical areas and the education and development of members of other professions.

With a background of research interests in both nutritional and anthropological topics, including a doctoral study of food and identity issues among Iranian migrants in Britain, the post holder has continued to develop the research component of this consultant post. She was awarded a local research bursary and conducted a pilot randomised control trial examining the effects of omega 3 supplements in the treatment of Alzheimer's patients. She has also led a review of the evidence supporting the use of nutritional supplements in depression on behalf of the Mental Health Group of the British Dietetic Association. Following this, she initiated a collaborative partnership with the Foundation of Mental Health and the Royal College of Psychiatry in order to produce practical evidence-based patient information booklets.

Role of the consultant dietitian in clinical nutrition

This post was established in 2001 and encompasses a broad strategic role in ensuring that the nutritional care of patients is seen as a high priority within the trust and that the same consistent high standards of care are provided across the primary care and secondary care interface. Liaising and working with multi-disciplinary teams across the interfaces to raise the profile of clinical nutrition is an important part of the role. The main focus of the post is on the prevention and management of malnutrition across a broad range of clinical areas including medicine, surgery, trauma, critical care and long-term care. Taking the lead on the development of appropriate standards, procedures, protocols and audit tools and evaluating progress is an integral part of this work.

Developing sustainable education and training programmes relating to the nutritional management of patients is a key part of the role and the post holder is currently working with the training teams across the health community to develop e-learning modules. She is involved in postgraduate and undergraduate training and is also a member of the editorial boards of several professional journals; she regularly submits articles for publication. She is actively involved with national committees. These include the Parenteral and Enteral Nutrition Group of the British Dietetic Association and the British Association for Parenteral and Enteral Nutrition (BAPEN). Recent activities include working on the development of a tool for nutritional assessment as part of the Malnutrition Advisory Group of BAPEN. She has recently been awarded the prestigious Professor John Lennard-Jones medal for her contributions to clinical nutrition.

Role of the consultant dietitian in gastroenterology

The consultant dietitian is an expert practitioner in gastroenterology, with a responsibility to facilitate strategic development across primary, secondary and tertiary care and with King's College London. She provides expert clinical practice and continuing care for people with inflammatory bowel disease and irritable bowel syndrome who attend Guy's and St Thomas' NHS Foundation Trust. She works with the clinical director of gastroenterology and primary care to provide direct access for patients with acute exacerbations of inflammatory bowel disease and acts as an expert dietetic resource for gastroenterology locally and nationally.

The post holder is involved in developing evidence-based protocols and standards of care and undertakes research and audit in the field of nutrition and gastroenterology. Her role has enabled her to provide leadership for all dietitians working in primary care and local acute trusts and, at the same time, to facilitate the organisational change necessary to deliver a dietetic consultant-led service for patients with irritable bowel syndrome in collaboration with medical, nursing and allied health colleagues.

Role of the consultant dietitian for intestinal failure

The Intestinal Failure Unit is one of two nationally funded National Specialist Commissioning Advisory Group (NSCAG) units in the United Kingdom. The team cares for 140 home parenteral nutrition patients from all over the country. The role of consultant dietitian encompasses expert practice in the dietetic management of short bowel syndrome and of surgical patients with complex needs. The consultant dietitian has published work on distal feeding and fistuloclysis as part of the surgical team on the unit and regularly presents at national conferences and study days. She also chairs the nutrition steering group across primary and secondary care and therefore ensures clinical nutrition is considered at a strategic level within both organisations. One of her key roles is education. She holds an honorary contract at Chester University and regularly contributes to under- and postgraduate dietetic modules. She has been nominated to join the BAPEN education committee this year to represent the Parenteral and Enteral Nutrition Group of the British Dietetic Association.

Professional leadership is an essential part of the role. The consultant dietitian works across primary and secondary care, providing leadership for some 20 dietitians, 3 assistant dietitians and an exercise trainer; a significant amount of her time is spent ensuring the department is meeting the challenges of working in the modern NHS.

The role of the consultant dietitian in public health nutrition

This consultant is responsible for the development, implementation, monitoring and evaluation of a public health nutrition and dietetic strategy for a region served by three local authorities, three community health partnerships, one acute unit and one primary care division. This post involves working closely with other agencies to raise the profile of public health nutrition and to ensure that nutrition issues are incorporated into relevant strategies. The post holder is involved in the education and development of staff regarding nutrition, research and the direct management of seven members of staff and a small budget.

Conclusion – the future for consultant dietitians

Non-medical consultant posts were established in a political context in which there was a strong focus on improving the quality of clinical services and patient experience and a drive to strengthen clinical leadership (DH 2000b). However, they are expensive in relation to other non-medical clinical posts and in a health service that is under constant financial pressure, may be difficult to justify unless their value is made explicit. The role of medical consultants is well recognised by the public, politicians and other health service staff; non-medical consultants need to ensure that their roles are equally clear to others especially in terms of cost-effectiveness and benefits to the organisation. In particular, they must make clear why these benefits cannot be achieved by other, less expensive staff.

Consultant roles were established to provide clinical leadership and influence decision-making at a strategic level while maintaining clinical contact without the additional responsibilities of management (NHSE 1999). Consultant dietitians' posts are usually graded as similar to heads of dietetic services and, therefore, as senior members of staff, they may be asked to take on responsibilities, for example, managing a budget or members of staff (DH 2003a). In deciding whether to take on these tasks, the consultants will need to determine whether they will enhance or detract from the central focus of their roles.

The nature of consultant posts means that post holders can be isolated from clinicians at a similar level. This is certainly the case in dietetics and, to help in this matter, the British Dietetics Association has supported the development of a clinical network for consultants. Such networks will be useful in terms of professional networking and development for consultant dietitians and create a forum to advance their roles. Networks also have an important role to play in helping those who aspire to become consultants. Currently, there are few suitable applicants for consultant dietician posts. It is essential that clinicians have the chance to develop to a stage at which they can embrace this excellent opportunity to strengthen professional leadership.

? Key questions for Chapter 7

In your field of practice:
(1)   What are the opportunities for creating consultant dietetic posts?
(2)   How would you convince commissioners and stakeholders of the need for a consultant dietetic post?
(3)   To what extent do you think consultant dietetic posts might differ from other advanced roles such as that of clinical specialist? What are your reasons?

Acknowledgements

Kristine Farrar, Consultant Dietitian in Intestinal Failure, Salford PCT

Miranda Lomer, Consultant Dietitian in Gastroentereology, Guy's and Thomas's NHS Trust and King's College, London

Vera Todorovic, Consultant Dietitian in Clinical Nutrition, Doncaster and Bassetlaw Hospitals, NHS Foundation Trust

Dr Lynn Harbottle, Consultant in Nutrition, Guernsey

Clare Shaw, Consultant Dietitian in Cancer, The Royal Marsden NHS Foundation Trust

Lindsay Oliver, Consultant Dietitian in Diabetes Care, Northumbria Healthcare Trust

Joyce Thompson, Dietetic Consultant in Public Health, British Dietetic Association

References

Benner, P. (1984) *From Novice to Expert: Excellence and Power in Clinical Nursing Practice.* Menlo Park, California, Addison Wesley.

Benner, P. and Tanner, C. (1987) Clinical judgment. How nurses use intuition. *American Journal of Nursing* **87** (1) 23–31.

Birmingham City Council Health Overview and Scrutiny Committee (2004) *Children's Nutrition – Obesity.* Available at www.birmingham.gov.uk/scrutiny.

British Dietetic Association (2007) *Dietetic Consultant Posts: Your Questions Answered.* Birmingham, Unpublished paper, British Dietetic Association. Available at http://www.bda.com.

Campbell, J. and Gavaghan, S. (2005) Outlining the essential attributes of a nurse/therapist consultant: a role analysis. In *Demystifying the Nurse/Therapist Consultant. A Foundation Text,* (eds R. McSherry and S. Johnson). Cheltenham, Nelson Thornes.

Castledine, G. (1996) The role and criteria of an advance practitioner. *British Journal of Nursing* **5** (5) 288–9.

Department of Health (1998) *A First Class Service: Quality in the New NHS.* London, DH.

Department of Health (1999) *Making a Difference: Strengthening the Nursing, Midwifery and Health Visiting Contribution to Health and Health Care.* London, DH.

Department of Health (2000a) *Meeting the Challenge; a Strategy for Allied Health Professionals.* London, DH.

Department of Health (2000b) *The NHS Plan. A Plan for Investment. A Plan for Reform.* Wetherby, DH.

Department of Health (2001) *Arrangement for Consultant Posts – Staff Covered by the Professions Allied to Medicine.* PT 'A' Whitely Council. Advanced Letter PAM (PT 'A') 2/2001, Leeds, DH.

Department of Health (2003a) *Agenda for Change – Proposed Agreement.* Available at http://www.dh.gov.uk.

Department of Health (2003b) *National Service Framework for Diabetes – Delivery Strategy.* London, DH.

Department of Health (2004) *Agenda for Change. Final Agreement.* London, DH. Available at http://www.dh.gov.uk.

Department of Health (2005) *Structured Patient Education in Diabetes. Report from the Patient Education Working Group.* London, DH.

Health Development Agency (2004) *Evidence for the Effective Prevention and Treatment of Obesity.* London, HDA.

Health Professions Council (2006) *Your Guide to Our Standards for Continuing Professional Development.* London, HPC.

Her Majesty's Treasury (2004) *Spending Reviews 2004: Public Services Agreements 2005/2008.* Chapter 3, London, DH. Available at http://www.hmtreasury.gov.uk/spending_review/spend_sr04/psa/spend_sr04_psaindex.cfm.

Manley, K. (1997) A conceptual framework for advanced practice: an action research project. Operationalising an advanced practitioner/consultant nurse role. *Journal of Clinical Nursing* **6** (3) 179–90.

Marriner Tomey, A. (1993) *Transformational Leadership in Nursing.* St Louis, Mosby Yearbook.

McEvoy, M. and Johnson, S. (2005) Exemplifying the nurse/therapist consultant: a practical approach. In *Demystifying the Nurse/Therapist Consultant. A Foundation Text*, (eds R. McSherry and S. Johnson). Cheltenham, Nelson Thornes.

National Health Service Management Executive (1999) *Nurse, Midwife and Health Visitor Consultants*. Health Service Circular 1999/217 September 1999.

National Institute for Health and Clinical Excellence (2006). *Guidance on the Prevention, Identification, Assessment and Management of Overweight and Obesity in Adults and Children*. National Institute for Health and Clinical Excellence Clinical Guideline 43.

Sackett, D., Rosenberg, W., Gray, J., Haynes, R. and Richardson, W. (1996) Evidence-based medicine: What it is and what it isn't. *British Medical Journal* **312** (7023) 71–2.

Watson, S. (2002) *Hunger from the Inside. The Experience of Food Poverty in the UK*. London, Sustain.

Whitley Council (2007) National Framework Agreement. *Newsletter* **3**. Available at http://www.admin.ox.ac.uk/ps/hera/wcnewsapr07-pdf.

World Health Organisation (1995) *Physical Status: The Use and Interpretation of Anthropometry*. Report of a WHO Expert Committee. WHO technical Report Series 854. Geneva, WHO.

Chapter 8

Advanced Practice in Occupational Therapy

Lynne Frith and Janette Walsh

Introduction

This chapter explores the development of advanced practice in occupational therapy. There have always been highly experienced occupational therapists who have built up knowledge and skills throughout their careers but until recently there were few opportunities available to those who wished to further their careers in clinical settings. This situation has now begun to change, with advanced practice developing along similar lines to that of nursing. However, there is little published material about advanced practice in occupational therapy and this chapter is one of the first to address this topic.

The chapter begins by examining the concept of advanced practice in occupational therapy with regard to the differences among clinicians, specialists and consultant roles; the drivers and strategic developments that have led to these roles are discussed. The chapter then goes on to address the roles of clinical specialist and consultant occupational therapist. The expectations of the various roles are considered alongside the knowledge and education required for each. The chapter closes by examining the future of advanced practice in occupational therapy.

Advanced practice in occupational therapy

Until very recently occupational therapists who wished to further their careers beyond senior I under the old Whitley Council pay scales (now band 6 or 7 following Agenda for Change, DH 2004, 2005) were faced with a straightforward choice of posts in management, research or education (Craik 2002). There were no opportunities to develop a career in clinical practice. Current health service reforms aim to retain experienced practitioners in clinical settings and enable managers to be creative and flexible in order to make the best use of experienced staff (DH 2000b). These reforms have opened the way for the development of new roles that cross traditional professional boundaries as a way of meeting the increasing demands placed on the health service, reducing waiting lists and improving quality. In particular, it is anticipated that, to achieve these aims, the provision of health care in the future will involve the crossing of professional boundaries (DH 2000a).

In this context the College of Occupational Therapists (COT) supports the idea of extending clinical roles, for example, in requesting and interpreting X-rays, using complementary therapies and prescribing and administering medicines. However, these new developments must be within the scope of law; recognised and supported by employers; based on post holders having adequate knowledge, experience and skills for what is required; covered by adequate liability insurance by the employer as the British Association of Occupational Therapists will not indemnify extended roles; accompanied by appropriate changes in pay and grading and supported with appropriate supervision and advice (COT 2006a).

The COT has not specifically defined advanced practice. The term *advanced practitioner* has been synonymous with that of *lead practitioner* or *higher-level practitioner* although it usually refers to clinical specialist and consultant roles (COT 2003). Expert clinical practice is clearly a major feature of both these roles but other competencies are also required. These include the ability to use evidence-based practice, clinical leadership, organisational skills, management skills and communication skills. Moreover, the practitioner must be able to manage change within the context of providing a high standard of skills within a specific clinical area to improve patient and carer experience (COT 2003).

Specialist roles in occupational therapy

The COT defines a clinical specialist as 'an OT who works within a specific clinical area of practice at a highly specialised and advanced level. He/she will have an expert body of knowledge and skill particular to that area of clinical care' (COT 2003, p. 2). The college goes on to outline the main components of the specialist role.

Clinical caseload and expertise

Clinical specialists use advanced clinical reasoning at a high level to manage a complex clinical caseload. They engage in evidence-based practice and demonstrate skills in reflection and critical thinking in a manner that improves the quality of service provision and enables them to contribute to research.

Clinical leadership

Clinical specialists are actively involved in influencing service improvement in their clinical areas, providing a source of leadership expertise and advice. They take an active role in clinical governance and quality issues demonstrating effective communication. Their role encompasses professional activities both within and outside the profession.

Clinical teaching and mentoring

Clinical specialists actively participate in training at local and, possibly, national levels in their own specific areas. This includes the supervision of students and qualified, but less experienced, occupational therapists and the provision of specialist in-service training to colleagues, including other members of the multi-disciplinary team.

Specialist advisory role

Clinical specialists take the lead in developing strategies related to enquiries made within the service and service initiatives. They promote the role of occupational therapy within the field of expertise (COT 2003). Becoming a clinical specialist requires individual practitioners to meet specified criteria that include several years of in-depth clinical experience at senior level, evidence of professional development and involvement in a specialist interest group within the COT (COT 2003).

Clinical specialists normally concentrate on one particular aspect of practice such as stroke or intermediate care. However, their skills and competencies and the promotion of changes in current ways of working in the NHS (DH 2000a, b) mean that they can widen their horizons and branch out into areas that have traditionally been in the sphere of nursing such as case management (DH 2006b). This involves assessing patients, developing therapeutic relationships and devising a plan of action for managing their needs, in coordination with other professionals. These skills form part of the core skills of occupational therapists (COT 2006b). They are based on a holistic view of the patient, in some ways not unlike that of nursing but with an emphasis on occupation. The additional experience, skills and knowledge of clinical specialists mean that they are well equipped for case management roles. Thus they are engaged in extending the traditional boundaries of occupational therapy practice in line with what is expected of advanced practitioner roles.

Consultant roles in occupational therapy

When consultant roles for allied health professionals were first announced it was envisaged that they would be working alongside senior medical and nursing colleagues in all health settings (DH 2000a, b). This multi-professional approach would enable teams to devise better ways of meeting the health needs of their communities. The benefits of these new posts were seen to be better patient outcomes through improved quality and service, retention of experienced clinicians through increased career opportunities and enhanced professional leadership (DH 2000b). An 'advance letter' provided guidance for those setting up consultant posts; this included defining the role and its functions (DH 2001).

The COT welcomed consultant posts and the first appointments were made in 2002. These posts focused on four key functions: 'expert clinical practice, professional leadership, practice, service development research and education, and education (and) professional development' (COT 2004a, p. 2). At least half of the appointees' working time was to be spent in clinical practice, the nature of which depended on the field in which the individual worked. Alongside this core of practice were education, professional practice and service development and research (COT 2004a). These functions were similar to the remit of other consultant posts in physiotherapy and bore a strong resemblance to the qualities of an expert nurse outlined by Benner (1984) and Chartered Society of Physiotherapists (2002).

The COT recently updated the core functions of the consultant occupational therapist, building on this evolving role outlining five key functions and a number of non-clinical activities such as modernising services and providing leadership (COT 2007a, p. 2).

Expert clinical practice

At least half of the consultants' working time continues to be in the clinical setting where they demonstrate expert clinical skills in their practice area, with advanced clinical reasoning and knowledge. In promoting best practice and developing best practice standards based on evidence, consultants develop client-centred services, which cross traditional boundaries. They achieve this maintaining high degrees of autonomy and following ethical standards (COT 2007a).

Practice and service development

Consultants are influential in initiating and developing policies from local to national levels. This involves developing collaborative partnerships with the multi-disciplinary/agency teams both strategically and operationally and facilitating service users' participation in service development (COT 2007a).

Professional leadership and consultancy

As visionary leaders, consultants inspire others at local and national levels. They provide clinical leadership to influence both strategic planning and service delivery, crossing all professional and organisational boundaries. For the profession of occupational therapy they are influential at national levels in clinical practice, service planning and policy (COT 2007a).

Research audit and evaluation

Consultants are involved in research through partnerships with higher education establishments. They disseminate research findings and clarify their relevance to clinical practice. They apply research evidence to policy and service development while identifying relevant areas for investigation to support clinical practice (COT 2007a).

Education, training and development

Consultants foster working environments in which staff members are enabled to identify their own learning needs in line with the needs of service users. While providing teaching for students and professionals across a variety of settings, consultants are able to influence education policy for pre- and post-registration students and take responsibility for the development of education initiatives for services users, staff and organisations (COT 2007a).

The qualifications required by occupational therapy consultants currently appear to be similar to those of the clinical specialist. These are based around the college's post-qualifying framework and code of professional ethics (COT 2004a, 2005, 2006c). A master's degree or working at master's level is desirable as this provides evidence of a willingness and ability to undertake further study and research (COT 2007a). PhD study is not considered essential for the role of consultant. However, some currently in consultant posts are undertaking research degrees in areas relevant to their specialist roles (COT 2007a).

The clinical specialist and consultant occupational therapist as advanced roles

The core purpose of the clinical specialist and the consultant occupational therapist is to provide high-quality, expert care directly to patients. Both possess specialist knowledge and skills relevant to their fields of practice and which are beyond those of an ordinary practitioner of occupational therapy (COT 2004a). These specialist skills and knowledge are achieved though post-qualifying education, possibly at master's degree level, and associated with a breadth of experience in different settings that enables them to develop a wide repertoire of responses to any situation (DH 2006a). Thus both are able to function as mature and sophisticated practitioners.

The criteria for specialist and consultant roles echo that of advanced practitioners in other professions, particularly nursing. Advanced nurses are also expected to spend most of their working time in clinical practice as expert practitioners. They possess a wide range of competencies appropriate to their fields of practice but with certain core elements (Box 8.1). The National Profile for Occupational Therapists highlights similarities and differences between specialist and consultant occupational therapy job

---

Box 8.1   Core competencies of advanced nursing practice

Direct and expert clinical practice
Coaching and guiding
Consultation
Research
Clinical and professional leadership
Collaboration
Ethical decision-making

Source: Summarised from Hamric, A. (2005) A definition of advanced nursing practice. Chapter 3 in *Advanced Nursing Practice. An Integrative Approach,* (eds A. Hamric, J. Spross and C. Hanson), 3rd edn. pp 85–108. St Louis, Elsevier Saunders.

---

statements (NHS Employers 2006). These suggest that the two types of therapist may be practising in ways that are comparable to those of advanced nurses but research is needed to determine whether this is actually the case, since a great deal hinges on the level at which the individual practitioner is able to function. This concept of level of practice is particularly pertinent as differences between specialist and consultant occupational therapy roles start to emerge (Table 8.1) (DH 2006a).

Table 8.1   A comparison of some of the attributes of specialist and consultant occupational therapy (OT) roles.

Attributes	OT advanced clinical specialist	OT consultant
Interpersonal skills	Handles and communicates complex information about conditions and progress to patients and relatives	Handles and communicates a wide range of information to patients, relatives and professionals
Policy and service development	Proposes and contributes to policy and service development in own field of practice. These may impact on the work of other professions and beyond immediate work area	Responsible for policy and service development in own field of practice. Implements and makes changes to policies
Finance	Can authorise small payments	Controls and is responsible for a designated budget
Staffing	Responsible for day-to-day supervision of staff	Responsible for managing staff, ensuring training takes place, identifying and delivering staff development
Research	Undertakes research activity in field of practice	Undertakes research

Source: Based on National Profile for Occupational Therapy (DOH 2006, pp 10,11 and 13). Available at http://www.nhsemployers.org/pay-conditions/pay-conditions-1988.cfm.

One of the current concerns is the issue of responsibility. Consultants have greater responsibility for strategic and organisational development combined with a higher degree of clinical responsibility than their specialist colleagues (COT 2007a). For example, specialists are expected to take part in research and clinical audits within their area but for consultants, conducting research and audit is a major part of their role. Consultants are expected to lead research programmes and to be regularly involved in other research activities. Another area where the difference in roles can be seen is the development of policies and procedures. Specialists are expected to contribute to the development of policies and procedures for their area, which may impact on the work of others, but the consultant will lead and implement such developments both locally and nationally (COT 2007a). Consultants, therefore, have responsibility beyond the usual line management structure (DH 2006a) and are expected to have a broader understanding of health and social care needs that enables them to challenge traditional boundaries (COT 2007a).

Current issues for consultant occupational therapists

Consultant posts for occupational therapists have been slow to develop but are beginning to grow in number (COT 2004a, b, Lovelace 2004). Each post has to be set up as a new venture, rather than an existing job, with clear criteria that employers must meet. A professional assessor must be available to advise on issues relevant to the profession (DH 2001). Detailed preparation is required. Managers have to clearly identify and explain why the post is needed and the ways in which patients will benefit; the place of the role in the organisation's strategic plan must also be clarified (COT 2004a, b). Such considerations allow for creativity and the exploration of new roles, for example, as joint appointments between the health service and higher education or social care (COT 2004a). These preparatory requirements mean that individuals cannot simply be promoted into a post because of long service or some other attribute.

There are currently 16 consultant occupational therapists in post; over half of these are in the fields of mental health and learning disabilities. Mental health services are currently involved in the introduction and implementation of new ways of working (DH 2007a); a whole system reform is taking place. This is creating opportunities for all health professions to develop and extend roles. Suitably qualified occupational therapists will be able to take advantage of this situation, possibly creating exciting innovative posts at consultant level (DH 2007a).

All occupational therapists have to be registered with the Health Professions Council in order to practice. At present there is no separate registration for occupational therapy consultants. Other health professions are grappling with the need to address registration for advanced and consultant practitioners; occupational therapists, as professionals, will need to debate this issue and make decisions about what is required.

Once in post, consultant occupational therapists can find themselves in a rather lonely position; they may be the only member of their profession at that level in the organisation. It is, therefore, vital to have external networks of peers who understand the demands and pressures of the role and who can advise the new consultant about particular difficulties. In response to this need the COT has set up a Consultants' Forum for post holders to share information and experience as they develop their new roles (Cusack 2007). This forum will be able to inform debate about the roles of consultants, as their experience develops, leading the way for the development of future generations. However, this can only be the beginning. As consultant roles become more established, post holders will be better able to articulate their needs and develop multiple networks that fulfil specific functions. Included here must be the issue of continuing education. Professional isolation and other's perceptions that the consultant has reached the pinnacle of the profession can lead to the assumption that there is nothing more to learn but the complexity of health care brings constant change. Consultant occupational therapists will have to ensure that they find ways of maintaining and expanding the expertise that made them suitable for appointment in the first instance.

The future for occupational therapists

Occupational therapists who wish to become consultants must also look to their personal and continuing professional development making use of the many opportunities available to help them prepare for such roles (Craik and McKay 2003). Consultants currently in post have highlighted areas in which it is essential to obtain experience; these include training and development, evidence-based practice, involvement in carrying out research and implementing results, teaching and being politically aware (COT 2004a). These factors mean that career planning must be a long-term strategy focused on gaining relevant clinical experience and training (COT 2007a) and acquiring a master's degree (Craik and McKay 2003).

There is a variety of master's degree courses available; many were initially developed for nurses but some are now validated to include allied health professionals. There are also profession-specific master's degrees, such as the MSc in Advanced Practice Occupational Therapy at Canterbury Christ Church University (COT 2007b) and clinically specific courses, for instance, in palliative care or rehabilitation studies. Thus, there are a number of different opportunities available and occupational therapists can choose whichever best suits their learning needs and career plans.

The COT is committed to assisting the development of master's and doctoral courses focused on the development of clinical specialist and consultant roles (COT 2004a). The college has also published a post-qualifying framework designed to assist occupational therapists in planning their learning and developmental needs (COT 2006a). This has recently been complemented by the Interactive Learning Opportunities (COT 2007b). These can be accessed via a link on the college's website and include continuing professional development tools, links to appropriate learning opportunities, templates for personal development plans and more to assist occupational therapists in developing their career path (http://www.cot.org.uk.).

An important part of that career path must be a change in thinking. Like all health professionals, occupational therapists' horizons can be limited to the setting in which they work. Those who aspire to become consultants must learn to look beyond this to a much larger and more complex picture. Political awareness in the community setting can be gained by getting involved in local Primary Care Trusts as clinician members of the Professional Executive Committee; in secondary care aspirant consultant occupational therapists can put themselves forward as members of the organisation's board, which has Foundation Trust status. Both courses of action will bring opportunities for involvement in the decision-making process of the whole organisation (DH 2007a, b). Line managers can help by creating working environments that facilitate a grasp of the organisation as a whole rather than the small section in which the individual is employed; they can also provide support and mentorship for the development of staff who wish to further their careers (Craik and McKay 2003).

Conclusion

This chapter has explored advanced practice and what this means for occupational therapy. It is clear that advanced practice is high on the agenda of the health service; occupational therapy is experiencing changes in its career structure enabling clinicians to be recognised for their expert clinical skills. New clinical specialist and consultant roles have been defined by the Department of Health (DH) and the COT. However, consultant posts are new and limited in number, with clinicians still finding their feet. It is certainly an exciting time for occupational therapy as a profession. The opportunities presented by these new consultant roles need to be grasped as they enable the advancement of the profession and the practitioner but more importantly benefit the service users (Craik and McKay 2003).

? Key questions for Chapter 8

In your field of practice:

(1) How can occupational therapists ensure that their role is sufficiently understood by other health professionals and commissioners to enable them to take on advanced practice roles?

(2) Taking the Ten Key Roles for Allied Health Professionals as a start, what areas could be considered for extended scope practice within occupational therapy?

(3) How can advanced practice occupational therapists cross the boundaries of professional groups to ensure a modern service, which is evidence-based and meets patient need?

References

Benner, P. (1984) *From Novice to Expert: Excellence and Power in Clinical Nursing Practice*. Menlo Park, California, Addison Wesley.
Chartered Society of Physiotherapists (2002) *Physiotherapist Consultant (NHS): Role, Attributes and Guidance for Establishing Posts*. Available at http://www.csp.org.uk.

College of Occupational Therapy (2003) *Occupational Therapy Clinical Specialist*. London, College of Occupational Therapy.

College of Occupational Therapy (2004a) *Consultant Occupational Therapist*. London, College of Occupational Therapy.

College of Occupational Therapy (2004b) Strategic vision and action plan for lifelong learning. *British Journal of Occupational Therapy* **67** (1) 20–8.

College of Occupational Therapy (2005) *Code of Ethics and Professional Conduct*. London, College of Occupational Therapy.

College of Occupational Therapy (2006a) *Extended Scope Practice College of Occupational Therapy*. London, College of Occupational Therapy.

College of Occupational Therapy (2006b) *Definitions and Core Skills for Occupational Therapy*. London, College of Occupational Therapy.

College of Occupational Therapy (2006c) *Post Qualifying Framework: A Resource for Occupational Therapists*. London, College of Occupational Therapy.

College of Occupational Therapy (2007a) *Consultant Occupational Therapist*. London, College of Occupational Therapy.

College of Occupational Therapy (2007b) *Interactive Learning Opportunities*. London, College of Occupational Therapy.

Craik, C. (2002) Consultant therapists-are you prepared? *Therapy Weekly* 13 June.

Craik, C. and McKay, E. (2003) Consultant therapists: recognising and developing expertise. *British Journal of Occupational Therapy* **66** (6) 281–83.

Cusack, L. (2007) *(personal communication)*. London, College of Occupational Therapy.

Department of Health (2000a) *The NHS Plan. A Plan for Investment. A Plan for Reform*. Wetherby, DH.

Department of Health (2000b) *Meeting the Challenge: A Strategy for the Allied Health Professionals*. London, DH.

Department of Health (2001) *Advanced Letter PAM(PTA)2//2001 Arrangements for Consultant Posts – for Staff Covered by the Professions Allied to Medicine PT ''A'' Whitley Council*. Available at http://www.dh.gov.uk/en/Publicationsandstatistics/Lettersandcirculars/Advancedletters/DH_4004127. Accessed 30 October 2005.

Department of Health (2004) Agenda for Change. Final Agreement. Available at http://www.dh.gov.uk.

Department of Health (2005) *Agenda for Change: NHS Terms and Conditions Handbook 3617*. London, DH.

Department of Health (2006a) *National Profile for Occupational Therapy*. Available at http://www.nhs.employers.org/pay-conditions/pay-conditions-1988.cfm. Accessed 18 March 2007.

Department of Health (2006b) *Caring for People with Long Term Conditions: An Education Framework for Community Matrons and Case Managers*. Available at http://www.dh.gov.uk/en/Publicationsandstatistics/Publications/PublicationsPolicyAndGuidance/DH_4133997. Accessed 11 July 2007.

Department of Health (2007a) *Guidance for the PCT Professional Executive Committee (PEC): Fit for the Future*. Available at http://www.dh.gov.uk/en/Publicationsandstatistics/Publications/PublicationsPolicyandGuidance/DH_073508. Accessed 11 July 2007.

Department of Health (2007b) *Membership of Foundation Trusts*. Available at http://www.dh.gov.uk/en/Policyandguidance/Organisationpolicy/Secondarycare/NHSfoundationtrust/DH_4095717. Accessed 11 July 2007.

Lovelace, N. (2004) Hutton probes disappointing take-up of consultant posts. *Therapy Weekly* 8 April 2004.

National Health Service Employers (2006) *National Profile for Occupational Therapists*. Available at http://www.nhsemployers.org/pay-conditions/pay-conditions-1988.cfm.

Chapter 9

Working as an Advanced Nurse Practitioner

Mark Radford

Introduction

Working as an advanced practitioner in a modern health economy is a rewarding experience but also a challenging one that provides opportunities for significant patient pathway improvements, develops the individual and enriches the organisation and nursing as a whole. However, advanced nursing practice roles are implemented in a challenging professional, financial and political climate, which, if coupled with an organisation that is not fully prepared for the role, may leave the appointed advanced nurse practitioner poorly supported, lacking direction, isolated, professionally challenged or compromised. Highly motivated clinicians may feel frustrated, devalued and leave little opportunity to truly optimise their impact for patients, the organisation or the profession.

This chapter draws on the experience of advanced practitioners and consultant nurses to provide an overview of those areas that are critical in maximising the potential of these roles. These areas include the importance of maintaining a focus on what the practitioner is to achieve, developing strategic influence and deliberately seeking out opportunities to deliver innovative models of care by reinvigorating the traditional and refocusing on efficient ways to deliver services. The advanced practitioner should aim to develop services in a commercially orientated market that delivers productivity, clinical excellence and offers value for money to the community that it serves. The context in which the practitioner operates is dynamic with the pace of reform often outstripping organisational and professional ability to proactively manage change. This change includes greater public involvement in service planning.

In the United Kingdom, health service reforms require a focus on productivity and efficiency, which offer significant opportunities to advanced practitioners in the new National Health Service (NHS) landscape of foundation trusts working with reconfigured strategic health authorities and primary care service providers including private companies. Looking to the future of the NHS, the introduction of new incentives to enable health-care professionals and NHS corporate teams to better respond and deliver to the needs of the local population are paramount. The programme of reform will continue to accelerate with new initiatives brought online from the Department of Health, Monitor and the Healthcare Commission requiring clinical nurses and more importantly advanced practitioners, to demonstrate how they deliver improved productivity, choice, quality and value for money.

Defining a need

There is little evidence in the literature to practically support organisations in developing advanced practitioner roles. Woodward *et al.* (2005) examined some of the organisational influences in developing ANP roles, identifying that these may have had a negative effect on the success of many of the roles. In the case of consultant nurses in the United Kingdom, simple central policy guidance (DH 1999) and monitoring processes were followed by devolvement to regional level, leading to significant variation in terms of delivering each of the roles.

The politicised nature of the health-care systems of the United Kingdom and the United States means that performing roles at the boundaries of practice will often ensure that, while developments such as advanced practice gain exposure, they can bring significant additional pressure. However, in some cases, political policy will prompt a rethink and be of significant benefit for the future development of advanced practice roles. This is particularly evident where traditional care models have failed to deliver expectations of the population, specific patient/client needs have emerged or have been identified following a central policy shift. The UK context has seen several policy initiatives where the development of advanced practice models has benefited, including the development of cancer services through the National Service Frameworks (NSFs) (Box 9.1) and, in primary care, case managers for those with long-term conditions. This has often been followed by economic support such as start-up capital to deliver programmes of training and development, providing a significant and welcome boost in achieving early impact.

The link between UK central policy in the development of market principles has led to many organisations rethinking how they can deliver their health-care portfolio in the most cost-effective way (Wells *et al.* 2006). This has involved a fundamental examination of what may be required from corporate nursing and

---

Box 9.1   National Service Frameworks

National Service Frameworks (NSFs) were identified in the policy document *The New NHS* (DH 1997) where the government set out plans to modernise the NHS. The concept of the NSF was to describe service models for defined care groups and put in place strategies to establish performance measures. The NSFs have been developed in partnership with professionals working within organisations in England and currently only apply to health services in that country. There are a number of NSFs including mental health, coronary heart disease, older people, diabetes, children's services, long-term conditions, renal services, cancer/oncology and paediatric intensive care.

---

clinical roles (Renshaw 2005). In addition, external societal and medical influences must be included as they have, historically, been potent catalysts for the development of advanced practice. Recent changes in the training of doctors in the United Kingdom have brought about another surge in specialist and advanced practice roles and this has been turned to the advantage of both nursing and organisations. However, Maylor (2005) suggests that, despite the successes of advanced roles, they are still implemented as local solutions and, other than, specific examples in cancer care, no coordinated strategy for advanced practice seems to exist.

Developing new roles must always begin with defining the needs of the patients and what they require in the clinical pathway or service. This is often the most challenging stage of role development as significant pressures and the conflicting priorities of the health economy, be they financial or operational, will often dictate how the roles are developed. The impetus for advanced roles may be partly driven by operational needs and therefore excludes certain key stakeholders who may guide and shape the development. In some cases, roles may be developed without input from established advanced practitioners, which may reduce the chances of shared learning particularly related to the pitfalls in role development. When considering the development of advanced roles, key stakeholder groups should be developed on a short-term basis with a clear remit for evaluating the health needs of the population. These groups should establish links with users and collect or interpret the data to support the need for a new role, taking into account the health economy context, outcomes of the patient population and needs analysis and the political context in which the role will work. Relevant local or national policies must also be considered. Alongside this, it is prudent to take into account the potential of the role to contribute in other domains such as the following:

- Organisational kudos
- Research development
- Teaching and education
- Potential political influence on nursing or health-care agendas at regional or national levels

Radford (2004) argues that this initial stage of role development should establish the nature and scope of the problem or population need. This should be followed by a thorough needs analysis as to whether the advanced nurse practice role is the most effective way of delivering to the population and to what extent the post holder will be engaging with the population. These clinical and economic perspectives inform robust business planning. It is imperative that the key stakeholder board examines these areas as a part of establishing the role and developing job descriptions, so that members are clear, from the outset, about what they are trying to achieve. Appropriate professional nursing advice should be sought to support their decision-making process.

Organisational preparation

For organisations, the development of advanced practice is a new and challenging process in which a clear understanding of the key professional issues involved will ultimately affect how the role delivers what is required (Box 9.2). A clear strategy must be in place to communicate and market the role within the organisation. Working as an advanced practitioner in an organisation that has no experience of or lacks clarity about such a role will lead to significant personal and political challenges that can, in some cases, leave both the organisation and the post holder frustrated.

Box 9.2   Checklist for the process of developing an advanced role

Attention should be given to the following:

- Role clarity
- Job planning
- Key stakeholder support including commissioners
- Medical management
- Nursing management
- Mentoring and professional development
- Funding and remuneration
- Organisational culture and experience of advanced nursing practice
- Practice authority and remit
- Legal review and assessment
- Additional activities including external consultancy
- Responsibility to the wider internal and external organisation and an evaluation process

---

Part of the organisational preparation is to identify the barriers that may affect the role. First, an advanced practitioner will be interacting with many professional groups, including medical colleagues and strategic or organisational managers. Ball (2005) suggests these are often the most influential stakeholders but it is ultimately nursing colleagues and nursing management who have the most significant influence on the acceptance. Second, there are often practical barriers, including funding streams for service development and issues about administrative support or office space. Finally, there may be legal considerations as advanced practitioners will often be working at the boundaries of traditional practice and, in some cases, in unique, innovative roles. Organisations must ensure that new posts are consistent with the law and that the appropriate insurance arrangements are in place.

Conflict can be pre-empted by clarifying the role, showing how the organisation is prepared for the new direction; thought should also be given to a communication strategy. Lack of preparation will affect the success or failure of the role (Redfern *et al.* 2003, Ball 2005, Woodward *et al.* 2005, Booth *et al.* 2006). Ultimately, lack of planning may leave the advanced practitioner unable to articulate what the role is about and what objectives it will achieve (Jasper 2006).

Job planning

Role clarity and definition will guide the ANP in the domains of operational and professional performance, but this needs to be supported through effective job planning. This is an area that is often neglected by organisations in supporting their advanced practitioners (Booth *et al.* 2006). In the United Kingdom, job planning is a process developed primarily with medical consultants (DH 2003) but it is one that has elements of benefit for advanced practitioners in that there is a far greater emphasis on service delivery, corporate goals and patient care. While the appraisal process will agree on the personal and professional development objectives, job planning will act as an interface to identify corporate objectives and how the advanced practitioner can develop services. It provides an important opportunity to review workload, balance internal and external commitments and provide a flexible objective setting for delivery. A robust job plan should include a prospective, focused and relevant review of current policy and the wider health-care agenda that offers an opportunity for the advanced practitioner to align local developments to this. Balance of workload is vital as the job plan offers and reflects a diversity of skill that is not solely related to clinical expertise but also includes research, leadership and change management. In some cases, without appropriate support, this large portfolio can lead to a dilution of the advanced practitioner's impact in the organisation. This can be offset by active timetabling that reflects patient and organisational needs, but which clearly links other professional activities. For some advanced practitioners this may mean fixed clinical sessions with protected time for administration, research, teaching and all external activities (Figure 9.1).

In the United Kingdom, consultant nurses are timetabled for at least 50% of the clinical time and other activities are divided in the remainder. The actual timetabling is often left to the discretion of the individual consultant which means that some elements can be moved depending on personal and professional needs. This flexibility allows the inclusion of external work that involves regional and national activities. It is advisable to ensure that this type of work is incorporated into the agreed job plan.

Overall, it is essential that the process of developing the job plan is transparent and that an audit trail provides evidence of how decisions are made and why. The aim

	8 AM–1 PM	1–6 PM
Monday	Clinical	Clinical
Tuesday	Admin and professional activities	Clinical
Wednesday	Clinical	Research and audit
Thursday	Research and audit	Clinical supervision/teaching
Friday	Clinical	Clinical

Fig. 9.1   Example of job plan timetable for an advanced practitioner.

of the job plan is to set out an agreement about areas such as activity efficiency and productivity, governance and quality, workforce development, education, service and clinical improvements. This agreement forms a statement as to what constitutes achievement.

Maintaining focus and delivery

There are many rewards and satisfactions from working as an advanced practitioner but equally there can be significant stressors, which culminate in a difficulty in maintaining focus on delivery. Part of the stress can come from work overload, spreading capabilities and resources too thinly or from clinical pressures associated with complex or difficult work. This stress also arises from managing expectations of the role; it is an individual process of developing personal and professional management strategies. However, there is also an organisational responsibility to ensure that the right support is in place for the advanced practitioner because there is a very real risk of burn-out if these stresses remain unchecked (Guest *et al.* 2004). Long hours coupled with working in isolation, in some cases without a team in which to delegate, are often compounded by high individual expectations to succeed. Importantly, consultant nurses in particular feel that the organisation has very high expectations and see those expectations as critical to its own success (Guest *et al.* 2004).

Linsky and Heifetz (2002) argue that the ability and capacity for reflection is an important tool for leaders in challenging political and industry roles if they are to maintain their focus. Advanced practitioners must observe their role in context by 'getting on the balcony' (Linsky and Heifetz 2002), that is to say, removing themselves from the challenge and taking a detailed observation of the scenario. The personal drive of many advanced practitioners can, in some circumstances, draw them away from delivery, preventing them from seeing a situation objectively. In such situations their attention may be diverted by those who regard the advanced practitioners' skills as a means of solving someone else's problems (Linsky and Heifetz 2002). It is easy to be drawn into this situation when the advanced practitioner is under significant political influence from administrators, professional colleagues, corporate nursing and external agencies to deliver too big a portfolio. To avoid this, advanced practitioners need to listen to the organisation, read the behaviours of other leaders, peers and coworkers and learn when to use their abilities to maximum effect.

Lack of role clarity and the absence of organisational professional support can leave the advanced practitioner an isolated box that attracts challenges from other professionals resulting in conflict situations. The ultimate expression of this will see others aim to discredit the role or the individual. Linsky and Heifetz (2002) argue that leaders have to master and control situations. However, in complex organisations this can turn into a need to gain more power and control than necessary or seek affirmation from those whose views conform to one's own; both will make advanced practitioners vulnerable, further isolating them away from the vision of their role.

One aspect of the role of advanced practitioner that is often neglected is personal and professional development. Advanced practitioners are often the leaders for many programmes of development and coaching for others, leaving little time or opportunity for making time for themselves. Nevertheless, it is crucial to ensure ongoing development from the start. Appointment marks the start of development further into advanced practice and requires support and coaching. Time must be set aside for educational and professional growth. The assumption that, since advanced practitioners are 'developed' and professionally at the peak of their clinical careers, development is no longer important means that it is forgotten, by both the organisation and practitioners themselves. Maylor (2005) rightly states that once in the post, the practitioner will take time to develop: from 2 to 7 years. He illustrates this with the Trent Cancer Nurses Allied Health Professions Advisory Group (TCN 2001) framework, in which consultants will move from probationary to proficient and towards expert, reflecting the model of Benner (2001). This formalises the clinical and emotional perspectives of many practitioners.

Developing strategic influence

One of the most important aspects of the advanced practice role is the ability to develop strategic influence through clinical credibility and visibility. This may take on many forms and reflects, partly, the role itself not only at the local level but also nationally and internationally in relation to clinical care or professional standards. Strategic influence is an often-quoted part of many advanced practitioners' job descriptions, although a definition is harder to come by. Stacey (2000, p. 43) suggests that strategic leadership is 'what the business of the organisation should be involved in and how corporate level manages that business'.

For advanced practitioners this part of the role will develop as they gain experience and confidence in operating at this level. Initially, developing strategic influence may take place through the provision of advisory support to the local health economy, for example, commissioning services, developing programmes of clinical support for patients, education, research or system redesign and clinical pathways. Later on this can lead to national influence with organisational bodies representing patients and professionals, to set out the vision for services and professional status. This may seem an enormous task on top of an already busy schedule but it is an important part of the role and one that in most cases is not provided for in training.

Coaching and guiding may assist the individual practitioner in developing skill and confidence (Booth *et al.* 2006). As Whitmore (2002, p. 23) states, 'The best way to develop and maintain the ideal state of mind for performance is to build awareness and responsibility continuously throughout the daily practice and the skill acquisition process ... Coaching is unlocking a person's potential to maximize their own performance. It is helping them to learn rather than teaching them'. Coaches and mentors who are experienced leaders can challenge and stretch the thinking of advanced practitioners, enabling them to see the potential in new situations. It must not be forgotten that achieving advanced practitioner status is only the start of developing leadership capability. The advanced practitioner must continue to move on, taking the organisation into new strategic directions.

Consultancy and entrepreneurship

Examination of the literature finds a prolific number of definitions related to the descriptive and process models of consultants. Until recently the terms *consultant* or *consulting* were synonymous with *medical practitioner*. The role of consultancy in relation to nursing and advanced practice is now more prominent but it is not always explicit in the contracts of UK advanced practitioners. Caplan and Caplan (1993) is considered the seminal source about consultation, describing a particularly relevant process framework that reveals a number of prerequisites (Box 9.3).

Box 9.3   Caplan's pre-requisites for consultants

- A request for consultation
- A person from whom to gain expert knowledge
- Encased in a problem-solving framework

Purchase consultancy and doctor patient consultancy both mirror established relationships of the consultation framework developed by Caplan and others. Expertise can be purchased or requested when the practitioner has amassed a level of knowledge that may be required by either an organisation or for the purposes of professional education. It is fundamental to an organisation to remember that the skills and expertise vested in an advanced practitioner are valuable commodities that can be used to develop consultancy internally and externally to an organisation for both financial as well as professional remuneration. As an example, commercial companies will often require input and advice in terms of product testing, research, education and advice. This can be provided, at a cost, to generate income for the organisation. This aspect of practice is not strongly represented in nursing although this situation is changing as legitimacy and currency of care is being established with other health-care providers. The UK context shows a significant shift from state to private providers and often advanced practitioners are moving between them. In addition to this, there will be national and regional bodies that are important areas where key strategic decisions are made. These decisions can be influenced and the advanced practitioner is ideally placed to provide this.

An entrepreneur is a person who is continually seeking out new opportunities to change and develop. The term is more often associated with industry rather than health but global changes mean that opportunities arise to provide new services or offer established services in innovative ways (Faugier 2005). The advanced practitioner is ideally placed to take up these opportunities in, for example, setting up new services, involvement in commissioning of services for health economies, developing national training or developing consultancy services to provide technical and intellectual advice to other organisations. In some cases this may mean developing a private practice model as an independent practitioner or generating income for a primary organisation through innovative health-care solutions. Patients, irrespective of the source of health expenditure, be it insurance, savings or state funding, are now consumers and are actively engaged in making decisions about which health-care provider they will access. The recent changes to NHS philosophy and direction mean that significant choice options are available both within the state system as well as the private sector.

In establishing an entrepreneurial model of advanced practice one area that has to be considered is marketing of both oneself and a more generic marketing approach to health. This is not just about advertising, a concept that has yet to take some effect in health care in the United Kingdom, due in part to legislation and also health service culture. The more conceptual ideas of marketing are important, as they are there primarily to educate people who might otherwise not understand the products or services available. For example, colleagues often do not understand the advanced role because advanced practitioners have not marketed what they are doing (Jasper 2006). A marketing approach may take many formats and should aim to identify and educate consumers about the unique points about advanced practice, demonstrate value for money and highlight quality and productivity. The aim of marketing is to inform the consumer, and this may include other health professionals and commissioners of services.

Marketing must be seen as a tool through which the advanced practitioner can educate and inform, develop networks of professionals and gain political support (Box 9.4). This is valuable in making the practitioner visible, giving credibility to the role and service, strengthening and maximising the personal and professional impact. Understanding marketing approaches also links well with the organisational objectives and planning as this may well influence the advanced practitioner's approach to specific issues. As Porter (1979) suggests in his seminal work on competitive markets this is especially important for 'new entrants', for whom understanding of market principles is vital for survival. A view more recently supported by Brandenburger and Nalebuff (1995) is that the 'business game' is one where you need to understand, not only your own contribution, but all the others who work in the same market. External marketing is also useful and can lead to new income streams, good publicity or influence in areas, such as, recruitment or retention of staff, particularly in economies where there is competition for resources. Advanced practitioners often function in niche areas or as part of larger services; both will provide significant marketing opportunities.

Box 9.4   Marketing strategies

- Newsletters to organisations and patient groups
- Organisational or individual web presence (interactive websites)
- Reports and publications within the organisation
- Publications of results in literature or professional conferences
- Presentations to corporate boards
- Presentations to local community, client or patient groups
- Portfolio of skills
- Tool kits for service development

Review and evaluation

The importance of a review and evaluation strategy for the advanced practitioner cannot be overstated. Regrettably, there is a lack of evidence to support the impact of advanced roles, despite a proliferation of advanced and specialist nursing practices. Organisations in the current health-care climate are taking productivity and value for money as key indicators when commissioning new services and practices, and the evidence must be in place to support innovative solutions for care. This requires advanced practitioners to think about their strategies and how they can align these with organisational goals and objectives, including cost-effectiveness. Traditionally, nursing has found difficulty in articulating its impact and many, including Fairley and Closs (2006), have suggested that the impact of nursing interventions is hard to quantify, or that the more qualitative elements of practice are difficult to present in a way that is meaningful to influential stakeholders such as administrators and medical colleagues in organisations. However, the advanced practitioner does have impact in a range of practice domains and must think laterally about how evidence about this may be gathered and communicated.

The primary question that the advanced practitioner must answer is 'what impact do I make on the patient/client in the healthcare system?' There may be subsidiary questions arising from this such as, 'what model of advanced practice best delivers to the patient/client or community?' 'What is the learning for others who set up future services?' However, the key question focuses on whether employing an advanced practitioner makes any difference to patient care. Evaluating the impact of the advanced practitioner can be a complex process that can be addressed with a variety of tools and techniques and is outside the scope of this chapter. There are several well-tested models that examine the impact of health-care interventions, including new role redesign or development. Radford (2004) has used work by Girouard (1996) and Ventura *et al.* (1991) to develop a continuum model that supports evaluation from the initial role conception and development (Figure 9.2). It links the evolutionary development of advanced practice to long-term evaluation, identified as the intervention impact becomes apparent.

The initial stages of this model work alongside the development of the role, as this is key in formulating the approach to evaluation. These stages are guided by the population and community assessment. Information at this stage may come from a variety of sources including research and clinical audit. Service user feedback may identify missed opportunities for care that can be addressed by an advanced practitioner. The clinical and economic development stage is an often neglected component but one that is vital in understanding the proposed model and its impact. This stage involves a number of key stakeholders and should aim to evaluate whether the proposed advanced practice post suits the identified health problem. It is also at this stage that assessments should be made with regard to the economic viability, sustainability and potential corporate risks of the new role.

Organisational functionality is often the first aspect of evaluative work undertaken by the advanced practitioner and this will examine and evaluate the initial 'honeymoon' period. During this initial period of work the advanced practitioner should

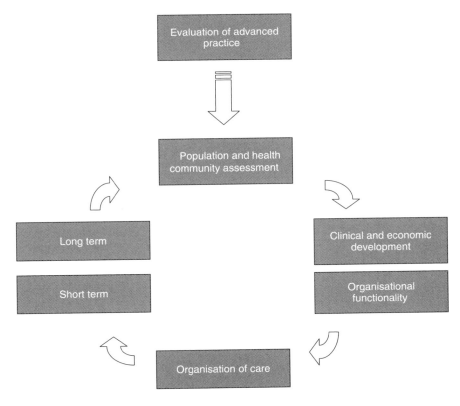

Fig. 9.2 Model of advanced practice evaluation.

aim to understand the role and workload, including types of work, the volumes and descriptors of clients or patients worked with and any potential for the role to move away from the original job plan. This honeymoon phase may last 6 months and it will help formulate a proposed research and audit plan for the advanced practitioner. It will also allow a much more directed approach to evaluation and prevent developing an ineffective and time-consuming programme that does not capture the true impact of the role. The most effective approach is a structured work diary that captures the essence of the experience and that may include qualitative and quantitative data. It is often the case, particularly in new roles, that the real impacts may be found in unexpected areas that differ from those that may be identified at the outset. This diary approach may seem to be rudimentary or basic but will give early indications as to what the advanced practitioner is facing in the new role, and if any additional workload is valuable to the overall goal. In addition, Radford (2004) proposed short- (Table 9.1) and long-term (Table 9.2) analyses utilising a similar structure of process and outcome assessment. They can be markedly diverse depending upon the nature of the work of the advanced nurse practitioner. However, the benefits link with job planning and a clear cyclical review to see if progress is being met and sustained.

Table 9.1 Short-term analysis of advanced practice.

Assessment	Plan	Examples of projects
Administrative assessment	• Target setting improvements with organisation and professional body • Meeting key national goals for population or profession • Assessment of job plan	• Reports to organisation • Clinical diaries • Competency documents • Portfolio development • Skills evaluation
Process assessment	• Impact on clinical teams • Impact on organisational care delivery • Service redesign and management of change	• Process mapping to identify how role has improved care • Audit examining department/hospital impact

Outcome assessment	• Patient pathway analysis
	• Care quality
	• Clinical effectiveness
		• Audit/research improving patient access and choice
		• Audit/research on care quality
		• Organisational key performance indicators
		• Clinical effectiveness audits on:
		  ○ Utilisation of resources
		  ○ Cost per intervention
		  ○ Complications
		  ○ Service provision
		  ○ Choice and access

Table 9.2   Long-term analysis of advanced practice.

Assessment	Plan	Examples of projects
Ongoing administrative assessment	• Target setting improvements with organisation and professional body • Meeting key national goals for population or profession • Reassessment of job plan	• Reports to organisation • Clinical diaries • Competency documents
Process assessment	• Whole system redesign • Influencing wider health community • Influencing profession • Education and development • Research portfolio	• Process mapping • Audit • Research studies • Publications • Presentations
Outcome assessment	• Patient morbidity and mortality • Quality and resource utilisation • Effectiveness and cost	• Audit/research improving patient access and choice • Audit/research on care quality • Adherence to national frameworks of care • Organisational key performance indicators

Career progression

The UK clinical nursing career framework has evolved to include a career progression ladder, with the role of consultant/advanced practitioner at the pinnacle. This provides a significant challenge for advanced practitioners and their career development. While there is a great deal of flexibility with roles to enhance clinical freedom, develop programmes of work and conduct research and education, career progression, where to go next, remains an issue (Woodward *et al.* 2005). Thought must be given to vertical and lateral progression.

Traditional models leave only a few opportunities open for advanced practitioners (Box 9.5). Most of these would require a reduction or complete cessation of activity in some of the advanced domains meaning that clinical expertise of the role would very likely be lost.

Box 9.5   Traditional models for career progression

- Corporate or executive roles with no clinical activity
- Academic or teaching roles
- Independent consultancy

The Modernising Nursing Careers framework gives a flavour of the future models that may be possible (DH 2006). These could create opportunities for advanced practitioners to continue to move forward allowing lateral moves into and out of clinical practice, shifting the emphasis into academic work, research, corporate or strategic responsibility without any loss of credibility or remuneration. This leaves open the possibility of hybrid models that draw upon the key domains of advanced practice to flexibly deliver a wider nursing agenda depending on the needs of the population served.

Advanced practitioners are recognised as a valuable asset because of their clinical visibility and credibility (Woodward *et al.* 2005). In medical practice, clinically credible leaders are utilised as senior corporate leaders such as medical directors of organisations. These individuals maintain a clinical workload and are, therefore, grounded in the practical considerations of service provision while also providing leadership and guidance to the organisation's corporate team. This approach could be used for and by advanced practitioners to formalise their strategic leadership function, extending their influence beyond the nursing domain into the wider health-care field. This would build upon key skills and expose them more widely to organisational experiences for the development of patient or client services (Box 9.6).

Box 9.6   Key advanced skills that could inform clinical leadership

- Research and evaluation
- Education and learning
- Workforce development
- Systems and service redesign
- Commissioning and clinical service coordination
- Professional and organisational leadership

If, as suggested by the literature, advanced roles are little understood, lack evidence of impact and are linked to individuals, there is a danger that as careers progress and practitioners move to new roles, they may leave significant gaps in service provision as organisations do not re-advertise posts. Crouch *et al.* (2003) found that recruiting to advanced and consultant posts was difficult. While there was a great deal of potential in the workforce, candidates often required significant development, up to 2 years, before being able to fully work in the role. Crouch *et al.*'s (2003) innovative solution involved a significant training and development programme. Organisations need to ensure that those they employ in advanced roles have the appropriate preparation, both academically and more importantly from an experience point of view, to function well (Ball 2005, Woodward *et al.* 2005). Those that are not prepared will experience the most frustration and struggle in their work.

Conclusion

Working as an advanced practitioner is a very rewarding job, one that provides significant opportunity for personal and professional growth. The impact these roles have on patients can be significant and this is well-recognised by employers. However, the health-care agenda is shifting significantly and this will require new and innovative models of nursing for a more consumer-orientated patient or client. Organisations are striving for excellence and affordability, placing an emphasis on added value to the patients' pathway. As we have seen in this chapter, organisations and health economies need to give significant time and effort to planning and implementing these roles to ensure delivery of the key objectives set. The period of preparation must establish not only the technical aspects of the role such as job description, referral mechanisms and remuneration but also the adaptive or cultural changes required to ensure that roles function appropriately in meeting the needs of patients and the organisation. The established advanced practitioner is in a good position to influence this agenda and also to set the pace of reform for patient services. Strategic direction and the ability to think laterally about the role within the context of the organisation, are essential. Advanced practitioners will have to ask themselves some fundamental questions on how they operate clinically, professionally and politically. To maximise the impact of their role, they must think beyond the traditional view of nursing and will need to embrace a range of new skills and tools.

 Key questions for Chapter 9

In your field of practice:
(1) What considerations should be taken into account by an organisation when developing an advanced practice role?
(2) Why is it important for the advanced practitioner to think about marketing strategies?
(3) How could advanced practitioners demonstrate their impact on patient care?

Acknowledgements

I would like to thank Barbara Beal, an inspirational leader who showed me how to 'lead on the line' and provided the opportunity for me to develop as an advanced nurse practitioner and Liz Lees, consultant nurse in Acute Medicine at Heart of England Foundation Trust, for her helpful comments as a consultant and advanced practitioner in the preparation of this chapter.

References

Ball, J. (2005) *Advanced and Specialist Nursing Roles: Results from a Survey of RCN Members*. London, Royal College of Nursing.

Benner, P. (2001) *From Novice to Expert: Excellence and Power in Clinical Nursing Practice*. 1st edn. Philadelphia, Prentice Hall.

Brandenburger, A.M. and Nalebuff, B.J. (1995) The right game: use game theory to shape strategy. *Harvard Business Review* July–August 57–71.

Booth, J., Hutchison, C., Beech, C. and Robertson, K. (2006) New nursing roles: the experience of Scotland's consultant nurse/midwives. *Journal of Nursing Management* **14** (2) 83–9.

Caplan, G. and Caplan, R. (1993) *Mental Health Consultation and Collaboration*, San Francisco, Waveland Press.

Crouch, R., Buckley, R. and Fenton, K. (2003) Consultant nurses: the next generation. *Emergency Nurse: The Journal of the RCN Accident and Emergency Nursing Association* **11** (7) 15–7.

Department of Health (1997) *The New NHS: Modern. Dependable*. London, DH.

Department of Health (1999) *Nurse Midwife and Health Visitor Consultants: Establishing Posts and Making Appointments*. London, NHS Executive.

Department of Health (2003) *Terms and Conditions of Service 2003. An Agreement between the BMA's Central Consultants and Specialist Committee and The Department of Health for Consultants in England*. London, Department of Health.

Department of Health (2006) *Modernizing Nursing Careers*. London, HMSO.

Fairley, D. and Closs, S.J. (2006) Evaluation of a nurse consultant's clinical activities and the search for patient outcomes in critical care. *Journal of Clinical Nursing* **15** (9) 1106–14.

Faugier, J. (2005) Developing a new generation of nurse entrepreneurs. *Nursing Standard* **19** (30) 49–53.

Girouard, S. (1996) Evaluating advanced nursing practice. In *Advanced Practice Nursing: An Integrative Approach*, (eds A. Hamric, J. Spross, C. Hanson and J. Spross). Philadelphia, W.B. Saunders.

Guest, D., Peccei, R., Rosenthal, P., *et al*. (2004) *An Evaluation of the Impact of the Nurse, Midwife and Health Visitor Consultant Role*. London, Kings College London.

Jasper, M. (2006) Editorial. Consultant nurses and midwives – are you making a difference? *Journal of Nursing Management* **14** (2) 81–2.

Linsky, M. and Heifetz, R. (2002) *Leadership on the Line: Staying Alive Through the Dangers of Leading*. Harvard, Harvard Business School Press.

Maylor, M. (2005) Differentiating between a consultant nurse and a clinical nurse specialist. *British Journal of Nursing* **14** (8) 463–68.

Porter, M. (1979) How competitive forces shape strategy. *Harvard Business Review* March–April 137–45.

Radford, M. (2004) Advanced and specialist perioperative practice. In *Advancing Perioperative Practice*, (eds M. Radford, B. County and M. Oakley). Cheltenham, Nelson Thornes.

Redfern, S., Guest, D., Wilson-Barnett, J., *et al*. (2003) Role innovation in the NHS: a preliminary evaluation of the new role of nurse, midwife and health visitor consultant. In *Leading Health Care Organizations*. pp. 153–72. Basingstoke, Palgrave Macmillan.

Renshaw, C. (2005) *Mapping Our Future – The Role of the Director of Nursing – A West Midlands Perspective*. Birmingham, BBC StHA.

Stacey, R. (2000) *Strategic Management and Organizational Dynamics*. 3rd edn. London, Prentice Hall.

Trent Cancer Nurses Allied Health Professions Advisory Group (2001) *Nurse specialists, nurse consultants, nurse leads: the development of new roles to improve cancer and palliative care. An advisory paper*. Leicester, National Health Service Executive/ Leicestershire Health Authority.

Ventura, M., Crosby, F. and Feldman, M., (1991) An information synthesis to evaluate nurse practitioner effectiveness. Military Medicine **156** (6) 286–91.

Wells, W., Moyes, B., Fry, M., *et al.* (2006) *The Intelligent Board.* London, Dr Foster.

Whitmore, J. (2002) *Coaching for Performance: Growing People, Performance and Purpose.* London, Nicholas Brealey.

Woodward, V.A., Webb, C. and Prowse, M. (2005) Nurse consultants: their characteristics and achievements. *Journal of Clinical Nursing* **14** (7) 845–54.

Chapter 10
Pioneering New Practice

Kate Gee

Introduction

As advanced practice roles develop, new opportunities arise and one of the key characteristics of the advanced practitioner is the ability to take advantage of these, especially when they require the individual to function at the boundaries of practice. In advanced nursing practice such ability is associated with confidence and expertise, rooted in a broad vision of health, in order to challenge traditional methods of providing care (Patterson *et al.* 2003). This chapter presents an exploration of this pioneering role using a model designed by the author (Figure 10.1). First, the model is explained. After that, each of the four sections is discussed using examples of practice advancement in providing treatment and care for patients with various types of heart disease. These examples are drawn directly from developments in technology, health policies and the ensuing changes in patient groups. The chapter closes with some key questions for further discussion.

Background to the quadrant model

In 2005 Zubialde *et al.* (2005) devised the quadrants of care model that used two important dimensions of health issues – complexity of care and illness duration, acute

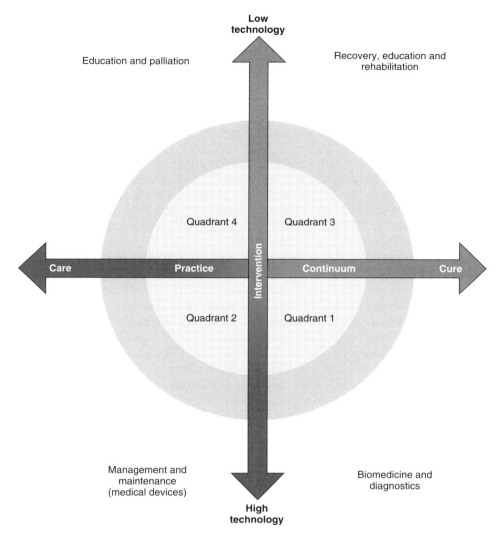

Fig. 10.1 The Quadrants of Cardiac Care Model (adapted from the Quadrants of Care Model for Health Services Planning model devised by Zubialde *et al.* (2005)).

or chronic – to create four quadrants that conceptualised health-care needs to support health service planning and management (Zubialde *et al.*, 2005). To discuss advances in cardiac nursing the author has applied the approach devised by Zubialde *et al.* (2005) to create a quadrant model that conceptualises patient needs and practice delivery. The two inextricably linked factors used to devise this quadrant model are technology and organisational culture. These factors have been chosen because of their strong association with the evolution and continued advancement of cardiac nursing practice (Sparacino 1994, Hamric *et al.* 1996, Greenhalgh 2000).

Technological innovations result from the growth in biomedical knowledge. These innovations extend the investigative and therapeutic options available to clinicians, and, in doing so, increase the complexity of their decision-making. Innovations, coupled with shifts in health-care focus by the Department of Health (DH) (as demonstrated by the 2006 White Paper of 2006, *Our Health, our care, our say: a new direction for community services* (DH 2006)), raise public expectations related to quality and length of life. These dynamics influence organisational culture and practice (Dowie and Elstein 1993, Doubilet and McNeil 1993). Changing political imperatives coupled with increased client expectations are altering the professional–client relationship and increasing the accountability associated with professional judgements and decisions (Dowie and Elstein 1993).

Within cardiology, one only has to consider the technical innovations of the oscilloscope and defibrillator to see the inextricable link between technology and organisational culture. By enhancing the clinician's ability to detect and treat life-threatening arrhythmias these innovations fundamentally changed clinical management of the acutely ill cardiac patient and subsequently the organisational cultures within which management was practised. The significant improvements in survival achieved with defibrillation prompted the national/international introduction of coronary care units (CCUs). As importantly, CCUs created new opportunities for advancing nursing since they required nurses capable of both identifying the arrhythmias and autonomously using their life-saving skills (Jowett and Thompson 1989). Paradoxically, 40 years later, the impact on survival attributed to such innovations has significantly contributed to the challenge now facing health-care organisations, which is how to manage survivors who now have chronic diseases. This situation has created new opportunities and threats to cardiac nursing.

The delivery of specialist skills such as defibrillation required organisational cultures focused on 'cure'. Such expertise facilitates 'accurate diagnosis, active intervention and rapid measurable changes in the markers of disease' (Greenhalgh 2000, p. 341). However, the pressing health-care needs of today are how to care for an aging population with chronic diseases. Chronic disease accounts for half the global health burden; 78% of all health-care spending in the United Kingdom (Murphy 2004). Stanley and Prasun (2002, p. 94) report: heart failure is, by all accounts, the most dramatic example of a chronic condition with a looming financial and resource burden, and a personal impact on society'. The national and international economic impact of this long-term disease is significant. Heart failure costs the National Health Service (NHS) an estimated £360 million per year (Swanton 2003). In the United States, the total cost of the disease is estimated at $21 billion every year (Stanley and Prasun 2002). Heart failure in the elderly has become one of the most common conditions accounting for almost one quarter of cardiovascular admissions. In the elderly, heart failure is the single most frequent reason for hospital admission and is associated with high resource consumption and costs (Liao *et al.* 2007).

The launch in 2006 of the White Paper: *Our Health, our care, our say: a new direction for community services* (DH 2006) heralds the need for organisational cultures to change to reduce the impact of chronic disease. Expertise is now required to focus practice on 'care' rather than 'cure' so that self-management and self-'care' are promoted (Astin and Closs 2007). Such expertise requires skills exemplified by 'support, empathy, effective communication and time'. Providing such expertise creates both opportunities and threats for cardiac nursing (Greenhalgh 2000, Astin and Closs 2007).

Astin and Closs (2007) describe this change from 'cure' to 'care' as a 'paradigm shift' for many health-care professionals where traditionally 'the prevailing model of medical education and, to a lesser extent, nurse education has emphasised an approach which focuses upon episodic care aimed at curing disease in individuals in an acute care setting' (Astin and Closs 2007, p. 105).

The quadrant model

As previously discussed, the quadrant model uses organisational culture as a horizontal axis and level of technology required to practice as the vertical axis. By these axes four traversing quadrants are created, each depicting a different dimension of practice (Figure 10.1). Along the horizontal axis (organisational culture) are two extremes, 'cure' and 'care' (Greenhalgh 2000, Astin and Closs 2007). The focus of nursing practice alters as it moves along the axis from left to right depending on the focus of care being delivered. The vertical axis represents the degree of technology required to deliver care. The extremes of the axis are 'high technology' and 'low technology'. This 'intervention continuum' describes the type of practice delivered based on the degree of technology applied to meet patient needs. The *high-technology* pole represents the application of technology in diagnostics, pharmaceutical products and other medical devices. The *low-technology* pole supports palliation or gives way to completely caring activities. The four quadrants created are as follows:

Quadrant 1 – 'High-Technology/Cure Culture Quadrant'. This quadrant represents the most technically advanced practice focused on cure. The type of practice can be either acute or non-acute but the emphasis is on the delivery of care in response to technological advances, for example, patients presenting to hospital with an acute myocardial infarction requiring thrombolysis (Figure 10.1).

Quadrant 2 – 'High-Technology/Care Culture Quadrant'. This quadrant represents practice where technology is still strongly evident but where the primary focus is providing support for patients, for example, following discharge after the implantation of an implantable cardioverter defibrillator (ICD) (Figure 10.1) (Jacobson and Gerity 2005).

Quadrant 3 – 'Low-Technology/Cure Culture Quadrant'. This quadrant reflects practice in a culture where non-technical strategies are required to support patients during the transition from diagnosis and treatment to life-long maintenance. Expertise is primarily focused on behavioural change, symptom management through education and rehabilitation programmes (Madan 2005, Myers 2005) (Figure 10.1).

Quadrant 4 – 'Low-Technology/Care Culture Quadrant'. This quadrant reflects practice focused on supporting patients for whom technical interventions are no longer effective. Emphasis is placed on providing expertise to optimise the patients' quality of life through symptom relief and education providing support for patients such as those with heart failure facing end-of-life decisions (Stanley and Prasun 2002, Laurent 2005) (Figure 10.1).

Quadrant 1: pioneering innovations in technical acute cure cultures

For this quadrant, coronary care and the management of non-acute arrhythmias provide exemplars of how the advanced practitioner can harness technology within an organisational culture focused on cure to pioneer new practice (Box 10.1).

Box 10.1   Examples of practice advancement in coronary care

Development of hospital protocols to support consistent clinical judgement in both nursing and medical staff (Hendra and Marshall 1992)

Advances in interprofessional teamwork that have supported developments of advanced electrocardiographic training programmes for nurses and paramedics (Gee 1998, Foster *et al.* 1994)

Recognition of the value of multi-disciplinary assessment, which has resulted in the acknowledgement of how nurses can support the diagnostic process in relation to symptom description, detecting electrocardiographic changes and clinical history taking (Alberran and Kapeluch 1994)

The introduction of a new nursing role: the thrombolysis nurse (Jones 2005)

Note: For full details of these examples please see reference list at the end of this chapter.

Chest pain is the most common symptom associated with acute coronary syndrome (ACS), the life-threatening clinical manifestation of coronary heart disease (CHD) that can result in an acute myocardial infarction (AMI) or unstable angina. The prompt detection and immediate treatment of ACS, which are critical in minimising its potentially catastrophic effects, have effectively led to a revolution in coronary care (Mant *et al.* 2004). Within the cure/high-technology quadrant, nursing competencies are focused essentially on the diagnostic/patient monitoring function, administering/ monitoring therapeutic interventions, the helping role and effective management of rapidly changing situations as outlined by Benner (1984) and Styles (1996).

In response to the dramatic reductions in mortality and morbidity associated with early thrombolysis (De Bono 1990, Ornato 1990), it became established as the major therapeutic intervention for AMI. The time-critical relationship between symptom onset and thrombolysis benefits required organisational cultures to change in order to achieve the mandatory targets introduced by the National Service Framework (NSF) for CHD (DH 2000a). Both hospitals and ambulance services were charged with the responsibility of minimising delays between symptom onset and thrombolysis. Nurses working in coronary care acquired new knowledge and skills and the new role of the thrombolysis nurses emerged as one model of support in minimising delays. Their duties varied from acting as coordinators of care to the administration of the thrombolytic agent, without the presence of a medical consultant, through the use of group protocols or patient group directives (Jones 2005).

In the author's organisation a different approach was used. Rather than appointing specialist nurses, emergency care nurses developed the skills to competently care for patients receiving thrombolysis. Action research was used to successfully facilitate the transition of responsibility for thrombolysis administration from CCU nurses to emergency care nurses. The approach empowered emergency care nurses because they determined the programme of education. This offered new practice opportunities for them to directly contribute to the care of the AMI patient (Gee 1998).

By using her clinical expertise the author guided and supported the practice of emergency care nurses so that they felt able to take responsibility for patients requiring thrombolysis. In addition, the author ensured that members of other disciplines were advised of proposed practice changes so that inter-departmental communication was effective. The audit process developed by the author remains instrumental in the measurement of organisational performance. The changes introduced by the author improved organisational performance, increased access to thrombolysis and, as importantly, were not associated with significant costs. Thrombolysis nurses were not required yet similar, and arguably more sustainable, outcomes were achieved (Gee 1998).

While there had been unquestionable patient benefits associated with minimising thrombolysis delays, the processes required to ensure effective implementation are complex. The introduction of paramedic-initiated thrombolysis and more recently primary angioplasty have required new skills acquisition and significant organisational reconfiguration (Quinn *et al.* 2002, Asseburg *et al.* 2007). Such initiatives are creating new opportunities for the pioneering advanced practitioner to challenge the boundaries of what is currently accepted and forge new forms of nursing.

Within the author's organisation the consultant's role continues to provide sustained direction for emergency care, and coronary care nurse practice and paramedics. The flexibility of the training programme originally developed for thrombolysis administration has facilitated practice change in response to new national imperatives, namely, paramedic-initiated thrombolysis and, more recently, primary angioplasty (Bjorklund *et al.* 2006).

Other examples of pioneering new practice can be found in the management of non-acute arrhythmias, atrial fibrillation and flutter in particular. Nurses with coronary care backgrounds and advanced life support skills are now undertaking elective cardioversion with patients as day cases (Currie *et al.* 2004, Shelton *et al.* 2006). Such nurse-led initiatives are reducing waiting times, reducing the requirement for hospitalisation and relieving pressure on both hospital beds and junior medical staff (Currie *et al.* 2004).

A variety of models have emerged. For example, the nurse may administer the synchronised electric shock while the patient is under a general anaesthetic administered by an anaesthetist (Currie *et al.* 2004, Shelton *et al.* 2006). Alternatively, the nurse may sedate the patient and deliver the electric shocks with a cardiology registrar being immediately available but not present (Boodhoo *et al.* 2004).

It could be argued that the real impetus for change has come from outside nursing. Certainly, reduction in junior doctors' hours and the increased demand for hospital beds created the opportunity for role expansion (Boodhoo *et al.* 2004, Currie *et al.* 2004, Shelton *et al.* 2006). Nevertheless, the pioneering work of practitioners such as Boodhoo *et al.* (2004) has contributed to the body of nursing knowledge. Their work has created safe frameworks that support the development of patient care outside the traditional model of a medically led service for patients with common arrhythmias associated with significant morbidity and mortality (Majeed *et al.* 2001). Thus the work of such pioneers has brought significant benefits for patients for whom the advanced nurse acts as a single point of contact, ensuring that problems are minimised and cancellations are reduced. As far as the organisation is concerned, such reductions, alongside improved resource management, are to be welcomed (Currie *et al.* 2004). Having a nurse consultant in control of the service supports improved multi-disciplinary team work because of the clinical and professional leadership provided by this expert practitioner (Currie *et al.* 2004).

Quadrant 2: pioneering innovations in high-technology/care cultures

Other opportunities for advancing nursing practice have been generated in the high-technology/care quadrant in response to initiatives such as the NSF for CHD and the reduction in junior doctors' hours. The focus of practice change is in response to technology. Here practice relates to the diagnosis and management of cardiac conditions, such as angina, via a rapid access chest pain clinic (RACPC), or associated with the early care required for patients who have specific care needs associated with insertion of a device such as a pacemaker or ICD (Jacobson and Gerity 2005). Practice takes place in non-acute settings where patients can be managed either as outpatients or day cases.

With regard to diagnosis and management of CHD, pioneers such as nurse consultant Alison Pottle, introduced nurse-led services for angina detection via the RACPC pathway, established in response to Standard 8 of the NSF (DH 2000b, Pottle 2005). Variability of medical input to the clinic within her organisation provided an opportunity for the nurse consultant to offer access to consistent nursing expertise, and promote clinical and professional nursing leadership that fostered multi-disciplinary teamwork. This vision broke the mould of traditional practice and established a credible nurse-expert-led service. The practice reflected the following domains of practice as advocated by Benner (1984):

- Using the consulting domain of practice improved the clinic profile and consequently enhanced communication with other disciplines, such as general practitioners (GPs), clinicians and managers, which increased patient referral rates.

- Within the diagnostic, monitoring and therapeutic domains of practice, expertise was available to interpret electrocardiographs, analyse exercise tolerance tests and prescribe medications via patient group directions.
- Organisational and work role competencies were achieved through rigorous audit and analysis, thus achieving the outcomes required by Standard 8 of the NSF (DH 2000b).
- Patient satisfaction questionnaires demonstrated that the service supported the helping domain by providing appropriate information and support.

Outcomes from a rigorous audit process established that this nurse-led approach facilitated early diagnosis of angina without an increased risk of incorrect diagnosis (Pottle 2005).

Another significant dimension of this pioneering work has been the proactive management of CHD. By having admission rights this advanced nurse has been able to arrange patients' admission for angiography thus reducing delays and minimising the risks to patients developing the more advanced manifestations of CHD (Mant *et al*. 2004).

In addition to diagnostic skills, new areas of nursing intervention have emerged that are associated with this high-technology/care quadrant, with the cardiac nurse specialising in the management of patients with ICDs. This role offers an exemplar of the ways in which the advanced practitioner can harness technology within an organisational culture, focused on care in response to high-technology innovations.

ICDs are considered the gold standard for the treatment of malignant tachyarrhythmias. In the past patients would have died. ICD implantation prevents sudden cardiac death and offers those with implants a second chance of life (Rao and Saksena 2003). There are however significant psychosocial and quality of life issues associated with ICD implantation (Jacobson and Gerity 2005). Nurses play a critical role in supporting patients and their families in adjusting to life with an ICD, for example, managing emergency situations and actions required when the device discharges and taking the necessary precautions to avoid environmental areas of risk such as magnetic fields (Jacobson and Gerity 2005).

Quadrant 3: pioneering innovation in low-technology/cure cultures – strategies for patient education and rehabilitation

This quadrant reflects the transition from high-technology/cure practice towards practice to support patients in the long term. While acknowledging that technology remains evident, its presence is less apparent as the direction for meeting patient needs moves towards clinical stability through maintenance and restoration of independence by follow-up care and rehabilitation.

Historically cardiac rehabilitation has been the focus of cardiac nursing in this quadrant. Here practice has advanced by the development of skills focused on limiting the physiological and psychological impact of cardiac disease. Symptom control, complication detection and, critically, facilitating behavioural change have been the key practice characteristics (Myers 2005). However, with recent innovations such as new pharmaceutical products and medical devices like pacemakers and ICDs, additional cohorts of patients require curative, low-technology nursing; this has, in turn, led to new nursing opportunities (Myers 2005). The role of the ICD and heart failure nurse specialists will be used as exemplars of how new practice has been pioneered within this low-technology/cure quadrant.

Development of ICD nursing expertise

Early ICD research focused on patient mortality (Tebbenjohanns *et al.* 1994). While evidence confirmed ICDs saved lives, outcomes revealed ICD patients experienced significant psychological problems adjusting to life with a device that would prevent their sudden death (Sneed *et al.* 1997, Sears and Conti 2002). As recently as 2004 a study reported that over 50% of ICD patients experienced severe psychological distress manifested as anxiety, depression, fear and anger (Dougherty *et al.* 2004). Service development attempting to address these issues has found nursing practice instrumental in delivering improvements. For example, ICD support group meetings following hospital discharge have been associated with significant improvements in patient acceptance of the ICD when compared to the traditional physician follow-up (Carlsson *et al.* 2002); ongoing nursing support after ICD implantation is now acknowledged as a critical component of care (Carlsson *et al.* 2002, Jacobson and Gerity 2005). The introduction of a telephone follow-up service provided by expert nurses has been found to reduce patient concerns regarding return to normal physical activities, which, in turn, significantly reduces anxiety and physical symptoms within the first month of implantation. This also leads to an overall improvement in reported health and quality of life (Dougherty *et al.* 2004).

There are challenges with this role; significant expertise and time are required to ensure effective long-term follow-up by ICD nurses (Jacobson and Gerity 2005). Deficits in nursing skills, particularly with regard to training in behavioural medicine, have been identified when trying to address the psychological distress experienced by patients and carers (Sears and Conti 2002). Recommendations have been made for the introduction of national standards of care for ICD patients (Tagney 2003).

Development of heart failure nursing expertise

Heart failure continues to carry a poor prognosis despite inotropic drugs, beta-blockers and surgical advances, which have increased treatment options and patient survival (Swanton 2003). Over half of heart failure patients die within 5 years (Zambroski 2006, Zapka *et al.* 2006), and the disease continues to be a leading cause of death in elderly and vulnerable adults (Miller and Froelicher 2005).

Innovations have moved heart failure 'from being a condition with a relentless downhill clinical course requiring frequent hospitalisations' to being a more manageable disease (Riegel *et al.* 2006, p. 149). Long-term management is now required for this patient cohort who can experience both distressing symptoms and considerable psychological problems (Reisfield and Wilson 2007). The needs of this group are complex. Patients are usually elderly, with coexisting conditions such as hypertension and diabetes, and have social and psychological needs associated with their increasing age (Miller and Froelicher 2005).

As the core elements of managing chronic heart failure are essentially non-technical, the general preference for cardiologists has been to remain in acute practice. This preference, coupled with the predominantly non-technical dimensions of practice, has created new opportunities for nurses (Rasmusson *et al.* 2005). Nurses are in an ideal position to lead practice and care delivery, not as medical substitutes, but as specialist clinicians with skills, firmly based in the concepts of traditional nursing practice, that utilise 'support, empathy, effective communication and time' as key aspects of practice (Greenhalgh 2000, p. 341) (Box 10.2).

Box 10.2   Seven key nursing functions in the care of patients with chronic heart failure

Monitoring signs and symptoms and reinforcing patients' self-management, identifying trends
Organisation, liaison and consultation with other health-care professionals to deal with changes in clinical status
Clarifying and re-enforcing patient self-care strategies
Assisting patients in their desire to avoid institutionalised care
Identifying patients' psychosocial issues, dealing with social isolation
Providing support; journeying with patients and their families
Helping patients and their families deal with death and dying

Source: Summarised from Davidson, P., Paull, G., Rees, D., Daly, J. and Cockburn, J. (2005) Activities of home-based heart failure nurse specialists: a modified narrative analysis. *American Journal of Critical Care* **14** (5) 426–33.

Evidence from systematic reviews indicates that multi-disciplinary working facilitated by specialised nurse follow-up in combination with patient education reduces both hospitalisation and prescribing costs (McAlister *et al.* 2001). The pioneering work of Linda Blue demonstrated considerable patient and organisational benefits when specialist nurses monitored treatment regimes and educated heart failure patients at follow-up. Nursing intervention reduced readmissions (28%), risk of readmission (62%) and length of stay as patients became more able to effectively monitor and manage their symptoms (Blue *et al.* 2001).

In 2002, McDonald *et al.* demonstrated significant reductions in death and readmission when specialist nurses intervened. Using a protocol-driven framework in combination with specialist dietitian consultation and nurse-led education/telephone follow-up, readmission rates were 7.8% in the intervention group compared to 25.5% in patients managed via traditional cardiology clinics (McDonald *et al.* 2002).

The ability of specialist nurses to convey information that supports behavioural change is critical as the cause of most readmissions appears to result from poor compliance with medication and dietary habits, factors that could be addressed through patient education (McAlister *et al.* 2004). As McAlister *et al.* (2004) report, hospital readmissions were reduced by 27% by heart failure nurses educating patients.

Heart failure nurse specialists can extend patient benefits beyond the simple organisational and clinical outcome measures of readmission and mortality. Using protocol-driven medical regimes, individualised education, counselling at monthly nurse-led clinics and weekly telephone follow-ups Kutzleb and Reiner (2006) established that nurse-led initiatives improved quality of life. By increasing the patients' ability to self-manage their diet and medications, independence was promoted. Through optimising compliance with both medical and non-pharmacological regimens, overall exercise tolerance and quality of life were improved despite no significant improvement in the patients' functional capacity (Kutzleb and Reiner 2006).

Organisational and clinical practice improves when specialist nurses work across boundaries. Home-based specialist nurses facilitated communication between professionals to support patients and families (Davidson *et al.* 2005). Strömberg *et al.* (2001) reported that when heart failure programmes are organised with specialist nurses central to care processes between primary care and hospitals, improvements in communication result. These improvements lead to greater coordination of services, increase access to essential diagnostic procedures, reduce delays in receiving results and promote greater consistency of heart failure information. Such benefits improve patient and clinician knowledge about the condition and establish closer contact among cardiologists, GPs and district nurses (Strömberg *et al.* 2001).

Quadrant 4: pioneering innovations in low-technology/care quadrant

This quadrant attempts to acknowledge a new dimension of nursing practice not normally associated with cardiac nurses. This dimension is the provision of palliative care for patients with chronic disease. The exemplar used for this quadrant is the care delivered by heart failure nurse specialists.

Unlike in cancer, there is no history of a synergy between cardiac nursing and end-of-life care. The past successes associated with acute cardiac care have meant that cardiac nursing has been predominantly perceived by patients and practitioners as a curative discipline (Hart 1988a, Jowett and Thompson 1989, Handberg 2006). However this is changing, in response to the growing care needs of patients with chronic heart failure. The expertise of heart failure nurses when meeting needs in both quadrants 3 and 4 are considerable (Laurent 2005). As Rasmusson *et al.* state,

> the foundation of heart failure care rests upon the cognitive aspects; identifying and diagnosing the problem, using evidence-based medications, maintaining appropriate intravascular volume status, educating patients about the disease process, and considering device-related and end-of-life issues. (Rasmusson *et al.* 2005, p. 1961)

When considered within Benner's (1984) model, the competencies required reflect several domains of practice; the teaching and coaching function, monitoring therapeutic interventions and the diagnostic and monitoring function (Styles 1996; Table 2.1, p. 32). Critically, the competency of consultation as described by Fenton (Styles 1996) is required as the specialist nurses have to use their expertise to act as communicators between the multi-disciplinary team and patients to ensure that, as the patients' advocates, patients' needs are met (Styles 1996; Figure 2.1, p. 33).

Bekelman *et al.* (2008) suggest that while heart failure patients may not be dying, palliative care skills can complement care at any point of the patient pathway. By offering such expertise, improvements in patient health status can be achieved through symptom management, relief of the psychological distress and effective goal-setting (Bekelman *et al.* 2008).

For heart failure patients, transition to low-technology care is insidious as the previously successful medical interventions gradually become ineffective. New caring skills are required to address the resulting physical deterioration and increasing complexity of the patients' growing social and psychological needs (Stanley and Prasun 2002, Miller and Froelicher 2005). The uncertainty of the clinical course of heart failure and the significant illness burden and risk of sudden death associated with the condition have created new opportunities for cardiac nurses within palliative care (Zambroski 2006).

Preservation of personhood for these sick, older patients is critical (Benner 1984). Expertise focused on the helping domain is required to provide specialist support directed towards meeting the caring needs of patients and carers when choosing treatment options and addressing end-of-life issues (Stanley and Prasun 2002).

Such caring skills as helper and educator become increasingly important with the progression of the disease. The transition from curative to palliative practice requires greater emphasis on non-pharmacologic clinical management practices such as sodium and alcohol management (Riegel *et al.* 2006). In the low-technology/care quadrant, there appears to be transference of the essential skills of monitoring therapeutic interventions from heart failure nurses to patients. Through enhancing patient knowledge, self-care is optimised and unnecessary hospitalisations avoided (Rasmusson *et al.* 2005). Careful integration of behavioural change into the patient's social circumstances requires expertise if the benefits are to be achieved. The language used must be clear, medical jargon avoided and the information must be delivered in a manner that supports patient engagement (Stanley and Prasun 2002).

To achieve behavioural change requires patients to feel able to openly express their concerns. This is particularly significant with heart failure patients, as they are likely to be from a generation where doctors were seen as figures of authority and not questioned (Hart 1988b, Stanley and Prasun 2002). The approach used by heart failure nurses appears to be one that promotes a therapeutic relationship by creating a relationship built on trust and respect as the elderly will frequently listen to a trusted friend (Stanley and Prasun 2002). Advanced nurses collaborate with patients, enabling them to understand how best to manage their condition in ways that suit their individual circumstances.

By acting as the expert interface among patients, carers and a multi-professional team, nursing skills promote the delivery of sensitive heart failure/end-of-life care. Such expertise has become pivotal in how the transition from curative treatment to palliative care is managed (Handberg 2006). By placing nurses at the centre of the multi-disciplinary team, patient and carer benefits are optimised in this multi-faceted dimension of low-technology care.

Conclusion

Critical to advancing nursing practice is having the vision to see what is needed to effectively deliver the nursing skills required to meet the needs of patients. Being aware of the context of practice provides essential information about the basic assumptions and unwritten rules by which individuals, teams and organisations operate (Handy 1993, Greenhalgh 2000). While the nursing skills required across the four quadrants described may differ, the pioneering elements remain similar. Trofino (1993) suggests that transformational leadership requires the development of synergistic relationships to promote education across professional boundaries in order to create professional relationships between groups that will propel practice forward (Trofino 1993). Advancing practice of whatever profession requires negotiation and effective mentoring with reciprocal communication including education that facilitates mutual learning sensitive to the contribution each discipline can make to the working relationship (O'Brien *et al.* 2008).

Pioneers need clinical and professional expertise to provide the leadership required to foster multi-disciplinary team work so that practice innovations occur. As the examples contained within this chapter illustrate, significant shifts in care delivery are taking place in the management of chest pain, angina detection, elective cardioversion, ICD implantation and heart failure. Each of the examples provides insight into how, as a cardiac nurse, our unique contribution can progress professional growth if given personal insight, the provision of opportunities and the courage and conviction to embrace change and explore new approaches to care.

There are challenges with these specialist roles. Advanced practice requires continuous reassessment as the work of Strömberg *et al.* illustrates. In her literature review of 2002 different perceptions of education needs were identified between nurses and heart failure patients (Strömberg 2002). These findings prompted her development of a CD-ROM. By using this technology, information and training was standardised to address the identified deficits to support both practitioners and patients. Evaluation of the CD-ROM indicated patients valued this educational medium. Access to information in their own time was welcomed. The information also appeared easier to understand, requiring less time to assimilate (Strömberg *et al.* 2002).

Application of old techniques in new situations is providing nursing opportunities where sharing of expertise and experience is required. For heart failure patients non-pharmacological regimens of exercise training and relaxation (usually associated with cardiac rehabilitation) appear to be improving both the psychological and physical health of older patients, offering new options for service developments (Yu *et al.* 2007).

Within the nursing profession specialist nurses need to ensure effective sharing of experience with their non-specialist colleagues. Outcomes from a study conducted by Wilson *et al.* (2006) suggest that significant challenges are associated with non-specialist nurses supporting expert patients with chronic disease. Lack of empirical knowledge tends to emphasise a relationship in which the patient is considered a passive recipient rather than active participant in care. In contrast nurse specialists have the expertise to discuss decision-making openly with expert patients (Wilson *et al.* 2006). Further work is required to examine how skills can be shared to support the needs of this growing cohort of patients.

In reality, the dimensions of practice are not as simplistic or as discreet as the quadrant model proposes. The author recognises that the transition from one quadrant to another is not immediate, and the transference of skills will occur at different stages depending on the condition of the patient. What is unique about the quadrant model is that it does allow both practitioners and organisations to examine care delivery from a different perspective; this in itself has the potential to advance health-care delivery. What is critical to the practitioner aspiring to become an expert is ensuring that amidst any change the humanity of nursing remains.

? **Key questions for Chapter 10**

In your field of practice:

(1)　To what extent might the elements of cure – care, technology – non-technology and organisational culture apply?

(2)　What factors are currently creating opportunities for new developments and why?

(3)　How might you ensure that the 'humanity of nursing' is retained in new developments?

References

Alberran, J. and Kapeluch, H. (1994) Role of the nurse in thrombolytic therapy. *British Journal of Nursing* **3** (3) 104–9.

Asseburg, C., Vergel, Y. B., Palmer, S., *et al.* (2007) Assessing the effectiveness of primary angioplasty compared with thrombolysis and its relationship to time delay: a Bayesian evidence synthesis. *Heart* **93** (10) 1244–50.

Astin, F. and Closs, S.J. (2007) Chronic disease management and self-care support for people living with long-term conditions: is the nursing workforce prepared? *Journal of Clinical Nursing* **16** (7B) 105–6.

Bekelman, D.B., Hutt, E., Masoudi, F.A., Kutner, J.S. and Rumsfeld, J.S. (2008) Defining the role of palliative care in older adults with heart failure. *International Journal of Cardiology* **125** (2) 183–90.

Benner, P. (ed.) (1984) *The Helping Role From Novice to Expert*. Menlo Park, California, Addison Wesley.

Bjorklund, E., Stenestrand, U., Lindback, J., *et al.* (2006) Pre-hospital thrombolysis delivered by paramedics is associated with reduced time delay and mortality in ambulance-transported real-life patients with ST-elevation myocardial infarction. *European Heart Journal* **27** (10) 1146–52.

Blue, L., Lang, E., Mcmurray, J.J., *et al.* (2001) Randomised controlled trial of specialist nurse intervention in heart failure. *British Medical Journal* **323** (7315) 715–8.

Boodhoo, L., Bordoli, G., Mitchell, A.R., *et al.* (2004) The safety and effectiveness of a nurse-led cardioversion service under sedation. *Heart* **90** (12) 1443–6.

Carlsson, E., Olsson, S.B. and Hertervig, E. (2002) The role of the nurse in enhancing quality of life in patients with an implantable cardioverter – defibrillator: the Swedish experience. *Progress in Cardiovascular Nursing* **17** (1) 18–25.

Currie, M.P., Karwatowski, S.P., Perera, J. and Langford, E.J. (2004) Introduction of nurse-led DC cardioversion service in day surgery unit: prospective audit. *British Medical Journal* **329** (7471) 892–4.

Davidson, P., Paull, G., Rees, D., Daly, J. and Cockburn, J. (2005) Activities of home-based heart failure nurse specialists: a modified narrative analysis. *American Journal of Critical Care* **14** (5) 426–33.

De Bono, D. (1990) *Practical Thrombolysis*. Oxford, Blackwell Scientific Publications.

Department of Health (2000a) Coronary heart disease national service frameworks. Chapter 3 in *Heart Attacks and Other Acute Coronary Syndromes*. London, Department of Health.

Department of Health (2000b) Coronary heart disease national service framework. Chapter 4 in *Stable Angina*. London, Department of Health.

Department of Health (2006) *Our Health, Our Care, Our Say: A New Direction for Community Services*. London, Department of Health.

Doubilet, P. and McNeil, B.J. (1993) Clinical decision making. In *Professional Judgement, a Reader in Clinical Decision Making*, (eds. J. Dowie and A. Elstein). Cambridge, Cambridge University Press.

Dougherty, C.M., Lewis, F.M., Thompson, E.A., Baer, J.D. and Kim, W. (2004) Short-term efficacy of a telephone intervention by expert nurses after an implantable cardioverter defibrillator. *Pacing and Clinical Electrophysiology* **27** (12) 1594–1602.

Dowie, J. and Elstein, A. (1993) *Professional Judgement a Reader in Clinical Decision Making*. Cambridge, Cambridge University Press.

Foster, D.B., Dufendach, J.H., Barkdoll, C.M. and Mitchell, B.K. (1994) Prehospital recognition of AMI using independent nurse/paramedic 12-lead ECG evaluation: impact on in-hospital times to thrombolysis in a rural community hospital. *American Journal of Emergency Medicine* **12** (1) 25–31.

Gee, K. (1998) The roles of consultant and researcher in Advanced Nursing Practice. In *Advanced and Specialist Practice*, (eds G. Castledine and P. McGee). Oxford, Blackwell Science.

Greenhalgh, T. (2000) Change and the organisation: culture and context. *The British Journal of General Practice* **50** 340–1.

Hamric, A.B., Spross, J.A. and Hanson, C.M. (1996) Surviving system and professional turbulence. In *Advanced Nursing Practice, An Integrative Approach*, (eds A.B. Hamric, J.A. Spross and C.M. Hanson). Philadelphia, W. B. Saunders.

Handberg, E. (2006) End-of-life issues in elderly patients with acute coronary syndrome: the role of the cardiovascular nurse. *Progress in Cardiovascular Nursing* **21** (3) 151–5.

Handy, C. (1993) *Understanding Organisations*. Harmondsworth, Penguin Books.

Hart, N. (1988a) Health and the mythology of medicine. In *The Sociology of Health and Medicine*, (ed. M. Haralambos). Ormskirk, Causeway Press Ltd.

Hart, N. (1988b) Medicine as an institution of social control. In *The Sociology of Health and Medicine*, (ed. M. Haralambos). Ormskirk, Causeway Press Ltd.

Hendra, T.J. and Marshall, A.J. (1992) Increased prescription of thrombolytic treatment to elderly patients with suspected acute myocardial infarction associated with audit. *British Medical Journal* **304** (6824) 423–5.

Jacobson, C. and Gerity, D. (2005) Pacemakers and implantable defibrillators. In *Cardiac Nursing*, (eds S.L. Woods, E.S. Sivarajan, S. Underhill Motzer and E.J. Bridges). Philadelphia, Lippincott Williams & Wilkins.

Jones, I. (2005) Thrombolysis nurses: time for review. *European Journal of Cardiovascular Nursing* **4** (2) 129–37.

Jowett, N. and Thompson, D.R. (1989) Introduction to coronary care. In *Comprehensive Coronary Care*. Harrow, Scutari Press.

Kutzleb, J. and Reiner, D. (2006) The impact of nurse-directed patient education on quality of life and functional capacity in people with heart failure. *Journal of American Academy of Nurse Practitioners* **18** (3) 116–23.

Laurent, D. (2005) Heart failure. In *Cardiac Nursing*, (eds S. Woods, E.S. Sivarajan Froelicher, S. Underhill Motzer and E.J. Bridges), 5th edn. Philadelphia, Lippincott Williams & Wilkins.

Liao, L., Anstrom, K.J., Gottdiener, J.S., *et al.* (2007) Long-term costs and resource use in elderly participants with congestive heart failure in the Cardiovascular Health Study. *American Heart Journal* **153** (2) 245–52.

Madan, S.K. (2005) Psychological risk factors: assessment and management interventions. In *Cardiac Nursing*, (eds S.L. Woods, E.S. Sivarajan Froelicher, S. Underhill Motzer and E.J. Bridges). Philadelphia, Lippincott Williams & Wilkins.

Majeed, A., Moser, K. and Carroll, K. (2001) Trends in the prevalence and management of atrial fibrillation in general practice in England and Wales, 1994–1998: analysis of data from the general practice research database. *Heart* **86** (3) 284–8.

Mant, J., Mcmanus, R.J., Oakes, R.A., *et al.* (2004) Systematic review and modelling of the investigation of acute and chronic chest pain presenting in primary care. *Health Technology Assessment* **8** (2) iii, 1–158.

McAlister, F.A., Lawson, F.M., Teo, K.K. and Armstrong, P.W. (2001) A systematic review of randomized trials of disease management programs in heart failure. *American Journal of Medicine* **110** (5) 378–84.

McAlister, F.A., Stewart, S., Ferrua, S. and Mcmurray, J.J. (2004) Multidisciplinary strategies for the management of heart failure patients at high risk for admission: a systematic review of randomized trials. *Journal of the American College of Cardiology* **44** (4) 810–19.

McDonald, K., Ledwidge, M., Cahill, J., *et al.* (2002) Heart failure management: multidisciplinary care has intrinsic benefit above the optimization of medical care. *Journal of Cardiac Failure* **8** (3) 142–8.

Miller, N.H. and Froelicher, E.S. (2005) Disease management models for cardiovascular care. In *Cardiac Nursing*, (eds S.L. Woods, E. Sivarajan Froelicher and S. Underhill Motzer). Philadelphia, Lippincott Williams & Wilkins.

Murphy, E. (2004) Case management and community matrons for long term conditions. *British Medical Journal* **329** (7477) 1251–2.

Myers, J. (2005) Exercise and activity. In *Cardiac Nursing*, (eds S.L. Woods, E.S. Sivarajan, S. Underhill Motzer and E.J. Bridges). Philadelphia, Lippincott Williams & Wilkins.

O'Brien, J.L., Martin, D.R., Heyworth, J. and Meyer, N.R. (2008) Negotiating transformational leadership: a key to effective collaboration. *Nursing and Health Sciences* **10** (2) 137–43.

Ornato, J.P. (1990) The earliest thrombolytic treatment of acute myocardial infarction: ambulance or emergency department? *Clinical Cardiology* **13** (8 Suppl 8) VIII27–31.

Patterson, C., Kaczorowski, J., Arthur, H., Smith, K. and Mills, D.A. (2003) Complementary therapy practice: defining the role of advanced nurse practitioners. *Journal of Clinical Nursing* **12** (6) 816–23.

Pottle, A. (2005) A nurse-led rapid access chest pain clinic – experience from the first 3 years. *European Journal of Cardiovascular Nursing* **4** (3) 227–33.

Quinn, T., Butters, A. and Todd, I. (2002) Implementing paramedic thrombolysis – an overview. *Accident and Emergency Nursing* **10** (4) 189–96.

Rao, B.H. and Saksena, S. (2003) Implantable cardioverter – defibrillators in cardiovascular care: technologic advances and new indications. *Current Opinions on Critical Care* **9** (5) 362–8.

Rasmusson, K.D., Brush, S.J., Hall, J.A., *et al.* (2005) Bridging the resource gap in heart failure expertise and management: the underacknowledged role of nurse specialists. *Journal of the American College of Cardiology* **46** (10) 1961–2.

Reisfield, G.M. and Wilson, G.R. (2007) Palliative care issues in heart failure #144. *Journal of Palliative Medicine* **10** (1) 247–8.

Riegel, B., Moser, D.K., Powell, M., Rector, T.S. and Havranek, E.P. (2006) Nonpharmacologic care by heart failure experts. *Journal of Cardiac Failure* **12** (2) 149–53.

Sears, S.F., Jr. and Conti, J.B. (2002) Quality of life and psychological functioning of ICD patients. *Heart* **87** (5) 488–93.

Shelton, R.J., Allinson, A., Johnson, T., Smales, C. and Kaye, G.C. (2006) Four years experience of a nurse-led elective cardioversion service within a district general hospital setting. *Europace* **8** (1) 81–5.

Sneed, N.V., Finch, N.J. and Michel, Y. (1997) The effect of psychosocial nursing intervention on the mood state of patients with implantable cardioverter defibrillators and their caregivers. *Progress in Cardiovascular Nursing* **12** (2) 4–14.

Sparacino, P.S.A. (1994) Issues and future trends for the critical care clinical nurse specialist. In *The Clinical Nurse Specialist Role in Critical Care*, (eds A. Gawlinski and L.S. Kern). Philadelphia, W. B. Saunders.

Stanley, M. and Prasun, M. (2002) Heart failure in older adults: keys to successful management. *AACN Clinical Issues* **13** (1) 94–102.

Strömberg, A. (2002) Educating nurses and patients to manage heart failure. *European Journal of Cardiovascular Nursing* **1** (1) 33–40.

Strömberg, A., Ahlen, H., Fridlund, B. and Dahlstrom, U. (2002) Interactive education on CD-ROM – a new tool in the education of heart failure patients. *Patient Education and Counselling* **46** (1) 75–81.

Strömberg, A., Martensson, J., Fridlund, B. and Dahlstrom, U. (2001) Nurse-led heart failure clinics in Sweden. *European Journal of Heart Failure* **3** (1) 139–44.

Styles, M.M. (1996) Conceptualisations of advanced nursing practice. In *Advanced Nursing Practice An Integrative Approach*, (eds A.B. Hamric, J.A. Spross and C.M. Hanson). Philadelphia, W. B. Saunders.

Swanton, R.H. (2003) Cardiac failure. In *Pocket Consultant Cardiology*. (ed. R.H Swanton), 5th edn. Malden Massachusetts, Blackwell Publishing.

Tagney, J. (2003) Implantable cardioverter defibrillators: developing evidence-based care. *Nursing Standard* **17** (16) 33–36.

Tebbenjohanns, J., Schumacher, B., Jung, W., *et al.* (1994) Predictors of outcome in patients with implantable transvenous cardioverter defibrillators. *American Heart Journal* **127** (4 Pt 2) 1086–9.

Trofino, J. (1993) Transformational leadership: the catalyst for successful change. *International Nursing Review* **40** (6) 179–82, 187.

Wilson, P.M., Kendall, S. and Brooks, F. (2006) Nurses' responses to expert patients: the rhetoric and reality of self-management in long-term conditions: a grounded theory study. *International Journal of Nursing Studies* **43** (7) 803–18.

Yu, D.S., Lee, D.T., Woo, J. and Hui, E. (2007) Non-pharmacological interventions in older people with heart failure: effects of exercise training and relaxation therapy. *Gerontology* **53** (2) 74–81.

Zambroski, C.H. (2006) Managing beyond an uncertain illness trajectory: palliative care in advanced heart failure. *International Journal of Palliative Nursing* **12** (12) 566–73.

Zapka, J.G., Hennessy, W., Carter, R.E. and Amella, E.J. (2006) End-of-life communication and hospital nurses: an educational pilot. *Journal of Cardiovascular Nursing* **21** (3) 223–31.

Zubialde, J.P., Shannon, K. and Devenger, N. (2005) The quadrants of care model for health services planning. *Families, Systems and Health* **23** (2) 172–85.

Chapter 11
Cultural Competence in Advanced Practice

Paula McGee

Introduction

Culture is a form of mental software that provides a way of living in, interacting with and experiencing the world (Hofstede 1994). This software is encapsulated in a set of values, attitudes and beliefs that we learn as children and which permeate every aspect of daily life: food, religious beliefs, dress, gender and age relations, language, manners, occupations, education, politics, health and medicine. This means that culture is an integral part of every one of us rather than a set of characteristics associated with those whom we regard as different from ourselves. One of the difficulties in thinking about ourselves as cultural beings is that what we learn in childhood becomes taken for granted. We assume that everyone shares the same values, attitudes and beliefs, the same outlook on life. It is only when we encounter people whose cultural values, attitudes and beliefs appear to differ that we begin to realise the power and influence of the mental software through which we have been programmed. Successful interactions among members of different cultures depend on our awareness of ourselves as well as our ability to understand other people's views of the world. In health care, understanding and working with the patient's view of the world requires a high level of competence, which must form part of the advanced practitioner's repertoire of skills. This chapter presents a discussion about the importance of culture in care. It begins with an explanation of the diverse cultures to which everyone belongs: personal, professional and organisational. This explanation leads into a discussion about equality in health care and current UK strategies intended to address the inequity experienced by many members of black and other black and minority ethnic groups. The chapter then moves on to outline the relationships among culture, health, treatment and care. This is followed by a presentation of three theories of cultural competence and the chapter closes by considering their relevance to advanced practice.

Culture and equality

Culture exerts an influence on every aspect of our daily lives, determining how we behave, dress, work, think and communicate with others. On a daily basis we each function in several cultures, moving competently but unconsciously between them (Figure 11.1). To explain this further, we each belong to the culture into which we were socialised as children and which gave us our initial values and beliefs. Going to school, joining clubs and taking part in other activities exposed us to other views of the world, other ways of living. In entering a profession we were again introduced to a particular way of being in the health-care world, for instance, as a nurse or an occupational therapist. Each profession has values and beliefs, traditions, standards, behaviours and education associated with its work and position in society and which can be summed up as *being a nurse, being an occupational therapist*. These ways of being are transmitted to new recruits both formally through professional codes of conduct and informally through the hidden curricula in educational establishments and practical placements (McGee 1998).

Finally, each health-care organisation also has particular values, traditions, standards and behaviours. This organisational culture is expressed in ways of working, procedures, the appearance and manners of staff, and through many other, more subtle means that determine how the organisation functions internally and how it relates to the external world (Gheradi 1995). As we move from one organisation to

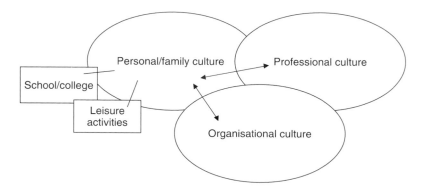

Fig. 11.1   Each of us belongs to multiple cultures.

another we have to learn how things are done in that place through both formal induction programmes and informal workplace orientation. Thus, organisational culture can be summed up as *the way we do things around here*.

Learning professional and organisational cultures can be unsettling. It takes time to become accustomed to what is required, to adapt to new ways of being. Reflection on this experience can be useful in opening the mind to what it means to be the outsider, the new person, the stranger and how easily problems can arise because of a lack of understanding of how the new workplace functions or the ways in which a member of a particular profession is normally expected to behave. The insights gained are transferable to situations in which professionals do not share the same personal culture either among themselves or with their patients. Drawing on experiences of what it means to be the new person can help professionals become sensitised to the needs and experiences of those who are unfamiliar with the majority culture.

Inherent in such situations are issues of power and inequality. Professionals and organisations need to examine their values and attitudes, be open-minded and flexible in their approach to people who differ and avoid blaming people for their differences (New Zealand Council of Nursing 2005). Numerous research studies have demonstrated that members of black and minority ethnic groups are disadvantaged in the UK health-care system (see, e.g. Evers *et al.* 1988, NAHA 1988, McGee 2000, Rabiee and Smith 2007, McGee *et al.* 2008, DH 2008a, b). Reasons for this include poor communication, lack of knowledge among health professionals (McGee 2000) and inappropriate services (DH 2008a, b). Racism, discrimination and stereotyping have also been noted in the behaviour of staff towards patients and each other (see, e.g. Beishon *et al.* 1995, McGee 2000, Notter and Klem 2001, Notter and Hepburn 2003).

In the United Kingdom, the inquiry into the death of Stephen Lawrence introduced the concept of *institutional racism* as 'the collective failure of an organisation to provide an appropriate service to people because of their colour, culture or ethnic origin. It can be detected in processes, attitudes and behaviour which amount to discrimination through unwitting prejudice, ignorance, thoughtlessness and racist stereotyping which disadvantage minority ethnic people' (Home Office 1999, para 6.34). Changes in UK legislation such as the Human Rights Act 1998, the Race Relations (Amendment) Act 2000 and the Equality Act 2006 represent current efforts to tackle all forms of discrimination. In particular, the Race Relations (Amendment) Act 2000 placed new responsibilities on employers and service providers not only to address inequalities but also to demonstrate evidence of practical changes in their ways of working. The established mechanisms intended to reduce inequalities; the Commission for Racial Equality, the Disability Rights Commission and the Equal Opportunities Commission were no longer appropriate. Consequently, these were amalgamated into the new Equalities and Human Rights Commission, which came into operation in October 2007. This new commission is intended to not only continue the work of the previous organisations but also take on responsibility for other issues including 'age, sexual orientation and religion or belief, as well as human rights' (Equality and Human Rights Commission 2007 http://www.equalityhumanrights.com/en).

As a result of these changes, the Department of Health (DH) introduced a number of strategies to address inequalities in health and social care for members of black and minority ethnic groups. These are implemented under the auspices of the Department's Equality and Human Rights Group (DH 2007). Two current examples are outlined here. The Pacesetters programme is based around local partnerships between disadvantaged minority communities, the National Health Service (NHS) and the DH. The intention is to involve patients, service staff and members of local communities in designing and providing services that meet their needs as a means of reducing inequalities in health, social care and working lives (DH 2008a). The programme provides a simple model for service improvement based on three key questions: 'What are we trying to achieve? How will we know if we have achieved? What changes will we introduce to bring about improvements?' While local partnerships are free to choose any aspect of a service that, in their opinion, requires improvement, each proposed initiative must undergo an equality impact assessment so that the anticipated benefits of a change are clearly articulated before work begins (DH 2008a).

The second example is Race for Health. This is an NHS programme, funded by the DH, which is focused on bringing about changes in primary care to improve the health of members of black and minority ethnic groups by modernising services, increasing choice and developing a diverse workforce (Race for Health 2007). The DH has identified ten aspects of primary care that require attention, including lack of understanding of the NHS, poor communication and inflexibility in the system (DH 2008b). As in the Pacesetters programme, Race for Health requires general practitioner (GP) practices to work collaboratively with local patient groups and their Primary Care Trusts to develop an accurate database about black and minority people and to bring about improvements in services. Trusts are charged with ensuring that service commissioning provides equitable access to appropriate services that are delivered by a suitably prepared workforce (DH 2008b).

Pacesetters, Race for Health and other such initiatives offer many opportunities to advanced practitioners whose role in direct care facilitates the development of a first-hand insight into the experiences of patients who have to cope with the dual demands of ill health and the health-care system. Advanced practitioners will be aware of patients' health needs, their frustrations, worries and fears. Advanced practitioners actively engage with underserved, marginalised and vulnerable people who might otherwise have limited or restricted access to health care because of some perceived difference that sets them apart from the majority. Identifying such individuals and communities is part of the advanced role in ensuring that services are acceptable, accessible and appropriate for patients' needs, both in terms of availability and patient experience. The collaborative working skills of advanced practitioners mean that they will already be part of local networks and know who to contact when help is needed. Even more importantly, advanced practitioners are in a position to provide clinical and professional leadership by challenging negative attitudes, recognising inequalities, developing standards and facilitating the development of members of staff, services and professional practice (Box 11.1).

Box 11.1　Key elements in meeting the needs of diverse individuals and communities

Identifying organisational factors that help/hinder appropriate, accessible and acceptable care

Recognising inequalities

Positively valuing people as individuals who differ from one another

Developing strategies that enhance the knowledge and skills of colleagues

Identifying diverse individuals and communities and developing accurate and up-to-date knowledge systems that are accessible and relevant to practitioners

Developing standards and systems of monitoring to ensure progress

Presenting evidence of achievements to internal personnel and external bodies such as the Healthcare Commission

---

Cultural relationships among health, illness, treatment and care

In providing such leadership, advanced practitioners will need to draw on an understanding of the relationships among culture, health, treatment and care. If culture provides a way of being in and experiencing the world then it follows that cultural values and beliefs will have an impact on ideas about health, what makes people ill and how that illness should be treated. For the majority of people, irrespective of their particular cultural background, the causes of ill health are rooted in social and supernatural explanations (Helman 2000). Illness is thus attributable to factors such as divine retribution for sin, curses or the actions of evil spirits. Similarly, disruptions in relationships, family tension, stress and other social or heritage factors may be blamed for causing sickness (Helman 2000). Health, in this context, is the absence of such negative events. In some instances, the conceptualisation of a particular health problem is entirely bound up with specific cultural beliefs. For example, the British concept of catching a chill is rather difficult to explain to other people but chills are, nonetheless, regarded by British people as real and debilitating. Similar, culture-bound ideas exist in many different cultures and have to be taken seriously as part of a patient's view of the world (Campinha-Bacote 1994, Echols 1998).

Patients' beliefs necessitate a broad, holistic approach to treatment and care that takes account of the meanings that they attach to their illnesses; focusing solely on the disease or symptoms is not enough. Thus, in providing direct care, the advanced practitioner works with the patient to determine what that person believes will help to restore health and, if possible, incorporate this into the care plan. Often, examples of what may be needed are couched in terms of religious and spiritual practices. While these are, of course, important to many people, beliefs about treatment and care may also include ideas about the relationship among treatment, food and medication. To explain this further, in Chinese tradition everything in the world is made up of two opposing but interdependent factors: *yin* and *yang*; illness is classified in terms of these two factors (Traditional Chinese Medicine Basics 2008). In Hispanic tradition this classification is expressed as *frio* (cold, *yin*) or *caliente* (hot, *yang*). Where such classifications are used, the underlying belief is associated with an imbalance in the body. Thus someone with depression or cancer has an excess of *yin* or *frio* and requires *yang* or *caliente* medicines, such as aspirin, and food, for example spicy dishes, to restore balance. Someone with a *yang* or *caliente* condition such as hypertension requires a *yin* or *frio* diet that includes green vegetables and dairy foods and medication (Echols 1998).

The advanced practitioner is able to incorporate such beliefs into patient care and help other practitioners to understand their importance. However, this may not always be possible. Some beliefs and practices may not be compatible with Western health-care treatments; some traditional remedies, for instance, may contain substances that interact negatively with prescribed medication. Such situations require the advanced practitioner to act as a cultural broker, explaining to the patient and relatives why certain practices are not advisable and helping staff to understand the patient's point of view. Ultimately, what matters most is the advanced practitioner's interpersonal skills in listening to all those involved and negotiating a satisfactory solution for the patient.

Achieving such a solution is not always easy. People can be uncooperative, unwilling to listen or to engage in negotiation. Rigid professional attitudes can present major difficulties in trying to find a way around a particular problem. It is, therefore, important that the advanced practitioner has confidence. Examination of theoretical ideas can help identify significant factors and support the advanced practitioner's efforts in establishing appropriate courses of action. However, it is worth pointing out at this stage that there is no one approach to the provision of culturally competent practice. Each theory offers a particular view of how such practice may be achieved but there is no 'right' way.

Theoretical approaches to culturally competent practice

Any serious study of culturally competent practice must include consideration of Leininger's highly influential theory of transcultural nursing (Leininger 1978, Leininger and McFarland 2002). She was the first to address culture and health in an academic way using anthropological methods (Leininger 1970). She defined transcultural nursing as 'a formal area of study and practice in nursing focused upon comparative holistic cultural care, health, and illness patterns of individuals and groups with respect to differences and similarities in cultural values, beliefs, and practices with the goal to provide culturally congruent sensitive and competent care to people of diverse cultures'. (Leininger 1995, p. 4). This definition of transcultural nursing drew heavily on anthropologically based knowledge and combined it with nursing. Leininger went on to propose that, in the provision of culturally competent care, the practitioner had three options. *Culture care preservation* meant working within the patient's frame of reference, for example, in helping people to lose weight or wean their infants. *Culture care accommodation* involved enabling people to cope with health changes, such as pregnancy, within their cultural framework.

Finally, *culture care re-patterning* involved helping people cope with imposed changes such as a stoma or diabetes (Leininger and McFarland 2002). More recently developed theories have all drawn to some extent on Leininger's ideas although all offer their own unique perspectives. Three theories are discussed here.

Papadopoulos, Tilki and Taylor's theory of cultural competence

Papadopoulos, Tilki and Taylor (Papadopoulos *et al.* 1998, Papadopoulos 2006) are a United Kingdom-based team that proposes an approach to culturally competent practice based on four factors: *cultural awareness, cultural knowledge, cultural sensitivity* and *cultural competence*. *Cultural awareness* asks the practitioner to focus on the self. Cultural values, beliefs and attitudes, all the taken-for-granted aspects of our daily lives, especially those about which we may hold strong views, are reflected upon in terms of their potential influence on practice (Papadopoulos *et al.* 2004). This reflection highlights individual differences; culture is not homogeneous or static. There are more variations between members of the same culture than between those from different cultural backgrounds (Helman 2000). Moreover, cultural values and beliefs change over time as individuals are exposed to life experiences that require them to adapt (Papadopoulos 2006).

Cultural knowledge refers to what is known about a culture and how. Professionals' knowledge is generated by many different academic disciplines: anthropology, sociology, psychology, history, medicine, nursing, the arts, politics, religion and science. This knowledge is often very detailed and interesting but it is, for the most part, a compilation of outsiders' views and opinions about a culture. It represents only one form of knowledge and 'it is important to balance – if not overturn – this domination of knowledge by enabling people to have a say in how they would like to see their world put together and run' (Papadopoulos 2006, p. 16). In making this statement Papadopoulos (2006) draws attention to the ways in which academically generated knowledge is valued and incorporated into the professional power base and argues for change. Papadopoulos *et al.* (1998) make clear that the development of cultural knowledge must include consideration of health inequalities and an understanding of the ways in which powerful institutions and professionals can, unwittingly, marginalise the very people they are trying to help. The knowledge possessed by patients, families and other members of a culture may be as valuable as academic perspectives, if not more and so 'whatever the source of the knowledge we access . . . must always ask ourselves: whose values were used to construct it?' (Papadopoulos 2006, p. 16). Thus, direct contact with members of black and minority ethnic groups is essential in ensuring that knowledge about cultural beliefs and practices is rooted in real and contemporary lives (Campinha-Bacote 2002, Papadopoulos *et al.* 2004).

Cultural sensitivity refers to interpersonal relationships between patients and professionals. Unless professionals regard and treat patients as equals who meet to address a specific health problem, effective therapeutic relationships cannot be established (Papadopoulos *et al.* 2004, Papadopoulos 2006). Inherent in such an emphasis on equality is a willingness to engage with different cultural values, beliefs, ways of living and conventions surrounding communication such as body language, greetings and the degrees of formality expected (Papadopoulos 2006). Interactional styles arise directly from cultural values and beliefs. For example, Western cultures tend to place a high value on individualism and interactional styles reflect that value. In contrast, patients from minority ethnic backgrounds may use the interactional styles of their own cultures or a composite of their own and the Western manner (Campinha-Bacote 1994). In both instances misunderstandings can arise, fuelling distrust and antagonism in both parties (Box 11.2). To sum up, advanced practitioners must examine their cultural values, attitudes and prejudices and recognise that their interactional styles may differ from those used by patients. Practitioners need to accommodate such differences in order to work effectively with patients and develop appropriate treatment plans (Campinha-Bacote 1994, 2002).

Box 11.2   Some examples of the ways in which interactional style can impact the effectiveness of interpersonal communication

Intonation

This refers to the ways in which the voice is used to emphasise a point, convey feeling or ask a question. For example, asking a question in English requires the speaker to raise the voice at the end of the sentence – don't we? In some other languages the voice is lowered. Using this pattern of intonation in English may, unintentionally, sound rude.

Eye contact

In Western cultures, looking straight at the speaker and engaging in eye contact is considered an important part of normal conversation. In other cultures, looking directly at the speaker, especially if that person holds an important position or is of the opposite gender, may be impolite.

Courtesy

In English, there are particular words for *please* and *thank you* and social rules about when and how these words should be used. In contrast, languages such as Urdu do not tend to use separate words in this way. *Please* and *thank you* are conveyed through other mechanisms such as intonation and the addition of a suffix such as *ji* to convey respect. Lack of understanding of this simple cultural difference may cause offence.

Note: For further information on these and other interactional issues see Andrews, M. (2003) Culturally competent nursing care. Chapter 2 in *Transcultural concepts in nursing care*, (eds. Andrews, M. and Boyle, J.), 4th edn. pp. 15–35. Philadelphia, Lippincott, Williams and Wilkins.

Finally, *cultural competence* requires the synthesis of the other three elements and their application to the assessment of patients, the formulation of diagnoses and the development of plans for treatment and care. These applications form practical demonstrations of the practitioner's abilities and understanding (Papadopoulos *et al.* 2004). Such skills develop over time, through stages, as the practitioner progresses from avoiding cultural issues in assessment to raising them confidently with patients. Competence is dependent on negotiating with the patient, particularly when there are difficult issues to be addressed. Papadopoulos *et al.* (2004, p. 110) make clear that competence is not solely concerned with clinical skills but also with the ability to 'recognise and challenge racism and discrimination and oppressive practice'.

Purnell and Paulanka's theory of cultural competence

This is a complex theory developed by American academics. Culture is presented as having 12 inter-relating domains, each of which is relevant to health (Purnell and Paulanka 2003). These domains include communication, high risk behaviour, workforce issues, differing patterns of health, family roles and customs surrounding major events such as birth and death. At the centre of these domains is an unknown zone, which represents those aspects of the culture that remain obscure to those outside the culture. Surrounding the 12 domains are 3 factors – the person, the family and the community. Ideas about the person reflect cultural values (Purnell and Paulanka 2003) (Figure 11.2). Western cultures tend to regard the person as a separate, independent entity who is able, and has the right to be self-determining; the person is expected to take responsibility for the actions of the self. This contrasts with cultures, such as those of Japan and China, in which the person is regarded primarily as a member of a group. Such cultures tend to emphasise group or family responsibility and prefer a collective, shared approach to decision-making and the care of group or family members (Maruyama 1997, Chen 2001). Purnell and Paulanka's concept of the family is very broad. A family unit consists of a minimum of two people who have emotional connections but who do not necessarily share the same living space or a

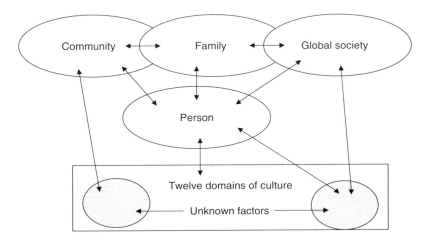

Fig. 11.2   The main features of Purnell and Paulanka's theory of cultural competence.

blood relationship. The family changes over time as members age, relocate or change their social status (Purnell and Paulanka 2003). Families exist within communities that are groups of 'people having a common interest or identity and living in a specified locality' (Purnell and Paulanka 2003, p. 9). Communities in turn exist within the overall society.

Purnell and Paulanka (2003) propose that cultural competence has seven elements. *Self-awareness* is an essential first step for practitioners in ensuring that their cultural values and beliefs do not intrude unhelpfully into interactions with patients. Practitioners who have achieved self-awareness are open to *cultural encounters*, that is to say, engagement with members of different cultural groups. Such practitioners recognise and *do not make assumptions* about cultural differences. They are able to *accept and respect patients' cultural values and beliefs* without agreeing with them or *making judgements about them. Knowledge and understanding* of the patient's culture, health beliefs and needs is necessary for the *adaptation of practice* in order to ensure appropriate care (Purnell and Paulanka 2003, pp. 3–4).

Becoming culturally competent requires change within the self. The individual begins as *unconsciously incompetent*, unaware of a lack of knowledge or skill. Developing self-awareness brings the practitioner to *conscious incompetence*, the realisation of ignorance and a gradual transition into *conscious competence* in which the practitioner strives to do what is needed but has to concentrate in order to achieve what is required. Gradually, this self-consciousness wanes into *unconscious competence* as the new knowledge and skills become integrated into the practitioner's regular repertoire. These four stages imply linear progress in a single direction but this need not be the case. Some individuals may learn faster than others. The achievement of *unconscious competence* in working with members of one culture does not necessarily mean that a practitioner is equipped to work in the same way with another (Purnell and Paulanka 2003).

McGee's theory of cultural competence

Cultural competence is an evolving state, a continuous process, of *learning, performing* and *reflecting* that can apply to both the individual practitioner and the organisation as a whole (McGee 2000) (Figures 11.3 and 11.4). For the individual, learning requires practitioners to develop self-awareness as cultural beings with their own beliefs, values and ways of being in the world. Part of this self-awareness is a growing understanding of the ways in which personal values and attitudes can be transmitted

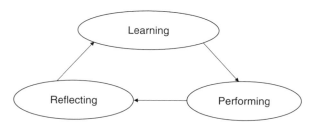

Fig. 11.3   Cultural competence is a continuous process of . . . .

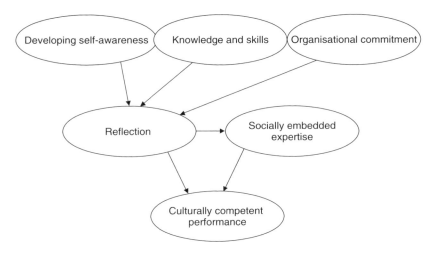

Fig. 11.4   A framework for cultural competence.

to patients. This is particularly important if such transmission is accompanied by negative judgements (Campinha-Bacote 2002). Health-care work inevitably brings practitioners into contact with habits or lifestyles of which they may disapprove. Frustration with a patient's refusal or inability to change is understandable but unhelpful in terms of providing treatment and care. Similarly, looking down on and blaming people for their culture as different and inferior will not contribute to improvements in their health or recovery from illness (New Zealand Council of Nursing 2005). Consequently, interpersonal skills form part of learning about culture. Practitioners need to be able to recognise the diverse communication styles used by patients and to adapt accordingly, observing the culturally based rules about greetings, courtesy and gestures.

Learning also requires practitioners to clearly identify and develop an understanding of their patients' cultures, their values, traditions and beliefs (McGee 2000). This involves moving beyond descriptive statistics towards professional knowledge based on direct engagement with patients, their families and appropriate contacts in the wider community. This may be complemented by academic studies where these exist. What matters most is that knowledge is accurate, useful and up to date as it will inform the adaptation of practice and thus the provision of treatment and care.

For the organisation, learning begins with the concept of institutional racism, the ways in which organisations can discriminate against certain members of the population and the legal responsibilities placed on employers by the Race Relations Amendment Act 2000 (Home Office 1999). Developing self-awareness requires a thorough examination of the structural processes, policies and procedures that govern the organisation and delivery of services. Reviewing these processes, policies and procedures will reveal the extent to which the organisation is really committed to addressing inequalities in access and patient experience. Organisations that are really determined to achieve equality are able to demonstrate how this takes place and have effective monitoring procedures in place to deal with lapses (McGee 2000).

Addressing inequality also requires knowledge about the cultures represented in the local population (McGee 2000). The organisation will need to develop strategies for engaging with local communities in a balanced way, ensuring that powerful and highly vocal groups are not privileged at the expense of those who are less assertive or articulate. This will require a review of the communication styles and media that are normally used and comparing these with local cultural values. For example, issuing written materials will make little impact on members of cultures in which it is important to visit in person if one has something important to say. Thus, effective engagement is dependent on an understanding of cultural mores and the avoidance of assumptions about those perceived as different. Finally, as knowledge about culture is generated, the organisation will need to ensure that it is applied at different levels, from service planning and commissioning to individual patient care.

An additional consideration for the organisation is the nature of the workforce. Managing a diverse workforce requires organisational commitment to recognise and value difference while taking account of the various ways in which that difference may impact on working practices through, for example, communication styles (Cornelius 2002). Organisations have to recognise that diversity can be a strength that makes good business sense. Staff can be recruited from a much broader range of people and bring with them diverse skills and abilities from which the organisation benefits (Cornelius 2002). Good diversity managers recognise that inequalities exist but seek to overcome these by creating a workplace in which both differences and sameness are valued. Their organisations have open channels through which individual employees can make their voices heard. There is transparency about how the organisation functions. For example, there are clearly established criteria for promotion and pay scales and access to training. The overall effect is a workplace that feels fair and equitable and in which all employees can attain their full potential (Cornelius 2002).

Performing care and enacting organisational strategies will enable practitioners and organisations alike to apply their understanding of cultural issues (McGee 2000). Reflection informs and refines learning, allowing competence to increase gradually, based on theoretical and experiential knowledge that is checked and tested through performance. In other words, practitioners and organisations are able to determine, in practical ways, what actually works. Even when mistakes arise, the processes of reflection can help to clarify what went wrong and what is needed to prevent a recurrence. Audit and clinical governance will provide some of the formal channels through which both practitioners and the organisation can monitor developments. Alongside these activities, practitioners' reflections could provide a starting point for staff to share learning experiences and build networks of socially embedded expertise in cultural care (Benner *et al.* 1996, McGee 2000). At present far too much depends on individuals; what is needed is an extension of the informal mechanisms through which practitioners normally share ideas and information in ways that help 'to limit tunnel vision and snap judgements' and provide 'powerful strategies for maximising the clinical knowledge of a group' (Benner *et al.* 1996, p. 205). Socially embedded expertise facilitates the development of shared competence so that patients receive the same standard of care irrespective of who is on duty and organisations are able to maintain a culturally competent service even if individual post holders change.

Relevance of theory to advanced practice

The theories presented here raise several issues for the advanced practitioner in terms of direct and indirect care activities (Koetters 1989). The advanced practitioner's role is primarily about providing direct care to patients, families and groups. In this context, all three theories emphasise the importance of developing an awareness of the self, of the ways in which personal values and attitudes can affect interactions with patients from diverse backgrounds. This self-awareness is closely linked to direct engagement with members of different cultures as the principal means of learning about difference (McGee 2000, Purnell and Paulanka 2003, Papadopoulos *et al.* 2004). The advanced practitioner is ideally placed to develop community-based networks as sources of information and, in return, offer culture-specific coaching and guiding that will promote health.

As a result of such engagement, culturally competent advanced practitioners develop knowledge and understanding of local cultures. They know how to behave appropriately with patients and how to respond to their communication styles. The advanced practitioner is able to accommodate difference easily; performance is unconsciously competent and practice is easily adapted to provide treatment and care that is meaningful and culturally acceptable to patients. Expertise in teaching and guiding means that the advanced practitioner is able to work appropriately with patients to facilitate changes in lifestyle that will benefit their health and accommodate changes such as aging or long-term conditions. Teaching and guiding skills can also be used in providing clinical and professional leadership to staff, enabling them to develop cultural competence in direct patient care. Once staff become confident, the advanced practitioner will be able to step back, acting as a consultant, should the need arise. To sum up, all three theories help the advanced practitioner to become culturally competent and facilitate similar development in others (McGee 2000, Purnell and Paulanka 2003, Papadopoulos *et al.* 2004).

However, there are differences between the theories, which means that the advanced practitioner may find it helpful to draw on more than one source of theoretical knowledge. Purnell and Paulanka's (2003) theory pays particular attention to specific differences that may affect health. Variations in patterns of health and disease are particularly are especially relevant. For example, there is a high incidence of coronary heart disease among South Asian people. In the United Kingdom, the mortality rate for South Asians, when compared to the white population, is 46% higher in men and 51% higher in women (Patel 2005). People of Caribbean origin are more likely to die from stroke than the rest of the population (Abbotts *et al.* 2004). They are also up to eight times more likely than members of other ethnic groups to develop severe forms of primary open-angle glaucoma (Cross *et al.* 2005). A study of such differences provides the advanced practitioner with opportunities to develop innovative approaches to practice that tackle inequalities in health and promote healthy lifestyles among members of black and minority ethnic groups. There is a sound business argument for this type of innovation. Current approaches are clearly ineffective and the refocusing of efforts and resources has the potential to reduce future demands on health-care services.

Similarly, Purnell and Paulanka's (2003) theory raises the issue of ethnic variations in response to treatment. This is an under-addressed area of health care but one that is important in ensuring that long-term conditions are managed correctly. To illustrate this point, Higginbottom and Mathers (2006) researched African Caribbean people with hypertension and found that many preferred to use traditional herbal remedies arguing that the Western medicine was too strong. Consequently, patients did not take their prescribed medication as directed but did not disclose this to practitioners.

A second area of difference between the three theories relates to workplace issues. Only Purnell and Paulanka (2003) raise the issue of the ways in which the health-care practitioner is perceived by those who access health care. Public images of a profession coupled with cultural beliefs and traditions about gender roles and status may have a profound influence on patients' attitude to staff. For instance, in Western societies, nursing has, in the past, been associated with a number of images associated with women: ministering angel, prostitute, doctor's handmaid and battle axe (Kalisch and Kalisch 1987). In more recent times, these images have been challenged through multiple channels that include improvements in professional education, changes in social status, the recruitment of men into nursing and television soap operas. However, in countries such as Saudi Arabia, changes are only beginning to take place. In a society in which gender segregation is an important cultural issue, women who decide to become nurses experience difficulties in working in an environment in which they have to mix with men. Pressure from families who fear that allowing a woman to become a nurse will render her unmarriageable, the attitudes of some male patients and long working hours that interfere with participation in family gatherings can all contribute to negative views about nurses, especially among those who regard caring as servants' work (Shalhoub 2008).

Other workforce issues are raised by McGee (2000) and Purnell and Paulanka (2003) both of whom recognise that cultural issues in health care are not confined to interactions between staff and patients. In the United Kingdom, the NHS has always relied heavily on staff from many different cultures but it is only recently that this multi-ethnic workforce has been regarded as a valuable asset rather than something to be exploited. There is still much work to be done in creating a fair workplace in which all staff feel valued and respected in cultural terms (Cornelius 2002). The indirect care role of the advanced practitioner provides opportunities to address inequalities among staff groups and promote culturally competent working practices. In particular, the advanced practitioner's ability to engage in critical thinking and ethical reasoning provides a basis for developing an ethical workplace in which staff feel that they are respected as cultural beings (Hamric and Reigle 2005). One aspect of ensuring such respect is to tackle discrimination. Papadopoulos *et al.* (2004) make clear that challenging prejudice is an integral part of cultural competence. The advanced practitioner, therefore, has a responsibility to ensure not only that anti-discriminatory policies are set in place but also that they are acted upon and that sanctions are applied to those who engage in racist or discriminatory activity.

Conclusion

This chapter has presented an overview of current ideas about cultural competence and related these to advanced practice. In a diverse society advanced practitioners must be capable of engaging constructively with cultural issues in health care. Their role as leaders in their respective professions means that they are ideally placed to act as role models for culturally competent clinical practice and facilitate the development of such competence in the workforce.

 Key questions for Chapter 11

In your field of practice:

(1)   What do you know about the cultural backgrounds of patients and how was this knowledge acquired?

(2)   How might an advanced practitioner promote the development of culturally competent practice?

(3)   What changes are needed in the organisation in order to promote cultural competence?

References

Abbotts, J., Harding, S. and Cruikshank, K. (2004) Cardiovascular risk profiles in UK-born Caribbeans and Irish living in England and Wales. *Atherosclerosis* **175** (2) 295–303.

Andrews, M. (2003) Culturally competent nursing care. Chapter 2 in *Transcultural concepts in nursing care*, (eds. Andrews, M. and Boyle, J.), 4th edn. pp. 15–35. Philadelphia, Lippincott, Williams and Wilkins.

Beishon, S., Virdee, S. and Hagell, A. (1995) *Nursing in a Multi-Ethnic NHS*. London, Policy Studies Institute.

Benner, P., Tanner, C. and Chesla, C. (1996) *Expertise in Nursing Practice. Caring, Clinical Judgement and Ethics*. New York, Springer Publishing.

Campinha-Bacote, J. (1994) Cultural competence in psychiatric mental health nursing. *Nursing Clinics of North America* **29** (1) 1–8.

Campinha-Bacote, J. (2002) Cultural competence in psychiatric nursing: have you asked the right questions? In *The Process of Cultural Competence in the Delivery of Healthcare Services: A Model of Care in Readings and Resources in Transcultural Health Care and Mental Health*, (ed. J. Campinha-Bacote), 13th edn. Available from Transcultural C.A.R.E. Associates at http://www.transculturalcare.net/.

Chen, Y. (2001) Chinese values, health and nursing. *Journal of Advanced Nursing* **36** (2) 270–73.

Cornelius, N. (2002) *Building Workplace Equality*. London, Thompson.

Cross, V., Shah, P., Bativala, R. and Spurgeon, P. (2005) Glaucoma awareness and perceptions of risk among African-Caribbeans in Birmingham, UK. *Diversity in Health and Social Care* **2** (2) 81–90.

Department of Health (2007) *The Work of the Equality and Human Rights Group (EHRG)*. Available at http://www.dh.gov.uk/en/Managingyourorganisation/Equalityandhumanrights/DH_077319.

Department of Health (2008a) *Making the Difference. The Pacesetters Beginner's Guide to Service Improvement for Equality and Diversity in the NHS*. Available at www.dh.gov.uk/en/publications.

Department of Health (2008b) *No Patient Left Behind: How Can We Ensure World Class Primary Care for Black And Minority Ethnic People?* Report of the group chaired by Professor Mayur Lakhani CBE, London, Department of Health.

Echols, J. (1998) Cultural assessment. Chapter 5 in *Health Assessment and Physical Examination*, (ed. M.E.Z. Estes), pp 101–27. New York, Delmar Publishers.

Evers, H., Badger, F., Cameron, E. and Atkin, K. (1988) *Community Care Working Papers*. Birmingham, Department of Social Medicine, University of Birmingham.

Gheradi, S. (1995) *Gender, Symbolism and Organisational Cultures*. London, Sage.

Hamric, A. and Reigle, J. (2005) Ethical decision making. Chapter 11 in *Advanced Practice. An Integrative Approach*, (eds A. Hamric, J. Spross and C. Hanson), pp 379–414. St Louis, Elsevier Saunders.

Helman, C. (2000) *Culture, Health and Illness. An Introduction for Health Professionals*. 4th edn. Oxford, Butterworth Heinemann.

Higginbottom, G. and Mathers, N. (2006) The use of herbal remedies to promote general well being by individuals of African-Caribbean origin in England. *Diversity in Health and Social Care* **3** (2) 99–110.

Hofstede, G. (1994) *Culture and Organisations: Software of the Mind. Intercultural Co-operation and Its Importance for Survival*. London, Harper Collins.

Home Office (1999) *The Stephen Lawrence Inquiry. Report of an Inquiry by Sir William Macpherson of Cluny*. London, The Stationery Office.

Kalisch, P. and Kalisch, B. (1987) *The Changing Image of the Nurse*. Menlo Park, California, Addison-Wesley.

Koetters, T. (1989) Clinical practice and direct patient care. Chapter 5 in *The Clinical Nurse Specialist in Theory and Practice*, (eds A. Hamric and J. Spross), 2nd edn. pp 107–24. Philadelphia, W. B. Saunders.

Leininger, M. (1970) *Nursing and Anthropology: Two Worlds to Blend*. New York, John Wiley & Sons.

Leininger, M. (1978) *Transcultural Nursing: Concepts, Theories and Practices*. New York, John Wiley & Sons.

Leininger, M. (1995) *Transcultural Nursing. Concepts, Theories and Practices*. 2nd edn. New York, McGraw-Hill.

Leininger, M. and McFarland, M. (2002) *Transcultural Nursing: Concepts, Theories, Research and Practice*. 3rd edn. New York, McGraw Hill.

Maruyama, T. (1997) The Japanese pilgrimage: not begun. *International Journal of Palliative Nursing* **3** (4) 203–8.

McGee, P. (1998) *Models of Nursing in Practice. A Pattern for Practical Care*. Cheltenham, Nelson Thornes.

McGee, P. (2000) *Culturally-Sensitive Nursing: A Critique*. Unpublished PhD thesis, University of Central England, Birmingham.

McGee, P., Morris, M., Nugent, B., *et al.* (2008) *Irish Mental Health in Birmingham: What Is Appropriate and Culturally-Competent Primary Care?* Report published by the Centre for Community Mental Health, Birmingham City University. Available at http://www.health.bcu.ac.uk/ccmh/ccmh_publications.htm.

National Association of Health Authorities (NAHA) (1988) *Action Not Words: A Strategy to Improve Health Services for Black and Minority Ethnic Groups*. Birmingham, NAHA.

New Zealand Council of Nursing (2005) *Guidelines for Cultural Safety, the Treaty of Waitangi and Maori Health, Nursing Council of New Zealand.* Available at http://www.nursingcouncil.org.nz

Notter, J. and Hepburn, B. (2003) *Improving the Representation of Black and Minority Ethnic Staff within Ambulance Services.* Report published by the Faculty of Health, Birmingham City University.

Notter, J. and Klem, R. (2001) *Recruitment and Retention in Nursing and PAM of Individuals from Black and Ethnic Minority Communities.* Final report published by the Faculty of Health, Birmingham City University.

Papadopoulos, I. (2006) The Papadopoulos, Tilki and Taylor model of developing cultural competence. Chapter 1 in *Transcultural Health and Social Care. Development of Culturally Competent Practitioners* (ed. I. Papadopoulos), pp 7–24. Edinburgh, Churchill Livingstone.

Papadopoulos, I., Tilki, M. and Lees, S. (2004) Promoting cultural competence in healthcare through a research-based intervention in the UK. *Diversity in Health and Social Care* **1** (2) 107–15.

Papadopoulos, I., Tilki, M. and Taylor, G. (1998) *Transcultural Care: A Guide for Health Care Professionals.* Dinton, Quay Publishers.

Patel, K. (2005) *Coronary Heart Disease in South Asian Populations*, editorial 12. Available at Cardiovascular Diseases Specialist Library at http://stage.library.nhs.uk/Cardiovascular/Page.aspx?pagename = ED12.

Purnell, L. and Paulanka, B. (2003) *Transcultural Health Care. A Culturally-Competent Approach.* 2nd edn. Philadelphia, F A Davis.

Rabiee, F. and Smith, P. (2007) *Being Understood, Being Respected.* Report published by the Centre for Community Mental Health, Birmingham City University. Available at http://www.health.bcu.ac.uk/ccmh/ccmh_publications.htm.

Race for Health (2007) http://www.raceforhealth.org.

Shalhoub, L. (2008) *Nursing a Change in Attitude. Arab News* June 25. Available at http://www.arabnews.com.

Traditional Chinese Medicine Basics (2008) http://www.tcmbasics.com/basics.htm.

Chapter 12

Leadership in Advanced Practice: Challenging Professional Boundaries

Sally Shaw

Introduction

Modern health-care environments are challenging, complex and changing, impacted by both globalisation and health sector reform. Today's health environment is international; issues and trends such as regional trade agreements, workforce diversity, cross boundary migration and growth in information technology and communications go beyond national boundaries. These developments provide both opportunities and pressures for health systems.

Health sector reform has been a global trend as organisations and countries have tried to provide the best possible health care within available resources. Some countries have focused more on restructuring health systems and organisations, whereas others have gone further and implemented major health policy changes. Others are struggling to come to grips with how to implement much-needed changes within traditional bureaucratic structures and mindsets. Globally, health systems are challenged to find acceptable ways of defining priorities in order to achieve equity, quality and efficiency.

Change can bring optimism, uncertainty and anxiety. The need for effective health professional leadership is acute. Leaders must help others make changes in thinking and behaviour while continuing to look for opportunities to offer quality care and excellence in their practice, even when issues such as resourcing seem enormous. They must manage change, be proactive rather than reactive, seek solutions to problems and be continually focused on, and responsive to, the external environment. They work with and through other providers, encouraging and supporting them, advocating for consumers, influencing health policy.

In summary, the importance of leadership in nursing and health care reflects its capacity to influence and create policy and systems that enable excellence in practice in a constantly changing environment and produce effective health-care outcomes. Health professional leaders become advocates for both their colleagues and for the consumers of health care. They lead practice teams. They practice and promote quality care in environments of cost constraint. They are outward looking, able to understand and manage their complex and often changing work environments. They are effective role models, and they support and encourage the development of leadership in others. This chapter is about effective clinical and professional leadership in *advanced practice*, a term that is used to refer to clinical, managerial, educative and other areas of practice. Although the chapter is based primarily on nursing, it is also applicable to other health professionals.

Leadership in advanced practice

Advanced practice often takes place in resource-limited health systems and settings. Despite this challenge, much can be achieved. Effective leaders look beyond their immediate boundaries and work environments. They assess potential impacts on health and the health sector. They are in tune with the socio-political environment and know how to use and influence it effectively. They are aware of positive and negative factors that influence the health sector, and develop appropriate strategies. They seek and maintain networks and partnerships in the broader environment. Through their leadership activities and their understanding of the broader health and politico-economic and social systems, health professional leaders influence both the environment of health care and the professional practice within it. They influence policy and management decisions.

Health has become highly political, closely linked to economic policies and national development. Strategies for change in health systems have been wide-ranging and include decentralisation, performance management, changes in the financing of health care, privatisation and various cost-containment strategies such as rationing and managed care. These strategies have a direct impact on health professionals.

While facing changes that may be threatening for some, leaders must find new ways of doing things in their clinical or leadership practice. They must help colleagues understand the changes and create new practice modalities. They advocate for patients and clients who may experience difficulties in accessing health care. They are required to be innovative and resourceful, and to have courage, confidence and perseverance.

Thus, nurse leaders and others in advanced practice must

- be aware of external influences;
- be able to use the benefits of technology;
- contribute to and influence health and public policy;
- motivate and encourage others to be positive;
- be well informed and strategic in their thinking and action;
- work with and through others to achieve common goals;
- communicate and network effectively;
- assess and develop new opportunities for nursing and health care;
- adapt and develop new roles and skills as health systems change;
- be proactive in implementing necessary training and education changes;
- help develop skills and attitudes that strengthen individual practitioners and professional associations.

These requirements, and the issues they relate to, are often global. To work effectively in national, international or clinical settings, leaders must make a commitment to themselves and to future leaders. They accept challenge and change as realities rather than barriers to practice, and are innovative and proactive in finding ways to work in this environment. They select and support other potential leaders and their development. They are lifelong learners.

Theories and characteristics of leadership

What leadership is not

It is not about position, or charisma, although successful leaders may have both. Holding a position of high status, power and authority does not necessarily make one a leader. Position and status should be less important than the actual leadership itself. Drucker (1992, p. 121) argues that leadership is not a rank or privilege, but responsibility; effective leaders are not afraid of strength in associates and subordinates, but encourage it. Similarly, charisma does not guarantee leadership effectiveness, and can in fact be the undoing of some leaders as it can make them inflexible, convinced of their own infallibility and unable to change Drucker (1992, p. 120). Charisma can however be used positively to motivate people towards a goal or vision shared by both leader and followers. Bethel (1990, p. 38) says that 'some people's missions have transformed them into charismatic leaders because of the depth and passion of their desire to make a difference'.

Leadership can be learned

Are leaders born or made? The research of Posner and Kouzes (1996, p. 3) has shown that leadership is an observable, learnable set of practices. This evidence is the basis for the many action-learning leadership development programmes that have appeared in a number of countries in more recent years. Attributes and behaviours can be developed, and new skills and behaviours can also be developed. Thus leaders can be 'made'.

What is leadership?

Leadership is not easily defined. Norton and Smythe (2005, pp. 9–10) state that 'seeking prescriptive formulas is like trying to pick up mercury with your fingers ... definitions can be confining and restricting ... '. Nevertheless, key elements of leadership can readily be outlined as follows:

- Having vision
- Being strategic
- Having confidence in self, and the ability to inspire confidence in others
- Establishing credibility and trust
- Having excellent communication skills
- Being responsive to and able to initiate change
- Motivating and influencing people towards shared goals
- Taking environmental, or situational, factors into account
- Fostering teamwork, collaboration and partnerships
- Continually challenging and developing self
- Fostering the development of others

So a simple way of describing leadership is that it is having vision, or a clear view of what future state to aim for, and then being able to inspire confidence and motivate others so they share the vision and goals and will work together to try to accomplish them. Leadership is about passion and commitment, and a strong belief in self and the vision or 'cause'. It is hard work. It might mean risk and sacrifice. But it can be immensely rewarding. However, leadership does not exist in a vacuum, and it is more than a list of traits or attributes. Some behaviours are more important in some settings than in others, and leaders must be able to adapt their style and strategies to suit different situations and the needs of different groups of 'followers'.

Theories of leadership

A review of theories of leadership logically leads to a framework of leader, setting and followers that is used in the rest of this chapter. This framework broadly encompasses the environment and the people in it that help shape and influence how a person exercises leadership.

Traits-based theory offers a universal set of ideal qualities, personal traits or behaviours. This theory is now considered too limiting to give a clear and balanced picture of leadership. Indeed, more recent literature warns against leadership models that are primarily trait-based, promoting more dynamic models that integrate *leader, setting,* or *situation,* or *environment* and *followers.* In particular, traits theory was criticised for failing to acknowledge the importance of the situation in which leadership occurs. Ahn *et al.* (2004, p. 112) say that traits-based models can create resistance to change and organisational myopia, and can focus leadership only on the leader at the top.

Situational theory attempts to deal with the need to take account of the *setting* of leadership. It highlights the importance of both the environment and the position held. In this context the leader is the individual who was in a position to initiate change when change was needed. However, *situational* theories do not sufficiently take account of followers.

Transformational leadership theory acknowledges the significant role of *followers* in the concept and practice of leadership. This approach holds that one or more persons engage with others in such a way that leaders and followers continually motivate each other to operate at higher levels. This is an important concept for advanced practice and is central to transformational leadership theory. Two examples illustrate the importance of followers. Research by Kouzes and Posner (1995, p. 67, 1998, p. 318) identified *five* types of key leadership behaviour:

- Challenging the process: searching for opportunities, experimenting, taking sensible risks
- Inspiring a shared vision
- Enabling others to act by fostering collaboration
- Acting as a model and setting shorter goals so the longer-term achievement seems more realistic
- Encouraging the heart, for instance, by celebrating achievements and recognising followers' contributions

Grossman and Valiga (2000, p. 15) also identified *five* recurring elements of leadership from the literature:

- Vision
- Communication skills
- Change
- Stewardship
- Developing and renewing followers

Key elements of leadership

A number of the *key* elements that relate to the person who is the leader, and also take account of the setting and the followers, are now discussed. Note this is not an exclusive list of all leadership elements.

(i) Vision and strategic thinking. Vision is the most important characteristic, regardless of the setting or the leadership style required. Indeed, Drucker (1992, p. 121) states that the effective leader knows that the ultimate task of leadership is to create human energies and human vision. Vision can be a dream that lifts people above their routine, everyday world. It introduces passion into leadership. Vision means having long-term thinking, and not being limited by the immediacy of current situations and events. It requires an ability to keep firmly focused on a long-term goal – even for years at a time. This means having a clear view of the future and potential opportunities, to look ahead, anticipate change and plan for it. A clear vision helps organisations, teams and leaders stay focused and avoid being side-tracked. Having a vision helps to determine the main goals to strive for along the way, and to set the short steps and strategies that will focus people on achieving the goals. Goals are usually shorter term, and allow clear plans to be made and achievable targets set. They help keep people on track, and also enable them to see how their activities fit into the broader picture. The vision should influence the entire constituency: staff, a clinical team, or members of a professional association. Kouzes and Posner (1995, p. 318) argue that leaders inspire a shared vision, meaning that they passionately believe they and others can make a difference. Leaders create an image of the future and help others to see future possibilities.

(ii) External awareness. Assessing how other factors in the environment might influence the vision and the journey towards this is no easy task. Today's health environment is often chaotic, uncertain, unpredictable and changing. Leaders need to take into account political and economic factors, demographic changes, new policies or new laws, health trends and issues, educational levels and other factors. There are a number of tools for developing both awareness and information about the external environment. Some examples are future think tanks, environmental scanning, environmental assessment, SWOT analysis, assessment of what helps and hinders, stakeholder analysis. These tools help provide data, facts, trends, ideas and opinions, on what the future might look like and what the key influences and driving forces might be. The environmental factors might cover a very broad range: economic development, political trends, social factors, trends in health and disease, labour market trends, new developments in information technology and new ideologies. Leaders with external awareness are informed on relevant laws, policies, health priorities and major decisions. They use this knowledge to help guide policies and planning. External awareness provides the context for strategic thinking, and is the key to the 'setting' component of transformational leadership.

(iii) Influence. Influence is the ability to help change the thinking and behaviour of others in order to achieve desired goals. It is the ability to help bring about change, in practice, in attitude, in policy and in law, and to help determine decisions and directions. It can involve the appropriate use of negotiation, authority or persuasion, or it can mean convincing others through well-researched arguments, debates and proposals. Influencing others is by using effective communication, networks and strategies to provide information and motivate others to change their thinking and behaviour.

(iv) Motivation. Motivation involves having and demonstrating commitment and energy to working towards the vision and achieving goals and targets. It means being able to communicate the vision to others and enlist their support. It is being able to take people with you towards key goals by generating in others an enthusiasm, commitment and sense of purpose. It gives followers both the desire and energy to help achieve shared goals. Motivation is having the will to succeed and generating this in others; it is providing the inspiration.

(v) Confidence. Confidence means having confidence in oneself and what one is doing, believing in the vision and making this belief clear and explicit to others. It involves making judgements and decisions in a way that gives other people confidence in their leader and in themselves. Kanter (2005, p. 21) argues that while many leaders have self-confidence, this is not the real secret of leadership. Rather, the more essential ingredient is whether they, the leaders, have confidence in other people and can, therefore, create the conditions in which the people they lead can get the work done. By believing in other people they make it possible for others to believe in them. Confidence is the expectation of success. It connects expectations and performance. It comes from experiencing one's strengths in action, and it grows with repeated experiences of success, because this makes it easier to use similar skills next time (Kanter 2005, p. 22).

(vi) Trust. When people are involved in planning and decisions that affect them, are clear about the strategies to achieve the goals and see these to be appropriate, they will trust the leader. Without trust in the leader, the ability for the leader to motivate others is extremely difficult. Kouzes and Posner (1995, p. 318) argue that mutual respect is what sustains extraordinary efforts, so leaders create an atmosphere of trust and human dignity and strengthen others, making each person feel capable and powerful.

(vii) Political skill. Political skill refers to understanding of and coping with the multiple and often conflicting goals, expectations, values, fears and behaviours of different people, groups and key stakeholders. Political skill involves valuing diversity in the people about you, and understanding the connections between different events and the factors that influence them. It means being able to plan and initiate effective, creative, proactive and appropriate strategies for different situations, using and fostering networks and strategic alliances and involving key people in strategies and decisions. Political skill extends to negotiating effectively, selecting and using the best mix of talent in a team to get things done, thereby empowering others to make decisions and take responsibility for their actions. It is appreciating there are different ways of doing things other than one's own way. It is managing rather than dismissing negative attitudes and people.

(viii) Review, change and renewal of self and others. Organisations, clinical leaders and followers need ongoing review. They must remain in tune with change and respond to new influences and pressures as they emerge. Effective leaders are proactive, initiating changes and new strategies as needed. They are always looking for ways to improve

things. They are creative and innovative, not afraid to try new ideas. This may mean taking risks, but effective leaders know this may be necessary, and if something does not work they accept that as learning, rather than as failure, and seek new or different ways forward. Leaders in situations of rapid or major change recognise the pressures this brings to individuals. They encourage people, celebrate achievements and give recognition to individual or team contributions.

Review and renewal also takes place on an individual level for leaders and others, and includes the following:

- *Mentoring:* encouraging, debating, challenging and pointing the leader/follower in the direction of new ideas, trends and literature
- *Peer review* and *performance-based performance appraisal systems:* to encourage leaders and followers to think broadly and relate their performance to the vision and goals
- *Retreats:* taking time out from the work environment for a few days to reflect on progress, strategies and results; it can be equally beneficial to the team and to individual team members
- *Formal and continuing education:* for the individual renewal of leaders and followers

(ix) Teamwork, partnerships, alliances. Teamwork is a critical part of effective leadership. It integrates the components of leader, setting and followers by using a diverse range of skills and ideas, ensuring effective collaboration with key stakeholders in different settings and environments. It invites participation and communication, and helps focus people on the mission and goals to be achieved. In particular, it helps empower those who might otherwise feel powerless or unimportant to the organisation or to those in authority. Teamwork means learning to work with others to achieve common goals. It is underpinned by a sense of shared destiny. It involves developing people, delegating authority and empowering and enabling others by listening to ideas, encouraging participation, removing barriers and obstacles, giving people the tools to do the job and encouraging and supporting creativity and imagination.

Some leaders find it difficult to encourage teamwork and empower staff. Advanced practice settings are probably not for them. The ability to collaborate, and form partnerships and strategic alliances, is critical to advanced practice. It enables sharing of new information and ideas, and allows different parties to work towards a common goal from a greater position of strength than one person or group alone might have. It requires flexibility in thinking and the ability to work effectively together. It brings different perspectives and skills to the development and implementation of strategies. It helps to share workload where there may not be sufficient resources.

Other important leadership characteristics

Different writers identify and discuss different lists, or emphasise different attributes, or express them in different ways. For example, Bethel's *Qualities That Make You a Leader* (1990, pp. 9–10, 12) talks about being a 'big thinker', having high ethics and using power wisely. She refers to being 'a magnet that attracts others', and talks about commitment as 'the glue to success'. Core competencies provide another way of describing the key skills of the leader. These can be summarised as follows:

- *Conceptual competencies*, such as systems thinking and acclimatisation to chaos
- *Participation competencies*, such as involvement, empowerment and accountability
- *Interpersonal competencies*, such as facilitation and coaching
- *Leadership competencies*, such as relationship dynamics, transformational style and technical expertise (Krueger and Porter-O'Grady 1999, p. 49)

Servant leadership was introduced by Greenleaf (1970). It puts service to the needs of others as the main goal of leadership; it later became a major part of many leadership writings. One example is Bethel (1993), writing about professional associations. She uses this concept in relation to the leadership of the association and its 'servants', promoting the idea of servant leadership as a vital quality for professional association leaders. Servant leadership in this context can be described as a commitment to serving others, for example, the members and the staff and boards of directors. The concept of servant leadership can also be applied to patients or consumers of health care.

Finally, it is important to maintain a sense of balance. The high-stress environment of constant change puts many pressures on a leader and can lead to burn-out. If leaders cannot control stress factors effectively in themselves, it can be more difficult for them to provide a stabilising influence for staff and others. Leaders must learn how to balance personal life and needs with business and professional demands. This recognises the development of the more turbulent environment described earlier, and emphasises the need to be able to cope with stress and conflicting demands.

Generally, more recent leadership literature puts the emphasis on human and personal qualities. Leadership is often viewed in a model, stressing learning, listening, coaching, experimenting and networking with other leaders. The ideas focus on personal attributes such as confidence, ability to earn trust and respect, having good listening skills, giving encouragement, empowering others, leading by example, networking, taking risks and developing others as leaders. Leadership attributes and behaviours, together with a sound knowledge and understanding of leadership theory and practice, will help ensure that the leader is perceived by others to have personal credibility and be successful in their particular setting.

The setting for leadership

The components, attributes and characteristics of leadership vary and are influenced by the settings in which leadership takes place: the type of organisation, the specific work setting such as a hospital unit or primary health-care practice, the political and policy environment, the education environment or an environment of change. Each of these can have a different social climate requiring a different leadership style and behaviour. Cammock (2003, p. 13) suggests that leaders, followers and their shared purposes are only part of the leadership system. He emphasises the fundamental importance of the social climate in bringing leaders and followers together.

To illustrate this point, changing work settings in hospitals influence nursing leadership. Nurse leaders have moved from an emphasis on operations and managing staff to advising and policy roles. These often include a greater focus on professional nursing matters such as setting and monitoring standards, fostering quality care, professional development, legal and ethical matters, developing new roles and models for nursing practice and demonstrating the effectiveness of nursing interventions.

Leaders in decentralised settings have special responsibilities. They must ensure the staff

- *are* and *feel* empowered to make decisions;
- receive appropriate training;
- understand the organisation's vision, so they have a context for decisions;
- know the goals and targets they are expected to achieve;
- know and are driven by the organisation's core values;
- give and receive appropriate information;
- are part of and contribute to performance measurement and monitoring.

The work setting can be influenced by external trends and factors in a number of ways. For example, the economic situation in the country can contribute to cost constraints and outward migration of nurses. This in turn influences conditions of work, staff shortages and difficulties in providing quality care.

The work setting can motivate or demotivate leaders by helping or hindering their activities. The leader can make a difference to the work setting by being aware of potential issues and constraints as well as potential 'helps', and by implementing appropriate strategies taking all environmental factors into account.

The policy environment is particularly relevant to nurse and other health professional leaders. Individually or collectively they can contribute significantly to regional or national health policy through their role or position, for example individually as the focal point for nursing in government or collectively through a professional association. In other instances some move into positions entirely related to the development of health policy. They are often attached to health programme areas in governments, governmental and non-governmental organisations, and in non-governmental organisations, including a variety of voluntary agencies. Because health is expensive, the allocation of resources often becomes a very political decision. Health professional leaders should be involved in influencing health policy and political decisions, such as the allocation of health resources and priorities for spending.

Changing work environments impact on leaders. For example, if leaders are to successfully initiate and manage change, they need to understand the key principles of change management, recognising that the staff are needed to make the change work and must therefore understand the purpose and outcomes to be expected. Change is also highly personal. Leaders must win their followers one by one. Duck (1993, pp. 109–18) says that for changes to occur in any organisation, each individual must think, feel or do something different. For some people change involves human reactions such as pain, anger, fear, uncertainty, and insecurity, while for others it means excitement, challenge and opportunity. The effective leader recognises and 'manages' the human, personal factors, using excellent communication, involving people in change that affects them, listening to concerns as well as to good ideas, supporting and encouraging people and demonstrating a caring and responsible approach. Hesselbein (2004) describes leading change as the great leadership imperative, where the challenges will be exceeded only by opportunities to lead, to innovate, to change lives and to shape the future.

The followers

Leadership involves leaders and followers interacting in particular social contexts (Cammock 2003, p. 27). Probably not enough attention has been given to the role of followers in effective leadership. They have an essential part to play in achieving outcomes in the work or professional setting. Followers need development to give them the confidence necessary to help achieve the desired outcomes. Followers, as well as leaders, can be developed by mentoring and other forms of support. This can help align them to the goals of a project, or specific work setting, or to an organisation's vision and goals. It will help bring people together and focus effort on aspirations and aims held in common.

A transformational leader motivates followers. Followers then become high performers who share the leader's vision and can help transform it into action. This clearly implies an active, dynamic interrelationship between leaders and followers, with each dependent on the other if leadership is to be effective. Thus, followers are an integral part of leadership, and the leader who tries to 'go it alone' is simply not a leader, however humbling it might be to appreciate this. Followers help to support the vision, and by their actions make it possible to achieve it. They work with the leader in a mutually reinforcing role that, together with the setting in which they interact, is what makes leadership work.

Thus an environment needs to be established in which followers can take even small steps and believe that these make a difference. They cannot wait for the big moves made by the leaders at the top, but must believe they are an important part of the system and that their contributions can – and do – make a difference. In this way they build their confidence in the system, in their colleagues and in their leaders.

So if these two roles are closely interrelated, how do we differentiate between them? Grossman and Valiga (2000, p. 52) identify the following:

Leaders	Followers
Study and create new ideas	Test new ideas
Make decisions	Challenge decisions
Assign responsibilities	Accept responsibilities
Create environment of trust	Use freedom responsibly
Take risks	Risk following
Are reliable	Are trustworthy and respectful
Are loyal to followers	Are loyal to the leader
Are self-confident	Know themselves well
Assume leadership	Follow as appropriate

Thus, leaders and followers interact together in mutually reinforcing and supportive roles that position them to create the most effective advanced practice outcomes in different settings.

Leadership styles and their relevance for advanced practice

There are many different work settings in health care and numerous situations arise that need different leadership styles. The term *situational leadership* has been used for almost four decades, and refers to leaders using a style based on their followers' ability to perform as required. Four styles were commonly identified: *directing, coaching, supporting and delegating*. It was argued that as followers (staff; employees) became more effective, the need for a *directive* style decreased along with an increase in *delegation*. This model was applied to business, but is less straightforward with health and other complex modern organisations. More recent literature offers a broader range of models and styles to suit different circumstances. All should be carefully considered for their relevance to, and potential impact on, advanced practice settings. Leaders can be grouped into one of several categories.

Autocratic. Leaders make decisions unilaterally without consulting others. They are more likely to be found in bureaucratic organisations and may utilise close supervision of followers, or give them some space within a prescribed framework to carry out their work.

Permissive. Leaders allow followers to participate in decision-making and usually giving them reasonable autonomy in their work. They are more likely to be found in open, flexible settings that are responsive to changing environments. These leaders encourage staff to develop knowledge and skills to be more innovative and accountable. However, some might use close supervision. A distinction, therefore, needs to be made between the nature of decision-making as unilateral or participative, and the nature and amount of autonomy given to followers, when describing leadership styles as autocratic or permissive.

Democratic. The term is often used to refer to permissive leadership when all employees have an equal voice and vote in the making of a decision. It is usually used either in organisations of professionals (such as health professional associations), or sometimes when there is a particular need to build effective leader–follower relations.

Laissez-faire. Leaders give little or no direction to group/individuals. No one person seems to be in charge. Ideas, opinions and support are offered when asked for, and so the style is or should be used mostly with competent, high functioning teams. This may be seen in some areas of advanced practice.

Change agents. With a particular set of skills, they are brought into some settings or organisations especially to bring about change. They have the strong leadership skills necessary for transforming the organisation. Sometimes they only stay until the change job is done, then move on to a similar challenge elsewhere.

The following six-category model (Coleman *et al.* 2002) incorporates many aspects of the above styles, and is more descriptive than the earlier model of *directing, coaching, supporting* and *delegating*.

Visionary leadership. Inspires followers. It is used when major changes or new directions are needed.

Coaching. Has strong elements of listening, helping and encouraging, and is used to help motivate already competent followers to improve their performance.

Affiliative leaders. Promote harmony and solve conflicts. This is a style used to heal team conflicts and to motivate followers during stressful times.

Democratic leaders. Listen and collaborate, and are used to build support or consensus, or to get input from followers and team members.

The next two categories can have negative impacts on the organisational culture.

Pace-setting leaders. Have a strong urge to succeed personally, and may be low on empathy and collaboration. They tend to micromanage, and strive to get high-quality results from a motivated and competent team.

Commanding leaders. Operate by giving orders, maybe threatening, and exerting tight control. They tend to drive away talent rather than welcoming it. Commanding is referred to as a 'militaristic' style, and can be used in times of grave crisis, or with problem employees, or to start an urgent organisation turnaround (Coleman *et al.* 2002).

For leaders in advanced practice, it is clear that there is no one leadership style to suit all circumstances. Different settings and situations require different leadership styles, characteristics and behaviours. Leaders may need to adjust their styles according to new or changed situations. This emphasises the critical importance of external awareness, so that leaders can assess settings and situations and respond to different needs in the most appropriate and effective ways.

Leaders in advanced practice must be externally aware and internally flexible. Their mindset should not focus on their preferred style of leadership, but on what is going to be the most effective style in any given situation. Leaders create effective work teams based on competent practitioners that are not dependent on receiving orders or directions from the top. They rely on the broad organisational vision and goals to give them the framework for their own leadership and practice. They develop and support people so that they can work more creatively within a framework of clear accountability. Staff at all levels become more performance- and goal-focused, accountable, open in their communication, good team players and able to assume leadership roles.

There are advantages and disadvantages in each leadership style. Clearly, being able to assess the needs of the environment and adapt one's style accordingly help set the leader on the path to success. A democratic style is of little use until the followers are ready for this, while an autocratic style with a competent, innovative team will breed resentment and can lead to diminished performance and loss of talent through resignations. For the setting and the followers, the leader must be clear on potential disadvantages as well as the advantages of each leadership style in the health sector, which can be listed as follows.

Autocratic. There may be times when unilateral decision-making and close supervision of followers is warranted. However, this discourages ideas and innovation in staff and a feeling of being valued. Competent staff are less likely to want to apply to work with this style of leadership. Staff performance and quality of care may be low, and apathy could be a prevailing feature of the organisational climate.

Permissive. The advantages are in shared decision-making and staff autonomy. The style relies on competent practitioners and, therefore, is inappropriate in settings where a high degree of staff development is required first, or where the organisation is still in transition from a highly bureaucratic model to a more modern organisation.

Democratic. This leadership style reinforces for followers that they are valued as important contributors. It brings new ideas to the table for discussion and debate, and helps build strong work teams that are oriented to the organisation's goals. One potential disadvantage is that it can hamper effective decision-making if it relies too heavily on getting consensus in all situations.

Laissez-faire. The key advantage is that it allows high performers to get on with the job without unnecessary interference. The disadvantage is that people may not get feedback on ideas and performance, and may feel the organisation is directionless.

Change agents. Leaders who understand the principles of change management should obviously be more effective in change situations than those who do not. A possible disadvantage is the potential to 'over-manage' some change situations, and to focus mainly on the positive, ignoring or putting aside some of the more negative aspects of change that emerge.

Visionary. This is inspirational and motivational, and a critical part of modern leadership. Its sets the direction and future path for organisations and teams, and is essential in times and environments of change. It focuses performance efforts. There should be no real disadvantages, unless the visionary leader neglects other leadership functions and activities that are necessary to turn the vision into reality, that is to say, the leader is perceived to be all ideas and talk but no action.

Coaching. This is usually focused on individuals or teams who are already competent, or need to develop their competence further. Advantages, therefore, lie in improving followers' performance and motivating them to achieve. There should be no disadvantages for these people, but if used as an all-encompassing style it can be irritating for those who are already high performers and may have their own mentor systems in place. It can also take time from other leadership activities and functions.

Affiliative. The advantage is in healing rifts in a team, or in conflict resolution, especially where these hamper standards of performance. However, as a style it should be regarded as situational, because on an ongoing and team or organisation-wide basis, it can use up time and energy that might be better directed to other leadership matters.

Pace-setting. The advantages lie in the high performance of the organisation and its staff, and its positive external image and credibility. Disadvantages are the possibility of 'burn-out' for both the leader and the followers, resistance by high performers to micro-management and the possibility of taking on more new initiatives than the leaders and followers have the capacity to work on effectively.

Commanding. The main advantage is the ability to deal with a major crisis by making policies, orders and rules explicit. However, it should only be used for a short term as it can create a negative organisational climate and lead to loss of talent from the team or organisation. Performance and outputs become poor; goals and targets are less likely to be met. This is particularly important in modern as opposed to traditional bureaucratic organisations.

In summary, the less successful approaches for advanced practice are the autocratic and commanding styles. Those that can have benefits in particular situations are the pace-setting, laissez-faire and change agent styles. Coaching and affiliative styles have clear benefits for individuals and teams. Visionary, permissive and democratic styles, properly used and modified as appropriate, are the most likely to have a broad positive impact, and be able to be sustained in the longer term.

Sustaining and nurturing leaders

Advanced practitioners need to be supported and nurtured if their leadership skills are to be sustained. To discuss this fully is beyond the scope of this chapter. A brief mention is made later of competencies and credentialing, to encourage the reader to recognise the importance of these to advanced practice and to read more on these topics. Reference is then made to mentoring as a strategy to nurture and sustain effective leaders.

Competencies. Competencies are behavioural descriptions of what effective leaders/practitioners do, and should be regarded as essential to both performance and leadership development. They are observable actions that can be assessed by both the self and others. They articulate the leadership behaviours that can be learned. Identifying and making explicit the competencies of the advanced practitioner helps provide a conceptual framework for practice, regardless of the setting or the degree of change in the environment. Performance review is usually based on established competency statements and can usefully be done as self-appraisal, appraisal by a supervisor or peer review. Competencies are also used as the basis for leadership development and career planning.

Credentialing. Competencies are the foundation of credentialing processes. Advanced practice is often recognised through some form of educational or credentialing process, which gives it legitimacy in the work and professional setting, and with followers. This legitimacy is especially important in rapidly changing health-care systems and environments. Advanced practitioners can be involved in teaching, management, research and policy. Whatever the setting, these nurse leaders interact with their broader environment and with other colleagues and followers. Competencies help identify the leadership knowledge, skills and behaviours that can be applied in any advanced practice setting, regardless of the different roles involved.

Mentoring. Mentoring nurtures and sustains leaders. It is part of both leadership and leadership development. A mentor is a person who agrees to take on protégés, and to teach, guide, sponsor, validate, protect and communicate with them, in order to encourage their professional growth, development and sometimes advancement. It helps develop potential, capability, judgement and wisdom. Grossman and Valiga (2000, p. 199) describe a mentor as a close, trusted and experienced counsellor or guide who is accomplished and experienced and offers advice, teaches, sponsors and guides through significant points in the mentee's career. Counsellors thus provide the following:

- Counsel during times of stress
- Encouragement during risk-taking endeavours
- Intellectual challenge
- Assistance in the development and enhancement of professional skills
- Honest feedback, both positive and negative
- See potential in people that the people may not see themselves

Some kind of mentor relationship is particularly important for top leaders who might otherwise be in rather lonely positions. Effective leaders often have a mentor to help expose their ideas to critical review and debate. Peer relationships are important alternatives to conventional mentors. They have the potential for providing support and sharing mutual concerns, plans and ideas during change, including career change. Such relationships can at times be career-enhancing.

Mentors can take on different roles according to the needs of the followers and the setting, or environment, in which it takes place. Some mentors focus on career counselling, some are coaches who help clarify performance goals and development needs for a specific work setting, and are role models for successful behaviours. Sometimes the mentors are advisors on employment and career progression; sometimes they link the mentee to networking opportunities, or to resources that might help their development. Additionally, a distinction between mentor and coach is sometimes made, with mentor being person-focused and coach being job-focused.

Some of the attributes of effective mentors are as follows:

Credibility in their professional role or work position; respected by others

A wide knowledge base that includes the job functions and expected performance of the mentee

Development skills that include teaching, advising and professional development

Vision, the ability to envision a future for their area of advanced practice

Role modelling of behaviours that others will want to follow, and an ability to encourage others to achieve high standards themselves

The ability to challenge and debate ideas, decisions, skills and strengths of the person being mentored

The ability to let the other person work things out for themselves by not imposing ideas, giving advice too early, or providing answers for the other person to adopt

Interpersonal skills such as being caring, encouraging, empathetic and non-judgemental; the ability to challenge, debate and help others develop a positive self-concept and be motivated to high standards of performance

Personal attributes such as being mature and wise, admired and respected, and considered to be both trustworthy and dependable

Professional competence evidenced by being both qualified and competent in their field, with the necessary experience to contribute to another. The mentor is willing to share personal and professional experiences; has accurate and up-to-date information that can benefit a mentee; remains professionally involved and active in his or her profession; is a person who continues to develop and learn.

Indicators of effective leadership

There are many different ways to categorise indicators of success for leaders. Shaw (2007) uses nine broad categories:

Contribution to health policy (ICN 2005)
Focus on quality
Impact on organisations
Networks, partnerships and strategic alliances
Community development

Ongoing education of self and others
Curricula change
Strengthening National Nurses Associations
Leadership behaviour and 'soul'

Each category has criteria in a check list format to make it easier for monitoring and review.

Conclusion

Health professionals in advanced practice have a particularly challenging role. They must meet and maintain minimum standards or competencies for advanced practice that go far beyond the minimum requirements for initial registration in their professional area. This extended development usually includes both education and practice, and is ongoing throughout the practitioner's professional career. In addition, if a practitioner moves to another area of advanced practice, such as from a clinical area into education and research, new skills and knowledge are usually required. This is in addition to sustaining knowledge and skills in the clinical area being taught.

With the challenges of preparing for advanced practice, and then sustaining it over time, come many opportunities and rewards. There are opportunities for contributing to education and policy development at national and international levels. There are rewards that come with helping nurture and develop others, and to see the results in terms of good outcomes for professional development and effective outcomes for the consumers of health care. When both are evident at the highest levels, we see the results of leadership in advanced practice at its very best.

? Key questions for Chapter 12

In your field of practice:

(1)   Are there styles and characteristics of leadership that you could integrate more into your practice?

(2)   What do you do to sustain your own leadership skills and qualities, and to nurture these in others?

(3)   What are the indicators of effective leadership in your area of advanced practice?

Acknowledgements

Much of the material in this chapter is adapted from Shaw (2007) *Nursing Leadership*. Oxford, Blackwell Publishing. Reproduced with permission from Wiley-Blackwell and the International Council of Nurses.

References

Ahn, M.J., Adamson, J.S. and Dornbusch, D. (2004) From leaders to leadership: managing change, *The Journal of Leadership and Organizational Studies* **10** (4) 112–24.

Bethel, S.M. (1990) *Making a Difference: 12 Qualities That Make You a Leader*. New York, Berkley Books.

Bethel, S.M. (1993) *Beyond Management to Leadership: Designing the 21st Century Association*. Foundation of the American Society of Association Executives.

Cammock, P. (2003) *The Dance of Leadership: The Call for Soul in 21st Century Leadership*. Auckland, Prentice Hall Pearson Education in New Zealand Ltd.

Coleman, D., Boyatzis, R. and McKee, A. (2002) Primal Leadership. *Primal Leadership*. Harvard Business School Press.

Drucker, P. (1992) *Managing for the Future: The 1990s and Beyond*. New York, Truman Talley Books.

Duck, J.D. (1993) Managing Change – the Art of Balancing. *Harvard Business Review* **71** (6) 109–118.

Greenleaf, R. (1970) Servant leader (1991, 2002). *The Robert K. Greenleaf Center for Servant Leadership*, New Jersey, Paulist Press.

Grossman, S.C. and Valiga, T.M. (2000) *The New Leadership Challenge: Creating the Future of Nursing*. Philadelphia, F.A. Davis Company.

Hesselbein, F. (2004) Leadership Imperatives in an Age of Change and Discontinuity. Paper presented at the *New Zealand Institute of Management Conference*, Auckland, October 2004.

ICN (2005) *Health Policy Package*. Geneva, ICN.

Kanter, R.M. (2005) How Leaders Gain (and Lose) Confidence. Interview in *Leader to Leader* **35** 21–7.

Kouzes, J.M. and Posner, B.Z. (1995) *The Leadership Challenge*. San Francisco, Jossey-Bass.

Kouzes, J.M. and Posner, B.Z. (1998) *The Leadership Challenge: How to Get Extraordinary Things Done in Organisations*. 2nd edn, San Francisco, Jossey-Bass.

Krueger, W.C. and Porter-O'Grady, T. (1999) Are your management skills obsolete? *Leading the Revolution in Health Care: Advancing Systems, Igniting Performance*. Gaithersburg, Maryland, Aspen Publishers.

Norton, A. and Smythe, L. (2005) *Not Just Another Book About Leadership*. Pre-publication draft.

Posner, B.Z. and Kouzes, J.M. (1996) Ten lessons for leaders and leadership developers. *Journal of Leadership Studies* **3** (3) 3–10.

Shaw, S. (2007) *Nursing Leadership*. Oxford, Blackwell Publishing.

Chapter 13

Management Issues in Advanced Practice

Paula McGee and Mark Radford

Introduction

The development of advanced practice is indicative of the constant evolution of health services to meet both the changing needs of their patients and the expectations of the society within which they are based. Advanced practitioners must be prepared to cope with the uncertainties that are generated by working at the forefront of their professions. *Professional maturity* is an essential feature of advanced roles: highly developed interpersonal competence and a broad repertoire of theoretical knowledge coupled with technical and clinical skills, honed in a wide range of settings with diverse patients, inform a flexible approach to direct engagement with patients as individuals. Inherent in this flexibility is the ability to focus on the patient's particular situation and select the most appropriate course of action quickly and without error. In a complex, modern health-care system, this can mean that advanced practitioners have to engage in *challenging professional boundaries* by working collaboratively with members of other professions or, if the situation demands, lead them towards new ways of working. It may even require advanced practitioners to *pioneer innovations*, develop new forms of practice based on critical appraisals of patients' needs based on direct engagement in care and a thorough understanding of what is practicable and achievable.

As leaders, advanced practitioners can provide a vision of what is needed in the clinical and professional domains of practice. This will inspire others to work together to achieve it using democratic processes in which power is shared rather than concentrated in one individual (Marriner Tomey 1993, McGee 2005, Hanson and Spross 2005). However, leadership is only one part of effecting change. To become a reality, leadership must be linked with a thorough understanding of the ways in which the organisation functions and why, and the ability to think and act politically (O'Grady 2005). In other words, advanced practitioners must have both leadership and management skills if they are to function effectively.

This chapter addresses a number of managerial issues that influence advanced practice and vice versa. It begins with management of the self. Working as an advanced practitioner can be very rewarding but it is a busy, demanding role that requires good organisational skills; without these the practitioner can easily start to feel overwhelmed by the responsibility and the volume of work. The chapter then goes on to discuss a number of management issues and their relevance to advanced practice. These include targets and standards for service provision, care and treatment and the impact of changes in career pathways. Finally, the chapter addresses the management of advanced practitioner posts, the advanced practitioner as a manager and the importance of evaluating the impact of the advanced role. The chapter closes with some key questions for further discussion.

Managing the self

Good management begins with the self, a view supported by many in the mainstream leadership literature such as Heifetz and Linsky (2002). Appointment as an advanced practitioner is an exciting and challenging step. The new post holder is filled with enthusiasm and determination to make a difference, a sense of idealism linked, quite possibly, to an awareness of being one of a small number of practitioners to reach this level (Woods 1998, 1999). While recent estimates suggest that there are between 3000 and 5000 advanced practitioners in the United Kingdom, these numbers are small compared to the overall size of the health-care workforce (Coombes 2008). The small numbers of advanced practitioners means that health-care organisations may employ only a few and, consequently, newly appointed advanced practitioners may not have a ready-made peer group, at local level, to which to turn for support. In this context, the multiple, and at times competing, expectations of patients, colleagues and managers can seem very daunting. Idealism and a genuine desire to do one's best make it difficult to refuse requests for work, particularly where there is opposition to the advanced role. There is a real danger that the workload will expand exponentially if the post holder feels unable to say *no* or feels uncertain about the boundaries of the job. Such uncertainties will lead to becoming over-stretched, burnt-out and thus ineffective.

To offset these possibilities, advanced practitioners can use the skills of *critical practice* outlined in Chapter 4 to analyse not only what is happening in patient care but also in their own workloads. Simple exercises, as identified in Chapter 9, such as maintaining a time management diary can help clarify how working time is being used and where changes may be required (Box 13.1). The first of these relates to the job

Box 13.1   Example of a time management diary

Activities	0700 to 0730	0730 to 0800	0800 to 0830	0830 to 0900	0900 to 0930	0930 to 1000	1000 to 1030	1030 to 1100	1100 to 1130	1130 to 1200	1200 to 1230	1230 to 1300	1300 to 1330	1330 to 1400	1400 to 1430
E-mails	30 min											10 min			
Phone calls					5 min		5 min								
Paperwork		10 min								10 min					
Wound care/dressings			30 min	30 min					15 min						
Advising staff						10 min									
Meetings													30 min		30 min
Ordering supplies											30 min				
Assessing patients						20 min				15 min					
Breaks							10 min							20 min	
Removing clips						10 min			5 min						

description that sets out the organisation's expectations of the post. Regular meetings with their managers will help new advanced practitioners to clarify their understanding of these expectations and the specific goals to be achieved through job planning as also highlighted in Chapter 9. Such meetings enable managers to keep abreast of advanced posts as they develop in the light of the post holders' experience, the context of the organisation and changes in practice. What this means is that the initial job description continues to evolve over time to meet the continuing needs of the organisation. Managers should be fully informed about clinical and practice developments and ensure that these are in line with organisational plans and insurance arrangements. For example, the terms of collaboration between advanced and medical practitioners, including protocols for scope of practice, referrals and prescribing require careful planning to ensure that responsibilities and lines of accountability are clearly set out (Shay *et al.* 1996).

The second consideration is the extent to which patients, colleagues and managers understand the concept of advanced practice. It is easy to feel frustrated by ignorance and mistake this for opposition. New advanced practitioners should not assume that everyone knows what they do or what they are able to contribute to the organisation. Advanced practitioners should be prepared to spend time in explaining the remit of their posts and how they make a difference to patient care.

The third factor to address is the need to establish a peer group to which the individual advanced practitioner can turn for reference, advice and support. A peer group within the organisation may develop out of collaborative working and the application of interpersonal competence. It may include people at different levels and in diverse occupations, but who are able to act as critical friends, providing a sounding board for new ideas and a trusted arena in which difficulties can be explored. External peer networks may be found in groups associated with a particular clinical speciality or in broader networks formed, for example, by non-medical consultants. These external networks serve a different purpose in enabling advanced practitioners to keep abreast of regional and national developments in their field. They also help contextualise local experiences within the broader picture of what is happening elsewhere.

The final consideration is the need for regular breaks away from work. Planning and taking regular holidays, maintaining interests and a social life outside of work are all essential strategies in avoiding burn-out and enabling the advanced practitioner to work effectively.

Management issues and their implications for advanced practitioners

Health service management is a constant juggling act that requires attention to multiple policies, targets and standards. Historically, nursing played a low-level role as a leader and manager of care, often that of the domestic servant to the sick in a strong patriarchal health-care system (Helmstadter 2008). In the UK National Health Service (NHS), the post-Griffiths management reforms (Griffiths Report 1983) saw an influx of management practices from industry, with nursing at the forefront of those who took up new management positions due in part to their knowledge, team working and wider person skills set, but also because of their previous hierarchical systems or organisational experience (Warren and Harris 1998). White's (1985) analysis of nursing culture argued that health professionals who progressed into management developed a different mindset in order to cope with the many demands on their time and attention. This view was shared by Kalisch and Begeny (2006), who identify that nurse managers remain concerned about the treatment and care of patients although their main focus is on getting through the work required in terms of meeting their targets. Anything not directly connected to these issues carries far less priority.

This section examines some of the current issues of concern to managers and highlights the ways in which advanced practitioners can contribute to managers' agendas. The key theme here is that advanced practitioners need to understand the organisational culture in which managers have to function and present proposals and arguments in ways that are in tune with their concerns. Thus, although the examples used are drawn from the United Kingdom's NHS, the underlying principles will be applicable in other health-care settings.

Current health service priorities

The NHS Plan set out a programme for a radical reform of the UK health service (DH 2000a). It aimed to reduce health inequalities and transform the experiences of service users by improving access to health care and making services more appropriate and responsive to local needs. This plan was further developed in subsequent years as priorities and targets were introduced to ensure that reforms were implemented. The most recent priorities focus on five key areas (Box 13.2): infection prevention and control, widening access to services, improving health, patient and staff satisfaction and large-scale emergencies (DH 2007a). The targets relating to each priority allow for flexibility at local level and can be linked to local plans dealing with specific needs. In addition, all NHS trusts are required to take action on other aspects of services where these fall short of the standards set: equality, mixed sex accommodation, people with learning disabilities, diabetic retinopathy, mental health, disabled children, older adults with dementia and disabled children (DH 2007a). The priorities and targets outlined here are due for completion by the end of 2009. They constitute only one aspect of the overall health service reforms and thus must be viewed alongside complementary developments such as the standards set out in the National Service Frameworks. These standards provide national, long-term strategies for specific areas of care such as coronary heart disease, cancer and diabetes (DH 2000b, 2003a, 2007b). National Service Frameworks provide a means of addressing health inequalities by attempting to ensure that patients receive the best care, irrespective of where they live or any other distinguishing characteristics.

An additional consideration is the recommendations put forward by the NHS review undertaken in 2008 (DH 2008a). This review drew on, but attempted to move beyond, recent health policies. The recommendations placed considerable emphasis on quality as a core feature of every aspect of the health service. Quality begins with 'getting the basics right first time, every time' and incorporates independent quality standards that should be set by the National Institute for Health and Clinical

---

Box 13.2   NHS priorities for 2008–2009

Infection prevention and control addressed the cleanliness of the care environments and the targets to be met in reducing the incidence of methicillin-resistant *Staphylococcus aureus* (MRSA) and *Clostridium difficile*.

Access to services
- Set a target of a maximum of 18 weeks between referral by a general practitioner (GP) and the start of treatment.
- Require GP practices to improve the availability of services in evenings and at weekends and improve response to patient need.

Improving health and reducing health inequalities focused particularly on improvements in cancer and stroke care, child health and maternity services.

Patient and staff satisfaction required organisations to do the following:
- Monitor, measure and demonstrate improvements in patients' experience and satisfaction.
- Demonstrate engagement with the wider public and incorporate their views into local planning.
- Engage with staff to ascertain what is working well and demonstrate improvements in staff satisfaction.

Large-scale emergencies focused on the preparedness of all NHS trusts to cope with major emergencies.

Source: Summarised from Department of Health (2007a) *The NHS in England: The Operating Framework for 2008–9.* London, DH.

Excellence (DH 2008a, p. 11) Quality includes enabling people to stay healthy and empowering them to have greater control of what happens to them. Thus the review recommends piloting personal health budgets and greater attention to personalised care (DH 2008a). These last two ideas are not new. Patient and public involvement in the health service and increasing patient choice have been important features of health service reform for some time but the review goes much further in recommending that patients be given their own budgets. Personal budgets were introduced in 2007 for adults as part of a strategy to improve social care. They allow individuals to decide how they wish to spend the money allocated to them for their care or that of a family member: the services they want to use and the carers they wish to employ (24dash.com 2007). It is as yet too early to comment on the success of this initiative but much depends on the ability and willingness of health service users to become budget holders. While some may find the experience liberating, especially in managing disabilities, others with severe health problems may find that employing people or services directly may be too much to cope with; time will tell.

The priorities, targets and standards outlined here have considerable implications for advanced practitioners and their managers. Managers are responsible for ensuring that reforms are implemented and that standards and targets are met within the appointed timescale and the available budget. NHS trusts have to demonstrate how they plan to achieve targets and standards and show real improvements. Clinical governance departments are responsible for ensuring that services, treatment and care meet what is required and that individual NHS trusts can demonstrate, to the Healthcare Commission, that the best possible outcomes have been achieved. Annual checks focus on key areas such as safety and medicine management. The commission publishes the outcomes of inspections using a 'traffic light' system of colour coding so that areas requiring improvement are easily identified; for example, green indicates excellent but orange means that an aspect of service provision is fair but could be improved (Healthcare Commission 2008 Available at http://www.healthcarecommission.org.uk/homepage.cfm).

The agenda put forward for the health service as a whole determines and dominates managers' priorities and the focus of their activities. Advanced practitioners need to understand this situation, regardless of the setting in which they work. Every health-care system, irrespective of how it is funded, will have targets and standards that have to be met. Consequently, advanced practitioners should familiarise themselves with what is required as well as the particular documents relating to their specific fields of practice, and identify the opportunities they present for demonstrable improvement, innovation or change in practice, service development or organisational systems. The advanced practitioner is able to draw together professional expertise and use collaborative working skills to develop proposals for action that are firmly linked to the priorities, targets and standards that the managers have to achieve. This will mean that proposals are more likely to be regarded positively and will help to demonstrate that the advanced practitioner has a central role to play in this sphere.

Modernising health professionals' careers

The NHS Plan not only addressed patient care and service provision (DH 2000a) but also put forward a proposal to change the working lives of those employed in health-care settings. This proposal was, in part, recognition of the need for new working practices to allow reforms to take place. However, it was also influenced by changes in working time regulations (DH 2007c), which will mean that, by 2009, junior doctors may not work more than 48 hours a week (DH 2007c). This was significant because, while other staff groups had contracts of employment that stipulated the number of hours to be worked each week, junior doctors had no such protection and could work as many as 100 hours at a time (Hooke 2007). Reductions in doctors' hours were, therefore, justifiable but created gaps in service provision that would have to be covered by other staff.

Other professions, notably nursing, took advantage of this situation, seeing it as a chance for professional development that provided greater autonomy in clinical practice through which nursing could reposition itself, within health care, as a better educated, more mature and independent body. Nursing had, for some time, been moving in this direction through the development of advanced practice courses that equipped nurses with increased capacity, capability and flexibility. Nursing did not only succeed in this bid for greater autonomy, it also managed to find a way of retaining experienced and able practitioners in clinical practice. The Modernising Nursing Careers Framework (DH 2006) developed senior clinical career routes that had previously been available only to doctors, and were now possible for nurses as advanced practitioners and consultants; similar opportunities began to develop for members of other health professions (DH 2000a, 2003b). These developments provided space in which medicine could develop a modern career development pathway for junior doctors based on a 2-year training programme followed by more specialised training (DH 2004).

Changes in doctors' hours and subsequent developments in other health professions have created challenges for managers responsible for service delivery. The reductions in the availability of doctors can create shortfalls that affect the quality of treatment and care given to patients. Managers therefore have to find ways of preventing this, for example, by introducing changes in working practices or staffing arrangements. The advanced practitioner is able to play a key role in this situation by managing caseloads autonomously and working across traditional professional and organisational boundaries. The advanced practitioner is also able to act as a consultant for other staff, providing an easily accessible source of knowledge and expertise to which staff can refer. In this context, the advanced practitioner may engage in coaching and guiding staff towards developing their own practice and use well-developed interpersonal skills in providing leadership that ensures high-quality treatment and care for patients (Spross 2005). However, following the election of the Labour Government in 1997, investment of funds into medical schools increased output to over 6000 doctors per annum (Goldacre 1998, Warden 1998). This has left an interesting paradox, in that, despite increased medical numbers, market demands are forcing a rethink on value for money and many hospitals have opted for nurse consultant-led and specialist/advanced nurse-run services where they can (Radford *et al.* 2008).

Patient and public involvement in health care

A key feature of health service reform has been the importance attached to engagement with patients and the public. This is rooted in the concept of personal autonomy, that all adult individuals have the right to make decisions, for themselves, about their own lives. This is particularly pertinent in health care where events may have a profound effect not just on the quality of life but on life itself. Patients, therefore, need to feel that they have been involved in decisions about their treatment and care; that they have had the opportunity to put forward their wishes and be listened to (DH 2004). In particular, patients need to feel that their wishes have been taken into account and that they are able to exercise their autonomy even if this means setting aside professional advice. Unfortunately, a great deal of activity about patient decision-making seems to focus on factors such as choice of hospital rather than later events that may concern patients (DH 2007d). However, this may, in part, be due to patients' uncertainties about exercising their autonomy. Understanding what health professionals are talking about and the plans they put forward for treatment is not easy for people who, in addition to being ill, are worried and unfamiliar with the topics under discussion. Being a patient is to be at a disadvantage in any discussion about treatment options because, inevitably, patients lack knowledge and, perhaps, confidence in asking questions or challenging proposals; a situation that may later give rise to complaints.

Public involvement is not only linked to the concept of autonomy but also, in the United Kingdom, to the idea that the health service belongs to everyone because it is publicly funded. However, public ownership does not automatically mean that the public really understands what the service is or how it functions (DH 2004). Recent health policy has sought to address this issue by encouraging anyone who is interested to participate in Local Involvement Networks, which are intended to provide arenas in which members of the public can learn more about the health service and make their views known directly to managers, commissioners and others responsible for services (DH 2008b).

The managerial responsibilities in patient and public involvement are considerable. The public image of the health-care organisation will affect people's views even before they have to use any of the services. The behaviour and attitudes of staff, patient environments and reports in the media are among the many factors that constitute the front door of the organisation and affect the judgements that patients and the public will make. Managers, therefore, have to ensure that the image of the organisation is balanced. Mistakes can occur, things do go wrong but constant negative publicity and public image is very destructive. One way in which negative publicity can be addressed is by ensuring a quick, effective and transparent response to complaints and setting improvements in place (DH 2008b).

Patient and public involvement creates many opportunities for advanced practitioners. Their involvement in direct care allows them to engage directly with patients and to facilitate their ability to make informed decisions. Coaching and guiding skills are particularly relevant here in enabling patients to make transitions, adapting to changes in their health or development (Hanson and Spross 2005). Transitions can also arise for staff as they adjust to changes in practice or technology and the advanced practitioner has the skills to help them cope with such developments (Elliot 1998, Gee 1998).

Coaching and guiding skills can also be used in the wider public arena through Local Involvement Networks, national and local patient organisations and local interest groups. One area of particular importance is the internet. The organisation's website is part of the front door of the organisation. Advanced practitioners could work with managers to exploit the potential of the website in providing easily accessible information to patients about, for example, common investigative and treatment procedures (McGee 2005). Recent research findings indicate that at least some sections of the population in general would welcome internet-based information about health from sites perceived as trustworthy, that is to say, recommended or provided by the NHS (Flynn and Flynn 2008).

The strategic and business plans

While targets and standards are set nationally, each health-care organisation is responsible for determining how they will be achieved. The organisation's intentions are expressed as a simple strategic vision or statement that sets out the direction of the organisation. An example from a leading NHS Foundation Trust organisation is 'to create a centre of excellence in the provision of healthcare and education' (Heart of England Foundation Trust 2007). Behind such visions are strategic documents sometimes called corporate plans, which set out aims and objectives for a finite period of time, normally about 5 years. These plans provide an overview of the current situation, a vision of the future 5 years ahead and the core values that underpin this. These statements are followed by a consideration of each objective in turn and information about how it will be achieved. Strategic plans are often not large documents but they should give a clear indication of the ways in which the organisation intends to progress.

The business plan sets out in more detail how the strategic plan will be achieved. This may include the policies and procedures needed to guide new working practices, building developments and strategies for meeting specific standards or targets. Business plans should draw on local consultations and reflect 'locally led decisions' and 'a strong emphasis on genuine partnership working between PCTs, local authorities and other partners (public, private and third sector – including social enterprise) to ensure that local health and wellbeing needs are better understood and addressed in partnership' (DH 2007a, p. 6). Thus business plans provide transparency for the organisation; they are not drawn up behind closed doors. Business plans are the basis for further activities that act as a series of checks and balances. For example, income and expenditure forecasts will have a major influence on events as the whole plan can only carried out within the budget available. Similarly, workforce planners will have to determine how many and what type of staff members will be needed to meet the requirements of the business plan which may, in turn, have an effect on how many are actually recruited.

Advanced practitioners must familiarise themselves with – and if possible help develop them as a key stakeholder – the strategic and business plans for their organisation and acquire a sound understanding of the constraints within which the organisation has to operate. Participating in discussions with managers will help both parties to clarify how the plans can be operationalised and enable advanced practitioners to focus on what is realistic and practicable in introducing improvement, innovation and change. Developing some business skills will help them cost initiatives accurately and, where appropriate, demonstrate savings that may be made. Thus managers and advanced practitioners can work together in developing services and patient care.

Managing advanced practice roles

The decision to employ an advanced practitioner depends on the development of a strong and persuasive business case. Presenting such a case requires consideration of a number of factors such as cost, need and benefits. Box 13.3 presents the topic areas that should be addressed in preparing any business case in order to make clear why whatever is proposed is necessary and why it is the preferred solution to the problem identified. An overall model for planning and evaluating advanced practice roles can be found in Chapter 9. In preparing business plans it is important to be aware that quite a number of the people who read them may not be fully aware of all the details associated with a particular service or clinical situation. They may not understand jargon or specialist clinical terminology so it is important to present the plan in plain, easily accessible language. Factual information is very important. For example, consider the next two paragraphs.

> We think that the incidence of head and neck cancers is increasing judging by the number of admissions. We think it will continue to increase over the next ten years.

> The population of the catchment area for this organisation is estimated to be 35,000 according to (source). The incidence of head and neck cancers has increased each year. Figures for the last 5 years are (graph) and projections for the next ten years indicate a rise of 30% (source).

The first is vague and provides no evidence of need whereas the second makes the situation quite clear and draws information from other sources to present a more convincing case, which stands a greater chance of success in trying to persuade an organisation to allow changes to take place.

Box 13.3   Factors to consider in preparing a business case for an advanced practitioner post

What is the background to this proposal? What is the current situation?
What is the problem?
What aspects of the strategic plan will this post help to address?
Are there other benefits?
Is there a clinical need for this particular post or could the work be done by existing staff?
Are there any other alternatives?
What role and functions will this post perform and are these consistent with the Agenda for Change national profile?
What are the proposed lines of accountability and management?
How will the post be monitored?
How will the post be evaluated?
What are the anticipated outcomes?
What are the criteria for success?
What are the costs and are they affordable? Is this value for money?
Is there support for this post, e.g. from the head of the service concerned, the Strategic Health Authority and other stakeholders?
Are there any risks and how will these be addressed?

Source: Summarised from *Nurse Practitioner Advisory Committee – New Zealand (2005) Business Case Tool Kit To Establish the Position of Nurse Practitioner.* Available at http://www.ngangaru.co.nz.

Once the business case has been approved managers are responsible for recruiting and appointing a suitable person, ensuring that the professional qualifications, registration, occupational health and criminal record checks have been carried out. They are also responsible for ensuring that the applicants understand what the job entails by drawing up a job description that clearly defines areas of responsibility and accountability. Once an appointment has been made, managers are responsible for organising a period of induction to the organisation for the new appointee regarding the values, policies and procedures in place. A productive relationship between the advanced practitioner, managers and the corporate/executive team is essential. Each individual in this relationship must have a clear understanding of the contributions made by the others. Thus, managers and executives should be clinically aware and knowledgeable about clinical issues and the advanced practice role; similarly clinicians must understand the perspectives and priorities of managers.

As the post becomes operational, it is managers who are responsible for ensuring that the advanced practitioner develops improvements, innovation and change in line with organisational policies concerning risk as well as clinical effectiveness and quality. Managers can provide guidance and advice about steering new developments through organisational processes and procedures as a way of checking that changes have been planned in sufficient detail and that resources are in place.

Finally, managers are responsible for ensuring that advanced practitioners meet the requirements of their posts, that their performance is satisfactory and that they engage in professional development. Inman and McGee have reported elsewhere in this book about the evaluation of the roles of advanced practitioners (see Chapter 15). Out of a total of 57, just under half of the respondents reported any formal evaluation by their managers. In the majority of cases, this took the form of appraisal or performance review but 17 reported the use of multiple evaluative strategies such as patient survey data, service audits and a reduction in patient waiting times. These findings support earlier work that suggests managers do not always evaluate advanced posts (McGee and Castledine 1999). If this is the case, then urgent action is needed to ensure that advanced posts are meeting organisational expectations and that advanced practitioners continue to develop. However, part of this responsibility lies with the advanced practitioner to help establish an evaluation approach with the management team. Traditional management key performance indicators may not demonstrate the full impact of the role. Instead, audit evaluation and the service capacity of the advanced practice role will be key factors in any evaluation strategy. Another consideration with new roles is that there may be a lack of understanding by managers on how to evaluate such roles, and examples identified in the model in Chapter 9 will be helpful.

The advanced practitioner as manager

Historically, the role of the nurse as a manager has been influenced by organisational structures, culture, behaviours and gender. Advanced practice roles in the United Kingdom are at an important transitionary point in their development. Traditionally they have been managed through nursing structures or by doctors in the same speciality. However, advanced practitioners are also now clinical leaders and managers, often coordinating the workload not just of nursing personnel but also medical staff themselves although often indirectly through managed care systems where they take a leading role as coordinator. There is some controversy as to whether advanced practitioners should have other practitioners reporting directly to them, as it is perceived that it could dilute their role as clinicians, educators or leaders (Humphris 1994). However, within the NHS, there will always be an inevitable crossover of advanced practice roles and management. The development from senior nurses or allied health professionals into advanced practitioners often means bringing along a wealth of managerial capability, that is used, developed or evolves with the role (Snaith and Hardy 2007). There remains limited published literature on the extent of the advanced practitioner as manager, and with increasing pressure on organisations to deliver value for money, the debate is likely to develop over time.

Conclusion

This chapter has highlighted a number of issues about health service management in relation to advanced practice. Advanced practitioners need the support and encouragement of managers; they may also need direction and guidance in meeting organisational targets and standards especially if they are new in post and unfamiliar with local procedures or policies. Advanced practitioners will continue over time and posts will evolve as individual post holders gain confidence and experience. Managers must ensure that the remits of advanced posts are reviewed regularly to ensure that the necessary safeguards are in place to protect both the advanced practitioner and patient care. Good relationships between managers and advanced practitioners are essential; the two roles complement one another as each benefits from learning about the other's priorities and perspectives.

 Key questions for Chapter 13

In your workplace:
(1) What are your manager's priorities?
(2) What improvements, innovations and changes might you, as an advanced practitioner, wish to introduce?
(3) How do these relate to your manager's priorities and the organisation's strategic plan?

References

Coombes, R. (2008) Dr nurse will see you now. *British Medical Journal* **337** a1522.
Department of Health (2000a) *The NHS Plan. A Plan for Investment. A Plan for Reform.* Wetherby, DH.

Department of Health (2000b) *Coronary Heart Disease: National Service Framework for Coronary Heart Disease – Modern Standards and Service Models*. London, DH.

Department of Health (2003a) *National Service Framework for Diabetes: Delivery Strategy*. London, DH.

Department of Health (2003b) *Implementing a Scheme for Allied Health Professionals with Special Interests*. London, DH.

Department of Health (2004) *Patient and Public Involvement in Health: The Evidence for Policy Implementation. A Summary of the Results of the Health in Partnership Research Programme*. London, DH.

Department of Health (2006) *Modernising Nursing Careers*. HMSO, London.

Department of Health (2007a) *The NHS in England: The Operating Framework for 2008–9*. London, DH.

Department of Health (2007b) *The Cancer Reform Strategy*. London, DH.

Department of Health (2007c) *European Working Time Directive*. Available at http://www.dh.gov.uk/en/Managingyourorganisation.

Department of Health (2007d) *Report on the National Patient Choice Survey, England – July 2007*. London, DH.

Department of Health (2008a) *High Quality Care for All. NHS Next Stage Review Final Report*. London, DH.

Department of Health (2008b) *Local Involvement Networks and NHS Complaints Processes Gateway Ref. 9697 Letter*. Available at http://www.dh.gov.uk/en/Publicationsand statistics/Lettersandcirculars.

Elliot, P. (1998) Advanced practice in the care of older people. Chapter 18 in *Advanced and Nursing Specialist Practice*, (eds G. Castledine and P. McGee), pp 207–14. Oxford, Blackwell Science.

Flynn, A. and Flynn, D. (2008) "Give us the Weapon to Argue": eHealth and the Somali Community of Manchester, *Diversity in Health and Social Care* 5 (4) 255–67.

Gee, K. (1998) The roles of consultant and researcher in advanced practice cardiology nursing. Chapter 16 in *Advanced and Nursing Specialist Practice*, (eds G. Castledine and P. McGee), pp 192–98. Oxford, Blackwell Science.

Griffiths Report (1983) *NHS Management Inquiry Report*. London, HMSO.

Goldacre M. (1998) Planning the United Kingdom's medical workforce. *British Medical Journal* **316** 1846–47.

Hanson, C. and Spross, J. (2005) Clinical and professional leadership. Chapter 9 in *Advanced Nursing Practice. An Integrated Approach*, (eds A. Hamric, J. Spross and C. Hanson), 3rd edn. pp 301–29. St Louis, Elsevier Saunders.

Heart of England Foundation Trust (2007) *Summary of the Clinical and Corporate Strategies*, Birmingham, HEFT, unpublished paper.

Heifetz R. and Linsky M. (2002) *Leadership on the Line: Staying Alive Through the Dangers of Leading*. Harvard, Harvard Business School Press.

Helmstadter, C. (2008) Authority and leadership: the evolution of nursing management in 19th century teaching hospitals. *Journal of Nursing Management* **16** 4–13.

Hooke, R. (2007) Junior doctors' hours and pay: a guide for foundation year doctors. *British Journal of Hospital Medicine* **68** (3) M38–M39.

Humphris, D. (1994) *The Clinical Nurse Specialist: Issues in Practice*. Houndsmills, Macmillan.

Kalisch B.J. and Begeny S. (2006) Nurses information-processing patterns: impact on change and innovation. *Nursing Administration Quarterly* **30** 330–39.

McGee, P. (2005) *Principles of Caring*. Cheltenham, Nelson Thornes.

McGee, P. and Castledine, G. (1999) A survey of specialist and advanced nursing practice in the UK. *British Journal of Nursing*, Specialist Nursing Supplement **8** (16) 1074–8. ISSN 0966 0461.

Marriner Tomey, A. (1993) *Transformational Leadership in Nursing*. St Louis, Mosby Yearbook.

Management Issues in Advanced Practice **191**

O'Grady, E. (2005) Advanced practice nursing and health policy. Chapter 15 in *Advanced Practice Nursing. Emphasising Common Roles,* (ed. J. Stanley), 2nd edn. pp 374–94. Philadelphia, F.A. Davis Company.

Radford, M., Denny, E., Williams, C. and Filby, M. (2008) 'Is the doctor still in the house?': a perspective on the contemporary organisation of care in uk acute hospitals. *Paper presented at the British Sociological Association: Medical Sociology Group Annual Scientific Conference,* September 2008, Brighton, UK.

Shay, L., Goldstein, J., Matthews, D., Trail, L. and Edmunds, M. (1996) Guidelines for developing a nursing practitioner practice. *Nurse Practitioner: The American Journal of Primary Health Care* **21** (1) 72–81.

Snaith, B. and Hardy, M. (2007) How to achieve advanced practitioner status: a discussion paper. *Radiography* **13** (2) 142–6.

Spross, J. (2005) Expert coaching and guidance. Chapter 6 in *Advanced Nursing Practice. An Integrative Approach.* pp 187–223. St Louis, Elsevier Saunders.

Warden, J. (1998) Extra 1000 medical school places by 2005. *British Medical Journal* **317** 300a.

Warren, J. and Harris, M. (1998) Extinguishing the lamp: the crisis in nursing. In *Come Back Miss Nightingale Trends in Professions Today,* (ed. D. Anderson), pp 11–35. London, Social Affairs Unit.

White, R. (ed.) (1985) *Political Issues in Nursing: Past, Present and Future.* Vol. 1. Chichester, Wiley.

Woods, L. (1998) Implementing advanced practice: identifying the factors that facilitate and inhibit the process. *Journal of Clinical Nursing* **7** 265–73.

Woods, L. (1999) The contingent nature of advanced practice. *Journal of Advanced Nursing* **30** 121–8.

24dash.com (2007) *Personal Budgets 'to Transform Social Care'.* Published by Webmaster in *Local Government* Monday 10 December 2007.

Chapter 14

The Preparation of Advanced Practitioners

Paula McGee

Introduction

Advanced practitioners are experienced and sophisticated professionals able to fulfil dual roles in direct and indirect aspects of health care. These roles require extensive preparation that equips the individual with the knowledge, skills and expertise needed in health care. This preparation must include practical, clinical experience with patients, in a wide variety of settings that expose the developing advanced practitioner to different client groups within the same field of practice. Such exposure facilitates the development of a broad repertoire based on paradigm cases that provide guidance for action and that are sufficiently varied to allow consideration of different solutions to clinical problems (Benner 1984). Flexibility is an essential ingredient of advanced practice because, while patients may share a medical diagnosis, they each present their symptoms and problems in unique ways.

However, to produce an advanced practitioner, this breadth of practical experience must be complemented by theoretical knowledge and associated skills because, without a theoretical base, practice descends into an incoherent series of tasks and rituals. This chapter considers the nature of this theoretical knowledge and associated skills and how these may best be acquired. The chapter begins with a short discussion on the nature of competence in health care, which is then applied to advanced practice. The chapter then moves on to consider the academic level of preparation required for advanced practice and how this might change in the future.

The concept of competence

The idea of competence underpins all aspects of professional development, at every career level, beginning with professional registration. This registration is, in itself, a statement of competence, made to the public, that suitably prepared individuals have attained a certain standard and are, therefore, considered safe to practise. Further professional education is deemed to enhance that competence and safety. In considering this emphasis placed on competence it is surprising to find many competing views and that there is no single agreed definition of what it means. For example, it may be regarded as the antithesis of incompetence: a make-or-break scenario in which the practitioner can either do something correctly or not (Lillyman 1998). This version of competence can be quite useful in determining whether someone can perform a practical skill such as giving an injection, passing a nasogastric tube or driving a car. Those learning the skill may be assessed against a specific taxonomy that helps to clarify the individual's knowledge as well as practical ability (see, e.g. Steinaker and Bell 1979).

Thus, a second way of thinking about competence is in terms of *stages* or *levels of performance*, a key element of Benner's (1984) theory about nursing. She proposed that the practitioner begins as a novice and progresses through various stages of development to become an expert. In this context, a beginner may be assessed as competent for novice-level practice but incompetent for the higher levels. Both these ideas about competence reflect rather simplistic views of professional practice. The idea that one is either competent or not ignores the complicated realities of dealing with patients. Their physical differences, individual needs, the environment for care and many other factors can all have an effect on how the practitioner performs an episode of care. Thus, a practitioner may be quite capable of performing a catheterisation, but individual anatomical variations in patients may challenge that capability. Moreover, the idea that one is either competent or not affects the ways in which practitioners are assessed. According to this thinking, competent practitioners should be able to perform the procedures and give care, at the same level, regardless of the situation. These one-off assessments may be effective in demonstrating certain types of learned skill but are quite limited when it comes to determining ability in relation to more complex issues. The assumption that the novice practitioner progresses in a linear fashion towards expert practice ignores the ways in which learning style and experiences impact on individual development. There may be times when individuals appear to regress to earlier stages in order to assimilate new learning. For example, in undertaking master's level study, student advanced practitioners may begin their courses feeling that they are experienced, competent professionals. However, as the course progresses, this certainty will be challenged as the students are exposed to new ideas, new ways of approaching clinical matters. This challenge can produce a crisis of confidence in which students begin to question everything that they initially took for granted.

Recognition of this complexity has encouraged a different way of looking at competence, that of critical thinking, the ability to question and analyse events (Brechin 2000). This view of competence is that of a complex web of attributes, knowledge and skills that inform the process of clinical reasoning and decision-making. In this context, competence is more elastic; there are more ways of achieving the desired standard and so practitioners can differ in how they do things but still be regarded as competent. Competence is more of an evolving state based on standards and criteria that anyone who undertakes a particular type of work might reasonably be expected to achieve. These standards and criteria are usually based on some sort of consensus or negotiation and specify what should happen, rather like benchmarking to determine best practice (Coleman and Fox 2003).

Competence as critical thinking has become associated with advanced practice, which requires individuals to possess a 'way of thinking and viewing the world based on clinical knowledge rather than a composition of roles' (Davies and Hughes 1995, p. 156). Thus, competence in advanced practice is about the type of person the individual is, the ability to think, to question and to reason. This view of competence is based in psychology and has been used in management to identify the best person for a job, the one who appears to stand out from the others as able to identify what is important in a situation and challenge weak or ill-founded proposals (Masterson and Mitchell 2003). From an employer's point of view, making use of such abilities makes good sense. In any organisation employees who stand out as having exceptional abilities may find that posts are created specifically for them and cease to exist once they move on (Toffler 1981). This may, in part, explain the development of some early specialist and advanced practice posts. However, if advanced practice is to be established as an accepted part of the health-care service, it will require far more than a few scattered individuals with outstanding or unique abilities.

Education is essential for advanced practice both in preparing practitioners for the role and in enabling them to develop further. This provides another view of competence as a *fusion of practice and academic study* that informs psychological processes and physical performance. The achievement of this type of competence depends on cooperation between various factions and agreement about the type of advanced practitioner they collectively need to produce: educationalists, academic institutions, commissioners, policymakers and service providers (Masterson and Mitchell 2003). Thus, competence is primarily about *fitness for purpose*, that purpose being defined by employers and health-care organisations with reference to the targets they have to achieve and the needs of their client groups.

What all this amounts to is the lack of a clear definition about the nature of competence and, even more importantly, who should formulate that definition. The result appears to be a situation in which everyone's view carries equal merit but no decisions are made. If advanced practice is to become fully accepted as a permanent feature of health care, the various professionals concerned must address three key points. First, each professional must examine the concept of competence in relation to advanced practice in its particular domain and clarify what is required. Second, health-care professionals must collaborate to determine the extent to which the various definitions of competence are profession-specific or common to all. Third, health-care professionals must decide how best to assess competence and how advanced practitioners should be expected to demonstrate their continued fitness to practice.

Competencies for advanced practice

A central feature of the discourse about competence in advanced practice is the issue of what, exactly, the advanced practitioner should be competent in; what the advanced practitioner should be able to do. This section compares a number of different sources about advanced nursing practice in terms of the competencies they propose for advanced practitioners (Manley 1998, Taylor 1998, Busby 2000, The Royal Marsden Hospital NHS Trust 2003, Hamric 2005, The Nursing and Midwifery Council 2005, The Royal College of Nursing 2008, International Council of Nurses 2008) (see Chapter 4 of this book; Table 14.1). These sources were selected for several reasons. There is a considerable body of literature and theoretical ideas about advanced nursing practice; other health professions have not yet generated anything comparable; what there is tends to depend heavily on developments in nursing. Manley (1998), the Royal Marsden Hospital NHS Trust (2003) and Hamric (2005) are quite influential sources used in the preparation of advanced practitioners in the United Kingdom. The Nursing and Midwifery Council (2005) and the Royal College of Nursing (2008) are examples, respectively, of a professional body and a professional organisation; the International Council of Nurses (ICN) is an example of an international professional body. Finally, Taylor (1998), Busby (2000) and McGee (see Chapter 4 of this book) represent the views of individual theorists and provide a balance between sources drawn from the United Kingdom and those from the United States.

All nine sources agree that the advanced practitioner must be equipped to provide expert care directly to patients and that this should form the main focus of the role (Manley 1998, Taylor 1998, Busby 2000, The Royal Marsden Hospital NHS Trust 2003, Hamric 2005, The Nursing and Midwifery Council 2005, The Royal College of Nursing 2008, ICN 2008) (see Chapter 4 of this book; Table 14.1). Direct care encompasses all activities that involve giving care to patients. It may involve sustained and regular contact with a particular patient, intervention to manage a crisis or the provision of specialist expertise (Koetters 1989, Brown 2005). It may also include working with less experienced practitioners, perhaps acting as a model for their performance or overseeing their activities in order to facilitate their development (Koetters 1989, Brown 2005) (Table 14.1). The ICN (2008) sets out three domains of advanced practice, the most extensive of which is care provision and management. Care provision refers to the direct activities involved in the nursing process: assessment, which includes making a diagnosis, planning, implementation and evaluation. Management refers to indirect care activities such as developing resources, participating in planning and 'establishing evidence-based implementation strategies for health promotion and accident prevention' (Koetters 1989, ICN 2008; p. 15). The Nursing and Midwifery Council for the UK (2005) and the Royal College of Nursing in the UK (2008) have also made specific statements about the inclusion of assessment using expert practice, while the Royal Marsden Hospital NHS Trust (2003) emphasises a particular field of care that reflects the hospital's client group. Hamric (2005) and McGee (see Chapter 4 of this book) both argue that expert care is the core feature of advanced practice. Thus, advanced practice is primarily about performance (see Chapter 4 of this book, Table 14.1).

All nine sources also agree that the advanced practitioner should be able to provide professional and clinical leadership (Manley 1998, Taylor 1998, Busby 2000, The

Table 14.1 Competences for advanced practice.

Competence	Manley 1998 United Kingdom	Taylor 1998 United States	Busby 2000 United States	Royal Marsden 2003 United Kingdom	NMC 2005 United Kingdom	Hamric 2005 United States	McGee 2009 United Kingdom	RCN 2008 United Kingdom	ICN 2008
Expert practice	√	√	√	Expertise in chronic illness, even for those in acute and critical care settings	Assessment and management of the patient in health and illness	√	Combined with interpersonal skills	Assessment and management of the patients' illness	√
Leadership	√	√	√	√	√	√	√	√ As part of the professional role	√ And management
Collaboration	√	√	√		√	√	√	√ But as part of other competences	√
Cultural competency		√	√ As part of other competences		√ As part of other competences	√ As part of other competences	√ As part of other competences	√	√ As part of other competences
Teaching and coaching	√	√	√	Role not explicitly stated	√	√	√	√	Role not explicitly stated

Ethical practice	Not explicitly stated	✓	✓	✓	✓	✓	Not explicitly stated	✓
Interpersonal skills	✓	✓	✓		✓ As part of teaching and guiding	✓ As part of professional maturity	Not explicitly stated	✓
Acting as a consultant for others	✓	✓	✓	Implied rather than stated	✓	✓	✓ As part of the professional role	
Research skills			✓ And evidence-based practice	✓	✓	✓	Evidence-based practice	Evidence-based practice
Partnerships	✓				✓			
Evaluation, monitoring and quality issues				✓		✓	✓	
Computer literacy	✓	✓	✓					
Inter professional health care								✓

Contd.

Table 14.1 *Contd.*

Competence	Manley 1998 United Kingdom	Taylor 1998 United States	Busby 2000 United States	Royal Marsden 2003 United Kingdom	NMC 2005 United Kingdom	Hamric 2005 United States	McGee 2009 United Kingdom	RCN 2008 United Kingdom	ICN 2008
Safe environment									✓
Quality issues									✓
Legal practice									✓

Source: Summarised from Busby (2000), Hamric (2005), The International Council of Nurses (2008), Manley (1998), McGee (see Chapter 4 of this book), The Nursing and Midwifery Council (2005), The Royal College of Nursing (2008), The Royal Marsden NHS Trust (2003), Taylor (1998).

Royal Marsden Hospital NHS Trust 2003, Hamric 2005, The Nursing and Midwifery Council 2005, The Royal College of Nursing 2008, ICN 2008) (see Chapter 4 of this book; Table 14.1). Moreover, several are quite clear that this leadership should be transformational in style, inspiring and empowering others (Manley 1998, The Royal Marsden Hospital NHS Trust 2003, Hamric 2005) (see Chapter 4 of this book). Manley (1998), Busby (2000) and Hamric (2005) associate leadership with acting as a change agent. This brings leadership into association with management, delegation of responsibility and supervision (Manley 1998, Taylor 1998, The Nursing and Midwifery Council 2005, ICN 2008, The Royal College of Nursing 2008). In contrast, other sources emphasise a distinction between leadership and other activities (The Royal Marsden Hospital NHS Trust 2003, Hamric 2005) (Table 14.1).

Eight sources reflect current health policy trends, identifying the ability to work collaboratively as a specific competence for advanced practitioners (Manley 1998, Taylor 1998, Busby 2000, Hamric 2005, The Nursing and Midwifery Council 2005, The Royal College of Nursing 2008, ICN 2008) (see Chapter 4 of this book). For Taylor (1998) and McGee (Chapter 4 of this book), collaboration is combined with creativity; the advanced practitioner works collaboratively with others to create new possibilities. For the Nursing and Midwifery Council (2005), collaboration is part of patient assessment and the management of health care. The Royal College of Nursing (2008) places it within the domain of the professional role. The ICN (2008) links collaboration to interprofessional working. In this context the advanced practitioner promotes collaboration through leadership that promotes trust and that is based on an understanding of the work of other, health-related disciplines and the ability to enable patients, families and carers to make their views known (Table 14.1).

Seven sources regard cultural competence as an important aspect of advanced practice (Taylor 1998, Busby 2000, Hamric 2005, The Nursing and Midwifery Council 2005, The Royal College of Nursing 2008, ICN 2008) (see Chapter 4 of this book). The Royal College of Nursing (2008) devotes the most attention to the subject and, like Taylor (1998), addresses it as a separate topic with specific requirements. The remaining sources place cultural competence within other domains such as leadership and direct care (Hamric 2005), challenging professional boundaries (see Chapter 4 of this book) or key principles of care (ICN 2008).

Six sources state that the advanced practitioner should be able to provide education. The terminology varies but the intention is that the provision of teaching, coaching and guiding is primarily aimed at patients, relatives and carers (Hamric 2005, Busby 2000, Manley 1998, The Nursing and Midwifery Council 2005, The Royal College of Nursing 2008, McGee 2008). Only McGee (see Chapter 4 of this book) appears to include the possibility of teaching, coaching and guiding for less experienced colleagues. The ICN (2008, p. 16) does not explicitly address this area of competence but does envisage that the advanced practitioner will be involved in health promotion by working with others to 'formulate strategies and mobilise resources'. The Royal Marsden Hospital NHS Trust (2003) and Taylor (1998) do not explicitly mention education as an aspect of advanced practice (Table 14.1).

Six sources make reference to the importance of the advanced role in promoting ethical aspects of practice (Taylor 1998, Busby 2000, The Royal Marsden Hospital NHS Trust 2003, Hamric 2005, ICN 2008) (see Chapter 4 of this book; Table 14.1).

The ICN (2008), Hamric (2005) and McGee (see Chapter 4 of this book) emphasise the importance of creating an ethical environment for care and stress that the advanced practitioner should be able to engage in and facilitate ethical decision-making in practice. The ICN's (2008) vision extends beyond the immediate work setting towards policy formation, monitoring situations in which patients' dignity may be compromised and ensuring that professional integrity is maintained when encountering marketing strategies for the prescribing of medication. Moreover, advanced practice must take place within the legal framework of the country concerned and so practitioners must be competent in their understanding of the law. Manley (1998) and The Royal College of Nursing (2008) do not explicitly discuss ethics but both make reference to the importance of valuing and respecting others, which may be considered the foundation of ethical practice.

Six sources make reference to the importance of interpersonal skills (Taylor 1998, Manley 1998, The Royal Marsden Hospital NHS Trust 2003, Hamric 2005, ICN 2008) (see Chapter 4 of this book; Table 14.1). However, in each case, these skills are addressed within the context of much larger topics. For example, Hamric (2005) locates interpersonal skills within the overarching competence of teaching and guiding and McGee (see Chapter 4 of this book) regards them as an integral part of expert practice. McGee's views in Chapter 4 are not too dissimilar to those of the Royal College of Nursing (2008), which places interpersonal competence within the nurse–patient relationship and monitoring quality. The Royal Marsden Hospital NHS Trust (2003) relates interpersonal abilities, particularly assertiveness, to providing patient care. The ICN (2008) places interpersonal skills within the overarching competence of care provision and management. Included here is the ability to communicate verbally, in writing and electronically. The advanced practitioner should be able to initiate, develop and end therapeutic relationships (Table 14.1). Manley (1998) and Taylor (1998) regard interpersonal competence as the key to advanced practice in terms of inspiring others, learning to challenge people in respectful ways through giving and receiving constructive feedback (Table 14.1).

Five sources include research skills as an important area of competence for advanced practice (Busby 2000, The Royal Marsden Hospital NHS Trust 2003, Hamric 2005, ICN 2008, McGee) (see Chapter 4 of this book; Table 14.1). These sources tend to emphasise the importance of research skills and the application of findings to practice although McGee (see Chapter 4 of this book), Busby (2000) and Hamric (2005) envisage that some practitioners will engage in more advanced forms of inquiry, conducting research projects or working as part of research teams. Hamric (2005) regards research skills as a separate area of competence but McGee (see Chapter 4 of this book) places them within pioneering innovations. Busby (2000), the ICN (2008) and the Royal College of Nursing (2008) concentrate attention on evidence-based practice as part of other broader areas of competence (Table 14.1).

Five sources state that the advanced practitioner should be able to act as a consultant for others (Manley 1998, Busby 2000, Hamric 2005) (see Chapter 4 of this book). The ICN (2008) and the Royal College of Nursing (2008) also make reference to acting as a consultant as part of the professional role and the Royal Marsden Hospital NHS Trust (2003) implies rather than states that the advanced practitioner will act as a source of expertise for others. Taylor (1998) and the Nursing and Midwifery Council (2005) do not seem to mention the consultant role in the context of being a resource for others (Table 14.1). For the council, consulting is more about advanced practitioners recognising the limits of their own expertise and then seeking help or advice from others.

In addition, certain sources mention other competencies. For instance, Hamric (2005) and Taylor (2008) discuss working in partnership with others (Table 14.1). The Royal College of Nursing (2008), McGee (see Chapter 4 of this book) and Busby (2000) emphasise the importance of monitoring and evaluating developments. Taylor (1998) regards computer literacy as an essential skill for advanced practitioners and the Royal College of Nursing (2003) makes reference to the need to incorporate new technology into care. The ICN (2008) includes several statements about ensuring that the environment for care is safe and emphasises personal, professional and quality development as a major area of competence (Table 14.1).

This comparison demonstrates that agreement on the competencies for advanced practice in nursing is still evolving. There appears to be agreement on several issues although terminology and the degree of emphasis vary: expert practice, leadership, collaboration, teaching and guiding, ethical practice, interpersonal skills and cultural competence. These are generic competencies that apply to advanced nursing practice in any situation and should be complemented by specific statements for each speciality. There is still a great deal of work to be done on clarifying specialist competencies for advanced practitioners as well as under-addressed aspects of care such as computer skills. Moreover, as theoretical ideas about advanced practice develop in other health professions, it is likely that new areas of generic and specialist competence will emerge.

Thus, while advanced practice has many strengths, it is still poorly defined, fragmentary and lacks political support. It is also still not clear where the advanced practitioner fits into the overall schema for health care. There are very real threats such as burn-out, apathy, the cost of insurance premiums and the low status of nursing and some other health professions in many societies. However, advanced practice does offer the opportunity of innovation and the utilisation of knowledge in meeting the rising demands of health care. It also offers women the possibility of a stronger public voice (Schober and Affara 2006).

The educational preparation of advanced practitioners

The ICN (2008) recommends that advanced practitioners should be educated at master's level (Box 14.1). This requirement is not surprising given the demands of the advanced role. The views of advanced practice put forward in this book indicate that practitioners must be able to function at senior levels in an organisation. They must have the professional maturity to cope with the complex demands of patient care, pioneer new developments and challenge professional boundaries. Performance of the advanced role requires practitioners to be able to move beyond degree level study that focuses on learning clinical and technical skills. Practitioners need to be able to think and reason in more sophisticated ways that serve different groups involved in health care: patients, relatives, carers, staff working with patients, managers, chief executives and others at national level.

Master's study provides aspiring advanced practitioners with the tools to build on what they have already learned, especially if their initial study for professional registration was at bachelor's degree level. They are able to identify their individual learning needs and deepen their understanding of clinical, professional and policy

---

Box 14.1   Educational standards for advanced practice courses

(i)   Courses should equip qualified nurses with the competence needed to work safely and autonomously in order to

fulfil the advanced role set out by the council;
provide sufficient practical experience to allow students to develop under supervision;
facilitate lifelong learning.

(ii) Tutorial staff should be appropriately qualified at a level beyond that of the students.

(iii) Courses should be approved by an appropriate national body.

Source: Summarised from International Council of Nurses (2008) *The Scope of Practice, Standards and Competencies of the Advanced Practice Nurse.* Geneva, ICN, p. 21.

---

issues of relevance to their fields of practice. Leadership, teaching and research skills can be developed and incorporated into their clinical portfolios. There is space and time in which to examine ethical, legal and policy issues arising from or having an influence on patient care. Master's level study facilitates access to experts outside the practitioner's workplace. This allows exposure to diverse points of view and the opportunity to discuss issues with prominent thinkers regionally, nationally and internationally. Contact with other advanced students from different disciplines helps to broaden horizons and encourage networking that informs future collaborative working. There are, therefore, considerable benefits in undertaking master's level study as an aspiring advanced practitioner and the status of the qualification obtained is instantly recognisable; thus the advanced practitioner with a master's degree has parity with other senior professionals.

However, preparing advanced practitioners at master's level highlights a number of problems. First, as far as nursing is concerned, it will be many years before all countries are able to meet the ICN's (2008) recommendation. Current evidence indicates considerable variation, sometimes within the same country. For example, preparation to become an advanced nurse practitioner in Taiwan takes about 4 months (Schober and Affara 2006). In Ireland, the National Council for the Professional Development of Nursing and Midwifery requires an advanced practitioner to have a master's degree or higher. The council also stipulates a number of additional criteria about length of practical experience, competence, certification and accreditation (http://www.nursingboard.ie). In Botswana, approximately 70% of the health-care workforce members are nurses and they represent patients' first contact with services at all levels. Nurses voiced their concerns about their lack of preparedness to cope with the responsibilities placed on them and consequently, family nurse practitioner programmes were developed with considerable assistance from nurses in the United States. The University of Botswana provides a course leading to Master in Nursing Science. This was established in 1996 with a US grant and the first students graduated in 1998 (Seitio 2000, The University of Botswana, Faculty of Education can be accessed at http://www.ub.bw/departments/education).

There are concerns that poorer countries may find it difficult to fund and support master's courses (Stark *et al.* 1999). For instance, in Fiji, an advanced practitioner programme was developed in 1998 but the first priority was to enable tutors to gain bachelor's degrees. Very few had undergone postgraduate education and it was not feasible to offer advanced practice courses before the tutorial staff were appropriately prepared (Downes 2007). Nevertheless, there is some evidence of success in that Fijian people living in remote areas welcomed and benefited from advanced nursing skills (Usher and Lindsay 2004). Such findings could no doubt be replicated in other remote and rural areas such as Australia, New Zealand and North America.

Even countries that have well-established postgraduate education systems seem undecided about master's level study. In Britain, the Department of Health (DH) has been consulting the nursing profession and stakeholders about nursing careers (DH 2008) (Figure 14.1). The department currently proposes five pathways to registration and three levels of nurse: associate, registered nurse and senior registered nurse. A senior registered nurse would be an advanced practitioner.

> A set of core competencies could be defined for each pathway and at different levels along that pathway. A number of competencies would be common across all pathways. Nurses who transferred across pathways would carry such competencies with them and an education and development programme could be planned to meet the new competencies required (DH 2008, p. 13).

These proposals will now go forward into the Next Stage Review (DH 2007), which will develop them in ways that ensure 'consistency with other healthcare professions for the benefit of patients and the public' (DH 2008, p. 4).

The regulation of advanced practice is being left to the United Kingdom's Nursing and Midwifery Council, which has consulted on issues such as whether initial nursing should be maintained at diploma level (The Nursing and Midwifery Council 2007). Progress on advanced practice issues varies between slow and non-existent. Although the council proposes to introduce regulation for advanced practitioners, this has not yet been developed and so decisions on master's level of education are unlikely to be taken soon (The Nursing and Midwifery Council 2007).

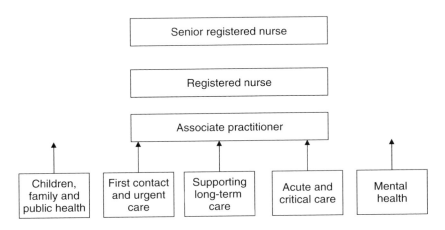

Fig. 14.1   Modernising nursing careers (adapted from DH 2008).

Mandatory master's education for advanced nurse practitioners would, inevitably, raise a number of questions about what should happen to those who lack formal qualifications but who are, nevertheless, fulfilling much-needed roles, especially if they lack the formal entry qualifications required for master's courses. Such concerns will also arise in poorer countries in which postgraduate study is still in its infancy. Where national health-care systems depend heavily on the nursing workforce to provide treatment and care, decisions that might result in a depleted workforce of experienced, capable staff may have far-reaching consequences for the whole country. Moreover, master's level study may raise nurses' expectations in ways that cannot be met. The result may be disillusionment and a possible loss of nursing staff who seek other outlets for their abilities through emigration.

Clinical doctorates

Despite the difficulties, master's level education has been established for nurses in a number of countries either formally or, as in the United Kingdom, by default through university courses. Where this has happened, there is now a growing opinion that continued development and change in practice and services mean that master's level study is no longer enough to meet the demands of the advanced role: 'Master's prepared advanced practice nurses identify additional knowledge that is needed for a higher level of advanced practice' and 'the time spent in Master's level nursing education is not congruent with the degree earned' (American Association of Colleges of Nursing 2004). In other words, curricula are over-crowded by the ever-increasing demands created by developments in practice and health care generally.

This may simply be a case of academic drift; curricula expand to fill the time available and tutors try to incorporate as much as possible to fulfil students' expectations. Once a novelty, master's level study is now far more commonplace and some people will always want a bit extra. About 20 years ago, even bachelor's degrees were rare among nurses in the United Kingdom. Now, a profession that previously had no experience of postgraduate study can count an impressive number of practitioners with master's and research-based degrees.

However, it would be unwise to dismiss out of hand the idea that master's level study is insufficient for advanced practice. Bachelor's and master's degrees are now accepted as essential professional currency and there is no reason able practitioners should not proceed into doctoral study. It is the form of that study which seems to concern those who want to see the level of advanced practice education raised.

Traditional doctoral study is a rather solitary affair. The individual student pursues a research investigation, over several years, under the supervision of senior and experienced academics, within a university. Health professionals who have pursued traditional doctoral study have contributed a great deal to our understanding of patients' and relatives' experiences of health and illness and the impact of treatment and care on people's lives. No doubt they will continue to do so but current ideas focus on the development of a different approach: clinical doctoral study (American Association of Colleges of Nursing 2004).

Clinical doctoral study has a large taught element that allows more time for the study of subjects already present in master's courses and the pursuit of clinical study in more depth (Box 14.2). When master's courses began in the United Kingdom, advanced health assessment was one of the principal components. This is now complemented by modules on formulating a diagnosis, developing treatment plans and prescribing. Clinical doctoral study would allow time for these modules to be more closely related to the students' fields of practice. Specific clinical knowledge and skills, for example, surgical practitioner work, could be included and assessed. This would have the added benefit of ensuring that practitioners who undertake new roles are assessed in a way that allows for national recognition and ensures parity, in standards of performance, between organisations. Expanded clinical knowledge and skill could also be linked more deeply and effectively with an understanding of health policy at national level and global health issues. This would help to broaden students' knowledge of their field beyond regional or even national boundaries.

Box 14.2   Clinical doctoral study

Extended study of physiology, pharmacology and prescribing
More attention to health policy, economics and global health issues
Business studies including financial management and insurance
Increased focus on altered states of health and disease processes
Specialist knowledge and skills
More time to develop expertise in advanced health assessment, formulating a
    diagnosis and treatment plans
Leadership
The health service and organisational processes
Collaborative working
Consultant working
Ethical practice
Legal aspects of practice
Research skills
Teaching and guiding skills
Employment issues such as developing a new role and job description

---

Clinical doctoral study would also allow a greater emphasis on organisational and business management skills. If they are to pioneer innovations and challenge professional boundaries, advanced practitioners need to know how organisations function and the processes through which change can be introduced. In this context, business skills are essential. Advanced practitioners need an understanding of sources of finance, how to develop a budget and how to plan and market innovations. Moreover, business skills would enable advanced practitioners to appreciate the perspectives of finance officers who are remote from service provision and work with them in making decisions that benefit patient care. Business skills might be combined with knowledge of the legal aspects of advanced practice to inform the development of sound business plans for the introduction of new roles. In addition, as advanced practice becomes more established, some practitioners may wish to develop businesses based on their field of expertise. Certain client groups or areas of practice may be particularly suited to this type of development: rehabilitation, continence management, stoma care, breast care and clients with mobility problems (Box 14.2).

Finally, clinical doctoral study would not preclude the conduct of research. There would be space for students to pursue investigations of clinical and professional issues. Thus doctorally prepared advanced practitioners would still be in a position to make contributions to knowledge. However, they would do this from a much broader knowledge base that equipped them to work as senior health professionals in all the indirect aspects of practice as well as expert practitioners in direct patient care (Koetters 1989).

Master's level study, therefore, appears to have some limitations. A comparison of the criteria for this and doctoral study suggests that the expectations placed on advanced practitioners exceed master's level work (Box 14.2). For example, the master's level student is expected to have 'a systematic understanding of knowledge, and a critical awareness of current problems much of which is at, or informed by, the forefront of their academic discipline' but advanced practitioners are required to be experts in their field and must, therefore, possess 'a substantial body of knowledge which is at the forefront of an academic discipline or area of professional practice' (Quality Assurance Agency for Higher Education 2001). Expectations are, therefore, those of doctoral study. Similarly, the master's level student is expected to show 'originality in the application of knowledge, together with a practical understanding of how established techniques of research and enquiry are used to create and interpret knowledge in the discipline' but advanced practitioners are expected to generate new professional knowledge and practice, which would seem to require the ability to 'conceptualise, design and implement a project for the generation of new knowledge, applications or understanding at the forefront of the discipline, and to adjust the project design in the light of unforeseen problems' (Quality Assurance Agency for Higher Education 2001) (Table 14.2). Once again more work is needed to determine whether these expectations are realistic and reflective of the true needs of current and future patient care or a sign of organisational behaviour, which seeks to offload too much responsibility onto individual practitioners.

Conclusion

There is clearly a great deal of work still to be done before there is complete agreement on how advanced practitioners should be educated. International bodies can only recommend what should happen; those responsible for the health service in each country have to make decisions that will best suit the needs of their populations and the size of their budgets. Thus, master's level preparation may not, at present, be practical in some settings; it is, nevertheless, a standard towards which health services are encouraged to develop. In addition, there are concerns that master's level study may not be enough, that it may not provide sufficient preparation for advanced practice. More work is needed to clarify the expectations placed on advanced practitioners and the level at which their educational preparation is best addressed.

Table 14.2   A comparison of master's and doctoral levels of study.

Master's study enables students to develop the following:	Doctoral study enables students to develop the following:
(a) The ability to demonstrate knowledge, understanding and critical thinking and apply these to the examination of a problem (b) A sound understanding of research methods and how to apply these in a research investigation (c) Understanding of how research methods have contributed to knowledge development in a particular field (d) The ability to critically evaluate research methodology and research investigations and propose alternative hypotheses	(a) A contribution to current knowledge, through original research or other advanced scholarship (b) A deep and coherent body of knowledge, which is at the forefront of an academic discipline or area of professional practice (c) The ability to plan and conduct a major investigation that generates new knowledge or examines a novel application of existing knowledge (d) A deep understanding of relevant research methods and the ability to apply these
A master's prepared practitioner should be able to perform the following:	A doctorally prepared practitioner should be able to perform the following:
(a) Collect and process complex information from different sources, make and communicate decisions to professionals and the public (b) Work independently in planning and conducting work (c) Continue to advance knowledge and understanding, and to develop new skills to a high level (d) Develop transferable knowledge and skills	(a) Take responsibility, make appropriate decisions, cope with uncertainty, handle unforeseen events and communicate findings to professionals and the public (b) Contribute to the development of research (c) Demonstrate transferable knowledge and skills

Source: Summarised from The Quality Assurance Agency for Higher Education (2001) *The Framework for Higher Education Qualifications in England, Wales and Northern Ireland - January 2001.* Available at http://www.qaa.ac.uk/academicinfrastructure/fheq/EWNI/default.asp#annex1.

?   **Key questions for Chapter 14**

In your field of practice:
(1) To what extent are the generic competencies, reviewed in this chapter, applicable and why?
(2) What specific competencies would be considered for advanced practice and why?
(3) Is master's level study the most appropriate level of education for advanced practitioners? Give reasons for your argument.

References

American Association of Colleges of Nursing (2004) *AACN Position Statement on the Practice Doctorate in Nursing* October 2004. Available at http://www.aacn.nche.edu/DNP/DNPPositionstatement.htm.

Benner, P. (1984) *From Novice to Expert: Excellence and Power in Clinical Nursing Practice.* Menlo Park, California, Addison Wesley.

Brechin, A. (2000) Introducing critical practice. Chapter 2 in *Critical Practice in Health and Social Care,* (eds A. Brechin, H. Brown and M. Eby). pp 25–47. Buckingham, OUP.

Brown, S.J. (2005) Direct clinical practice. Chapter 5 in *Advanced Nursing Practice. An Integrative Approach,* (eds A. Hamric, J. Spross and C. Hanson), 3rd edn. pp 143–85. St Louis, Elsevier Saunders.

Busby, A. (2000) Diversity: a call for culturally competent practitioners. Chapter 11 in *Advanced Practice Nursing. Changing Roles and Clinical Applications,* (eds J. Hickey, R. Ouimette and S. Venegoni), 2nd edn. pp 252–68. Philadelphia, Lippincott.

Coleman, S. and Fox, J. (2003) Clinical practice benchmarking and advanced practice. Chapter 5 in *Advanced Nursing Practice,* (eds P. McGee and G. Castledine), 2nd edn. pp 47–58. Oxford, Blackwell Publishing.

Davies, B. and Hughes, A. (1995) Clarification of advanced nursing practice: characteristics and competencies. *Clinical Nurse Specialist* **9** (3) 156–60, 166.

Department of Health (2007) *Our NHS Our Future: NHS Next Stage Review – Interim Report,* London, DH. Available at http://www.dh.gov.uk/en/Publicationsand statistics.

Department of Health (2008) *Towards a Framework for Post-registration Nursing Careers. Consultation Response Report,* London, DH. Available at http://www.dh.gov.uk/en/Publicationsandstatistics.

Downes, E. (2007) *Fiji.* ICN/ICP Network Bulletin Issue 7 May. Available at http://www.icn.org.

Hamric, A. (2005) A definition of advanced nursing practice. Chapter 3 in *Advanced Nursing Practice. An Integrative Approach,* (eds A. Hamric, J. Spross and C. Hanson), 3rd edn. pp 85–108. St Louis, Elsevier Saunders.

International Council of Nurses (2008) *The Scope of Practice, Standards and Competencies of the Advanced Practice Nurse.* Geneva, ICN.

Koetters, T. (1989) Clinical practice and direct patient care. Chapter 5 in *The Clinical Nurse Specialist in Theory and Practice,* (eds A. Hamric and J. Spross), 2nd edn. pp 107–24. Philadelphia, W. B. Saunders.

Lillyman, S. (1998) Assessing competence. Chapter 7 in *Advanced and Specialist Nursing Practice,* (eds G. Castledine and P. McGee), pp 119–31. Oxford, Blackwell Publishing.

Manley, K. (1998) A conceptual framework for advanced practice: an action research project operationalising an advanced practitioner/consultant nurse role. Chapter 8 in *Advanced Nursing Practice,* (eds G. Rolfe and P. Fulbrook), pp 118–35. Oxford, Butterworh-Heinemann.

Masterson, A. and Mitchell, L. (2003) Developing competencies for advanced nursing practice. Chapter 4 in *Advanced Nursing Practice,* (eds P. McGee and G. Castledine), 2nd edn. pp 31–46. Oxford, Blackwell Publishing.

Nursing and Midwifery Council (2005) *Implementation of a Framework for the Standard of Post Registration Nursing.* Agendum 27.1C/05/160 December. Available at http://www.nmc-uk.org.

Nursing and Midwifery Council (2007) *Review of Pre-registration Nursing Education.* Available at http://www.nmc-uk.org.

Quality Assurance Agency for Higher Education (2001) *The Framework for Higher Education Qualifications in England, Wales and Northern Ireland.* January 2001. Available at http://www.qaa.ac.uk/academicinfrastructure/fheq/EWNI/default.asp#annex1.

The Royal College of Nursing (2008) *Advanced Nurse Practitioners. An RCN Guide to the Advanced Nurse Practitioner Role, Competencies and Programme Accreditation.* London, RCN.

The Royal Marsden Hospital NHS Trust (2003) *Advanced Nursing Practice. A Consensus Document.* London, The Royal Marsden NHS Trust.

Schober, M. and Affara, F. (2006) *International Council of Nurses: Advanced Nursing Practice.* Oxford, Blackwell.

Seitio, O. (2000) The Family nurse practitioner in botswana: issues and challenges. *Paper presented at the 8th International Nurse Practitioner Conference*, San Diego, California. Available at http://www.icn.org.

Stark, R., Nair, N.V.K. and Omi, S. (1999) Nurse practitioners in developing countries: some ethical considerations. *Nursing Ethics* **6** (4) 273–7.

Steinaker, N. and Bell, M.R. (1979) *The Experiential Taxonomy: A New Approach to Teaching and Learning.* New York, Academic Press.

Taylor, D. (1998) Crystal ball gazing: back to the future. *Advanced Practice Nursing Quarterly* **3** (4) 44–51.

Toffler, A. (1981) *The Third Wave.* London, Pan in association with Collins.

Usher, K. and Lindsay, D. (2004) The nurse practitioner role in Fiji: results of an impact study. *Contemporary Nurse* **16** (1/2). Available at http://www.contemporarynurse.com.

Chapter 15

The Careers of Advanced Practitioners

Chris Inman and Paula McGee

Introduction

Becoming an advanced practitioner is an important and exciting step in a professional career. Experienced practitioners who have worked hard to achieve their qualifications will feel a sense of fulfilment in obtaining an advanced post which, they hope, will bring multiple rewards in terms of better patient care and services, enhanced practitioner status and remuneration. At first, the newly appointed practitioner will be filled with enthusiasm, confident that all difficulties can be overcome. Everything, it seems, will be well. However, gradually, the realities of the situation become apparent (Woods 1999). Perhaps some members of staff are uncooperative or obstructive; the parameters of the post are not as clear as first thought; new directions force a change of direction. Alternatively, it is possible that the newly appointed advanced practitioner becomes more aware of his or her limitations. The opportunities afforded by an advanced practice post can be exhilarating but the accompanying responsibility may seem daunting, especially for those who lack colleagues at a similar level in the organisation. Whatever the reason, exposure to reality has a sobering effect characterised by the recognition that success must involve negotiation with managers, colleagues and others. The advanced practitioner has to learn to fit in with these other roles, establish a credible position in which mutual respect and trust in one another's judgement foster collaborative working. One of the key issues here is the concept of autonomy: who has power and authority to act and in what ways. In health settings, the professional autonomy of nurses and allied health professionals has tended to be viewed comparatively with medicine. In this context doctors are seen as having considerable power and authority, others less so; advanced practice is, therefore, a means of reducing inequality. This is unsound. What really matters is not the autonomy of others but the extent to which the advanced practitioner can act without deferring to a member of another profession (Baer 2003). Inevitably the advanced practitioner comes to realise that the exercise of autonomy involves a constant process of negotiation between the self and others who also claim autonomy within the context of an organisation that ultimately controls what can and may happen.

As the advanced practitioner settles into the role it becomes clear that getting a post is only the beginning. Master's courses may prepare professionals to become advanced practitioners but further development is necessary to sustain and enhance the practitioner's knowledge and skill within constantly changing health-care environments. Thus what seemed at first as the pinnacle of a career becomes a stepping stone in a continuing professional life. How such lives may unfold is the subject of this chapter, which presents the findings of a recent survey of graduates from a Master's in Advanced Practice programme in a UK university. The chapter begins with an explanation of the context of the survey. This is followed by a presentation of the findings in which comparisons are made, where appropriate, with earlier studies by Ball (2006) and McGee and Castledine (1999). The chapter closes with key questions for further discussion.

Context of the survey

McGee and Castledine's (1999) survey showed that advanced practitioners were employed in only 21% of responding NHS Trusts ($n = 283$); of these 11.4% of posts were graded at H and a further 10.3% at G (bands 7–8). Advanced practitioners were employed in 60 different fields with the most common being hospital-based in accident and emergency, night duty, mental health, ophthalmology, paediatrics and orthopaedics. However, it was far from clear whether these posts were truly examples of advanced practice or an organisational response to other factors such as the reduction in the junior doctors' working time or the Allitt inquiry into children's deaths in Grantham and Kesteven Hospital (NHSE 1991, DH 1994). It was also unclear how many post holders had undergone a recognised course of study to become advanced practitioners as opposed to a short, in-house preparation. Regardless of the preparation, trusts expected advanced practitioners to be able to undertake advanced assessment of patients, make referrals, run nurse-led clinics, prescribe, treat minor injuries and alter medication. Advanced practitioners were also expected to teach, promote research-based care, act as a source of advice both within and outside the trust and provide clinical and professional leadership. The perceived advantages of advanced practice centred on the potential for improving patient care and pioneering new ideas but there was limited evidence about whether these advantages were achieved. Very few trusts seemed to have a systematic approach to evaluating the impact of advanced posts and those that attempted to do so relied mostly on patient satisfaction surveys and individual performance reviews (McGee and Castledine 1999).

A more recent postal survey by the Royal College of Nursing for the Nurse Practitioner Association ($n = 1021$) showed that some changes have taken place (Ball 2006). According to the findings, nurse practitioners are now typically women in their mid-forties, two-thirds of whom work in primary care, in posts in which the grading varies from F to H, bands 6–8; the remaining one-third are referred to by Ball (2006) as Nurse Practitioner Specialists and are predominantly employed in secondary care. Practitioners are highly qualified, 35% at master's level and view the core elements of their role as making autonomous decisions, assessing the health needs of patients, undertaking physical examinations, making new or initial diagnoses and making differential diagnoses. Nevertheless, difficulties remain. For example, 44% reported that referrals to other clinicians and for X-rays were refused, especially among those working in general practices. Many, particularly those who worked in hospitals, felt that their jobs were under threat – a situation fuelled by the introduction of the physician's assistant role (Ball 2006).

In the survey reported here, the aim was to investigate what was happening to advanced practitioners with regard to career development with particular reference to the nature of their current roles and employment; their perceptions of their roles; the extent to which their preparation helped them in fulfilling the requirement of their posts and their perceived need for further development. A postal questionnaire was designed, based on McGee and Castledine's (1999) survey tool. Questionnaires were posted to 121 graduates who had completed a part-time, postgraduate diploma or master's degree in advanced nursing or midwifery practice, in a single university between 1997 and 2007. All respondents had achieved the postgraduate diploma and 29 had progressed to the MSc award. Responses were completely anonymous and so no reminders were sent. A 48% response rate was obtained with 57 completed and useable questionnaires and 1 blank returned.

Findings

Employment issues

All respondents gave their job titles. These were grouped into four categories drawn from the data: posts with the title *advanced nurse practitioner*, (13 responses) *nurse practitioner*, (6 responses) *clinical specialist* (12 responses) and *other* (26 responses) which included nine with the title of *consultant*. The majority had been in post for between 2 and 4 years. Three were recent appointees and a further three had been in post for more than 11 years. A total of 49 respondents gave information about the grade of their post. This showed that the majority of posts were at band 7 with a smaller number at band 8. No post was graded lower than band 6. One respondent's post was graded half at band 9 and half at band 8. One post was reported to be graded at G and two at H. Six respondents were in the process of appealing for the grading of their posts to be raised. One respondent was self-employed.

Respondents were based in a wide variety of practice settings – 15 were based in primary care or community settings; 13 worked in hospital wards or departments that included gynaecology, operating theatres, a medical admissions unit, trauma and orthopaedics. Five worked in specialist NHS trusts, one was self-employed, one worked in education and another for a Strategic Health Authority. Twenty respondents had posts that did not fit neatly into any specific category. Of these seven, divided their time between two or more settings and three indicated that their posts had trust-wide remits. The remainder did not give sufficient information. Between them, respondents represented 45 specialities (Table 15.1). The majority

Table 15.1   Respondents' range of specialities.

Acute services included	Services for children included
Acute medicine Acute medicine and infectious diseases Cardiology Medical Colorectal surgery Critical care ENT Fertility Orthopaedic and trauma Perioperative care Respiratory Respiratory/medical oncology Surgical Urology*	Neonates Children's services/child development Clinical education Community children's nursing Paediatrics* Paediatric cardiology Paediatric oncology* Paediatric oncology/haematology
Women's health services included	Primary care/community-based services (non-mental health) included
Gynaecology Maternity services Midwifery/midwifery-led care Acute trust midwifery Midwifery* Obstetrics	General practice* Health promotion primary care Practice nurse School health nursing/public health Urgent primary care
Haematological conditions included	Mental health services included
Haemoglobinopathies Haematology Haemato-oncology	Mental health Mental health services for older adults Child and adolescent mental heath
Cancer and palliative care included	Other included
Oncology Palliative care*	Clinical education Learning disabilities Minor injury and out-of-hours care Older adults

*More than one respondent working in this field.

specialised in hospital-based fields such as acute medicine and colorectal surgery. Paediatric services and women's health represented the next two most common areas of speciality followed by primary/community-based care.

Perceptions of the role and its effects on practice

Respondents were asked to identify which aspects of the role they found most enjoyable. A total of 111 statements were identified. Of these the largest category, 37, concerned involvement in direct patient care or contact and clinical teaching. The remaining statements covered indirect care activities such as developing new ideas, dealing with critical incidents and supporting colleagues. Five statements indicated a general enjoyment of the role, the freedom to work autonomously and the variety of the work (Table 15.2).

Respondents were also asked about those aspects of their work that they least enjoyed. Of 93 statements identified, almost half were about management issues and the politics of trying to provide a service and meet government targets within a context of constant change. Managing staff, beds, violence and aggression, having to attend meetings and plead for whatever was needed all detracted from advanced practitioners' enjoyment of their posts. There was pressure to squeeze more and more out of limited resources. Closely allied to these frustrations were 18 statements about administration, meetings, paperwork and the financial situation in the National Health Service (NHS). Frustrations also arose because organisations did not seem to accommodate the new, advanced role or were reluctant to try new ways of working. Dealing with all of these issues meant that there was less time to do things. In contrast to these indirect care activities, seven statements reflected dissatisfaction with aspects of clinical work – reasons included non-compliance among patients and, according to one respondent, *the effect this role has on the general practitioners (GPs) is negative*. Other comments concerned working conditions and dealing with day-to-day problems at work.

Fifty-five respondents stated that their roles had brought improvements in patient care (Table 15.3). The 150 statements on this topic showed that respondents believed that they were responsible for many improvements particularly with regard to

Table 15.2   The most and least enjoyable aspects of advanced practice roles.

Most enjoyable	Least enjoyable
I love my job. I get to do everything I love. First time in clinical practice, second in education and research	Solving everyone's problems
	Sometimes overwhelming responsibility
Being able to have freedom to develop services I have identified needs change	Unrealistic expectations
	Working in isolation
More autonomy when working with children and families and the positive feedback from providing a better service	Working without peers
	Lack of support from secondary care colleagues
Diversity of my role	
Caring wholeheartedly for my patients	

Table 15.3   Practitioner's role in improving patient care.

Category	No. of statements	Examples
Improvement in patients' experiences	41	Continuity of care as patients move through A&E (Accident and Emergency) to other areas especially when doctors change Increased understanding of the needs of children and young people
Direct care	19	Telephone triage for patients with toxicities of treatment Telephone follow-up for patients 6 years post haemo-oncology
Education	19	Developing training packages for carers, users and professionals
Developing new services/practice	17	Development of a short stay rapid access to diagnostics, treatment and early discharge Developed an integrated care pathway for natural birth
Leadership and management	13	Quicker turnaround – freeing up beds for urgent admissions Representing the service at stakeholder meetings
Standards and quality	9	Part of my role is specifically about improving cancer standards and service improvements
Encouraging others to develop	9	Listening to practitioners and facilitating the changes they come up with
Research and audit	8	Questioning custom and practice and looking for evidence Experience and critical thinking makes me look for different solutions
Multi-disciplinary working	8	Assertive liaison with other professionals
Being a resource for others	6	Providing easily accessible information and advice

patients' experiences of care, through, for example, providing more accessible services, reducing waiting times and cancellations, having more time to spend with patients, providing better continuity of care and a more consistent approach through integrated care pathways. Empowering patients and providing specific help by listening to their concerns were also relevant and contributed to better therapeutic relationships. Respondents saw themselves contributing to improvements through specific, clinical activities, such as nurse-led clinics and patient assessment. Seventeen statements focused on developing new services or practice such as a midwife-led birth centre. None of the responses stated that respondents' roles had not improved care (Tables 15.3 and 15.4).

Table 15.4   Practitioner's role in improving patient care.

Category	No. of statements	Examples
Developing new practice	22	Introduction of new nursing practices that have transferred to other units Involvement in initiative to improve services for Irish led to development of outreach services
Education	20	Have been involved in teaching colleagues about memory clinics and dementia medication Developing the education and clinical competence of nursing staff
Improving patients' experiences	18	Increasing the number of patients able to return home with nursing care Improving the health of those who are able to give up smoking (with my help)
Staff development	14	Encouraging nurses to question practice Providing clinical supervision
Audit/research	13	Analysis of practice and its implications Application of research process to clinical issues
Standard setting and policy issues	9	Setting up robust policies/standard operating procedures Understanding wider impact of services
Advanced health assessment	9	Advanced clinical skills Clinical decision-making
Collaboration with other disciplines	9	Improving relationships with primary care Improved communication between medics and nurses
Leadership	8	Leading multi-professional clinical practice protocols Leading practice developments
Personal/professional attributes	8	Specialist knowledge of the area More accessible than medical staff
Holistic care		

The 144 statements about more general improvements in practice showed that respondents were involved in a broad range of activities providing education for colleagues, other staff, patients, carers and students. Creating an appropriate psychological environment for care in which people felt encouraged, supported and empowered to develop was part of promoting evidence-based practice, challenging outmoded ways of working. Respondents made indirect contributions to care through setting standards, writing care pathways, which suggested that they appreciated the need to consider the issue outside their immediate spheres.

Evaluation of the advanced practice role

Twenty-seven respondents stated that their roles had been formally evaluated by their employers. Responses indicated that employers used a number of strategies (Table 15.5). Seventeen respondents reported the use of multiple evaluative strategies and two respondents had undertaken their own evaluation. One focused on education and the other on service audits. A third stated that an individual appraisal had taken place but felt this did not amount to a full evaluation of the role. Twenty-five respondents stated that their employers had not carried out any evaluation although one stated that they were involved in regionally based learning sets and another, who worked in research, stated that their role was measured by the clinical trial coordinator in terms of the number of patients recruited. Three respondents did not know whether or not their employers had evaluated the role.

Perceived helpfulness of the preparation for the advanced practice role

Respondents stated that all the topics covered in the preparation were helpful (Table 15.6). However, they also identified a number of additional topics that would be helpful in their current roles. Seventeen responses indicated that more teaching about management would be welcomed, especially with regard to financial issues such as writing a bid or managing a budget. Twelve responses stated that nurse prescribing was particularly useful and several respondents had undertaken training about this since completing the MSc course. Ten responses stated that the module on advanced health assessment could be improved by more emphasis on physiology and

Table 15.5 Employers' evaluative strategies.

Patient survey	11	Reduction in treatment costs	3
Performance appraisal	22	Commission for Health Improvement inspection	3
Reduction in admissions to hospital	–	Service audits	4
Reduction in waiting times	10	Benchmarking	9
Reduction in complaints	5	Other – please specify Department of Health Clinical negligence scheme for trusts (CNST) assessment CNST Feedback from organisations in the Strategic Health Authority	

Table 15.6   Topics covered in preparing to become an advanced practitioner.

Topics covered in preparation	Additional topics that respondents felt would be useful
Analysis of advanced practice Advanced health assessment	More physiology and practical assessment (10 responses)
Teaching and guiding Supervised practice Ethics and legal issues Research methods Undertaking a research project and dissertation Health policy Practice facilitator Leadership and management of change	More about management and financial issues (17 responses)
Physiological issues Interprofessional working Critical thinking Decision-making	
	Prescribing (12 responses)
Other individual responses	Other individual responses
Networking with other advanced practitioners Counselling and psychotherapy module Socio-economic module	Diagnostic reasoning More about the political and economic contexts of advanced practice Interpreting laboratory results More about radiology Workforce redesign and development Report writing and writing for publication

practical assessment. Other individual responses provided a range of suggested topics including diagnostic reasoning, the political context of health care and interpreting laboratory results. Only eight respondents expressed the view that the topics covered during preparation had been sufficient (Table 15.6).

One topic that appeared to be particularly important to respondents was advanced health assessment. A total of 51 respondents stated that they had undertaken the module on this topic and provided 112 statements about factors that had enabled them to learn to carry out advanced health assessment (Table 15.7). The first category contained 68 statements about the usefulness of supervised clinical practice in the workplace. This was an important opportunity that gave them time to learn and practise the skills required and the chance to observe others in real situations. All those who undertook this module were assigned to a practice facilitator, usually a doctor, and a mentor in their workplace. The knowledge, support and enthusiasm of both the practice facilitator and the mentor were greatly appreciated. However,

Table 15.7　Benefits of supervised practice.

Category	No. of statements	Examples
Supervised practice	68	Opportunity to observe others Time to be able to practice the new set of skills
Practice facilitators	30	Excellent mentorship from GP Enthusiastic facilitator Being overseen at regular intervals and being told you are doing right
Other staff	5	Discussing the experiences, fears, findings, etc. with registrars – they were much more hep than consultants because they had more recent generalist experience and less specialist
Teaching in the university	24	Detailed anatomy and physiology lectures Instruction about practical skills
Critical thinking	3	Thinking critically and holistically Hands-on practical sessions
Personal issues	10	Increased confidence (3) The support of my peers (2)
Specific aspects of assessment	6	Physical examination Differential diagnosis Systematic assessment skills

the availability of practice facilitators varied. Thirty respondents rated the availability of their practice facilitators as excellent or good, but for the remainder this had not been the case. A similar picture emerged in relation to support from employers with 13 respondents stating that this was either good or excellent and 19 expressing the opposite view.

Career development

Forty-six respondents stated that their careers were developing to their satisfaction; only seven reported that this was not the case. A total of 124 statements concerned factors that had the most positive effects on respondents' careers once they became advanced practitioners. Of these, 31 statements concerned an increase in knowledge, skills or experience as a result of undertaking the course. A further 27 statements were about relationships with colleagues. Respondents reported feeling more respected, having better relationships with medical and other staff and the importance of positive feedback. Three cited their mentors as particularly important. Twenty-six statements concerned employment factors. The support of managers, opportunities for promotion and job satisfaction were all considered positive influences. Twenty-one statements concerned personal qualities with 17 respondents identifying an increase in their confidence as one of the main influences on their careers. Eighteen statements concerned working in practice and reflected feedback from patients, advanced health assessment skills and autonomous practice as important positive influences. The remaining categories contained small numbers of statements about the development of consultant roles, developing a profile outside the employing organisation, teaching and supervising others and leadership.

This picture was balanced by 97 statements about negative influences on respondents' careers. Of these, 11 statements indicated a lack of support from managers and others; one respondent described this as *being kept down instead of having knowledge and skill used*. Another 11 statements were about workload factors especially the unrealistic expectations that respondents felt were placed on them. Ten statements concerned negative attitudes among staff, with particular reference to doctors, although some nurses were also deemed to be at fault. Another ten statements reflected personal factors such as depression, the demands made by the job on personal time and having to change employers. Ten more statements focused on practice and, in particular, the lack of opportunity to practise practical skills. Nine statements concerned financial constraints; six focused on employment factors, particularly the lack of jobs available when respondents graduated. Six other statements reflected a lack of recognition of the advanced role.

Despite this rather mixed set of influences, 43 respondents had completed some form of further professional development, mainly in leadership, prescribing, management and specific clinical issues. Seventeen respondents were currently undertaking a course, four at PhD level. Topics included *midwifery, nursing* and *nurse colposcopy*. Respondents reported that they were undertaking courses for a variety of reasons that included career development and the need for more qualifications. However, no particular pattern emerged from the data.

Consultant practitioners

Ten respondents stated that they were consultant practitioners. Of the remainder, 22 planned to become consultants, 12 had no plans to do so, 11 were unsure and one did not reply. A total of 41 statements were identified regarding factors that, according to respondents, had prevented them from becoming consultants. Fifteen of these statements concerned policy decisions in NHS trusts, some of which had elected not to create consultant posts. These decisions were complemented by a perceived lack of understanding about advanced roles and the financial situation in the health service. Ten statements were about the lack of job opportunities in the areas in which the respondents lived. Six statements reflected a lack of confidence, of respondents not feeling ready to be a consultant – it was a step that required preparation in a wide range of topics including leadership, research, teaching, business planning, prescribing and clinical skills (Table 15.8). Two statements suggested that two respondents were in an ambiguous position of thinking that they were doing the work of nurse consultants but without the formal acknowledgement that this was the case.

Table 15.8 Topics recommended for inclusion in preparation for consultant practice.

Leadership
Research/audit
Research and development
Health assessment
Ethics and law
Health policy
Strategic awareness and influence
Policy development
Updating with the latest technology
Supervised practice
Teaching and coaching
Health economics and policy
Governance
Advanced clinical skills and experience
Presentation skills
Prescribing
Making a differential diagnosis
Management, finance and business skills

Discussion

These findings show first that advanced practitioners continued to be employed in a wide range of specialities. The grading of posts was similar to the findings of Ball (2006) with the majority of respondents in both studies employed at bands 7 or 8. In both studies, the majority of practitioners had been in post for less than 5 years. The range of specialties had altered since McGee and Castledine's (1999) survey and showed considerable increases in posts in the community, mental health and midwifery. However, the specialities continued to reflect medical interests. This finding is consistent with McGee and Castledine's (1999) survey and requires further investigation. It may be that funding for advanced posts has been concentrated in clinical fields that have been subject to considerable change. Advances in technology, changes in medical practice and health policy may have created situations in which advanced roles are more likely to be financed and supported. It may also be the case that these factors have coincided with the presence of practitioners with aspirations towards high-level clinical careers. However, it remains to be seen whether advanced practice must always be co-dependent with medicine. Allied health professions have quite different historical relationships with doctors and may find that these are reflected in their advanced roles. Moreover, certain groups of patients with long-term conditions are now living for longer than was previously thought possible. While their initial survival may be due to technological improvement, their continuing care is dependent on education and regular monitoring, both of which can be provided by an advanced practitioner. In some circumstances, the links between medicine and advanced practice may become quite distant. One example is the patient who has had a cerebro-vascular accident. Medical care will have been instrumental in confirming the diagnosis and providing interventions that help to alleviate symptoms or prevent additional problems. However, recovery will be facilitated by a combination of nursing and allied health therapies with little input from a medical practitioner. Situations like this have the potential to give rise to new forms of advanced practice, which are more independent of medicine.

Second, respondents perceived their roles as having brought about improvements in care largely through direct involvement with patients. This, they reported, enabled them to improve patient experiences, perform care activities such as assessment and develop new services/practice. Teaching also played a part in these improvements as did indirect care activities such as leadership, multi-disciplinary working, research and being a resource. However, such perceptions do not automatically translate into actual changes in health care. There is limited research on the effectiveness of advanced practice although a few studies have explored this issue (see, e.g., Woods 2006). Far more needs to be done to clarify what such expensive and highly-qualified practitioners contribute that could not be done by other, less costly grades. Closely allied to this issue of effectiveness is that of evaluation by managers. Only 27 respondents stated that their roles had been formally evaluated by their employers; of these, two-thirds reported the use of multiple strategies. While this indicates some improvement since McGee and Castledine's (1999) survey, when only a small number of trusts conducted evaluations, it also suggests that it is time for NHS trusts to pay more attention to this issue and develop some clear criteria for assessing the impact of advanced practice.

Third, all respondents had completed a postgraduate diploma and 29 had also completed a master's degree in advanced practice. This finding contrasts with Ball's (2006) nurse practitioners; while all of them had completed a first degree, only 18% had completed master's study. Thus it is necessary to question whether Ball's (2006) respondents can be seen as a match for those in the survey reported here. Teachers with experience working on master's courses will know that students in possession of bachelor's degrees are rarely able to demonstrate 'master's level thinking' (The Nursing and Midwifery Council 2005) in their reflective critical thinking and decision-making skills until they have successfully completed a structured and rigorous master's programme. Thus, it is a matter of concern that, in Ball's (2006) study, some respondents appeared to have been in post for more than 5 years and lacked study at postgraduate level.

Furthermore, a study of 16 consultant practitioners in Scotland revealed a similar picture. Seven had master's degrees and six held postgraduate diplomas (Booth 2006). Thus, as in Ball's (2006) study and the survey reported here, a significant number of respondents did not hold the minimum qualification for advanced practice, that is to say a master's degree. This minimum qualification was suggested by the Department of Health (DH) and is recommended by the International Council of Nurses (ICN) (DH 1999, Schober and Affara 2006). This situation is replicated in the United States, where nurse practitioner roles developed as a consequence of innovations in practice in rural areas, especially in public health nursing and nurse midwifery. Increasing emphasis on primary health care, a shortage of doctors and social changes brought about by the war in Vietnam also contributed to the development of this role. Nurse practitioner courses began in 1965 outside mainstream nurse education as a 4-month certificate course, run jointly by a nurse and a doctor, to produce nurse practitioners for paediatrics (Keeling and Bigbee 2005). Lack of integration with nurse education adversely affected the consistency and academic level of courses for some time. In the last 20 years, courses have become part of nurse education and there has been a marked shift towards master's degree courses for nurse practitioners. However, some certificate courses continue to exist, especially in women's health and neonatal care, where a shortage of nurse practitioners has led to service needs taking precedence over education (Keeling and Bigbee 2005, Woods 1997).

These discrepancies in qualifications highlight the need for professional regulation. In the United States, while the legislation pertaining to advanced practice differs in each state, specific titles such as clinical nurse midwife and nurse practitioner are protected in law; these titles are associated with certain clinical rights. For example, in Alaska, the Board of Nursing recognises nurse practitioners and clinical nurse midwives as advanced practitioners. Such practitioners are allowed to make medical diagnoses, prescribe medication and, in certain circumstances, admit patients to hospital; they can also bill insurance companies for their services (Phillips 2006). In contrast, in the state of Virginia, advanced practitioners are regulated jointly by the Boards of Nursing and Medicine and have to be supervised by a doctor. Nevertheless, they may prescribe, including controlled substances, bill insurance companies and admit patients to hospital (Phillips 2006).

In the United Kingdom, nursing is attempting to lead the way in professional regulation in proposals to open a section of the Register of Nurses in order to ensure professional standards and protect the public (NMC 2006). If the proposals are implemented, it is likely that allied health professions will follow suit. Much depends on decisions relating to the future regulation of medical and non-medical staff and where advanced and nurse practitioners are positioned in the new regulatory framework (DH 2007). Many of these practitioners are carrying out advanced health assessments and prescribing at a similar level to GPs and middle grade doctors, and so will be held accountable at the same level of competence as medical practitioners (Tingle 1998, Dimond 2003). Consequently, it may be necessary to have a system of regulation based on knowledge, skill and level of responsibility as well as membership of a specific professional group.

Updating the regulation of health professionals will include reducing the size of regulatory councils so they become less cumbersome and 'dispersing the perception that councils are overtly sympathetic to the professionals they regulate' (DH 2007, p. 5). In addition a 'General Pharmaceutical Council' is required for pharmacy and the regulation of counsellors and psychotherapists will be addressed. A rigorous and long-lasting system is planned to strengthen the existing clinical governance processes and safeguard patients (DH 2007). Furthermore, the power of the overarching Council for Healthcare Regulatory Excellence will be strengthened, making it more independent in its role of providing expert advice; it will also ensure parity between regulatory councils.

Finally, the majority of respondents had undertaken some form of professional development after graduation. The two most popular subjects were leadership

(17 respondents) and prescribing (14 respondents), which indicates the importance that the respondents and their employers attached to both. Management training followed close behind (12 responses). The emphasis on prescribing is understandable if advanced practitioners are to meet the everyday health-care needs of people by using nursing expertise and referring patients to a doctor only if the need arises (Smith 1995). In such contexts advanced practice must be seen as part of the front-line provision of health services. Prescribing is also appropriate in acute settings in which urgent decisions may have to be made regardless of whether a doctor is present or not. Patient group directions enable suitably prepared practitioners to meet the immediate needs of patients and indeed save lives. However, prescribing carries with it a new set of responsibilities, accountabilities and a requirement for regular updating. As the numbers and types of practitioners qualified to prescribe increase, so too must the professional and organisational regulations that govern standards and ensure individual competence.

The issue of prescribing highlights how much things have changed in 10 years. Advanced practitioners are now prepared to openly take on responsibility for a full episode of patient care in terms of assessment, diagnosis and treatment. The findings presented here indicate that while some are happy to do so, others lack confidence, suggesting a need for some sort of ongoing support. It is clearly important to look beyond graduation and the first few years of practice towards further career development. Being an advanced practitioner is a satisfying role centred around patient care. The problem is that there is no model for this type of high-level practitioner. The rhetoric of health policy emphasises the need for clinical careers, to retain competent and experienced professionals in practice settings but it has given little thought to what to do with them once they have arrived. Logic dictates that an experienced advanced practitioner will need professional development, not only to meet patients' needs but also to ensure that today's bright pioneer does not become a faded star left over from the past. Advanced practitioners will have to ensure that they use their collective power to retain and develop their roles. In this context, Ball's (2006) findings raise a matter of concern. The majority of her respondents were women. In the survey reported here, information about gender was not requested but the course concerned routinely recruits far more women than men. Further investigation is needed to establish whether, nationally, advanced practice is attracting significantly more women than men and why. If men are not attracted to advanced practice, if they prefer the more traditional career options of management or teaching, there has to be a reason which may, in the long term, have an impact on the status and future of advanced practice itself.

It is instructive to look at what is happening in the United States with regard to the long-term development of advanced practice. In 2007 many states enacted legislation that has removed barriers to advanced practice but progress has not been uniform. Two states, Alabama and Florida, have introduced new laws to restrict practice. For instance, in Alabama, there is new legislation governing the collaborating doctor's principal and remote practice sites. According to Phillips (2007, p. 16), such legislation reflects new efforts on the part of the American Medical Association 'to restrict the practice of physicians who collaborate with or supervise APRNs'. Phillips (2006) previously reported a move towards national certification but there is no evidence in her latest report that this has been sustained (Phillips 2007). If the United Kingdom is to avoid repeating the US experience, advanced practitioners must learn to collectively negotiate a position, within the health-care system, in which their roles are seen to tessellate with those of colleagues. In this way they will become an essential part of the health service and be able to develop their careers accordingly.

Conclusion

This chapter has shown that advanced practice continues to be an evolving concept in the United Kingdom. The lack of formal regulation in nursing has led to piecemeal development in terms of the preparation of practitioners, their employment, work roles and long-term career prospects. There is no doubt that many enjoy the freedom and opportunities afforded by advanced roles and believe that they are making a positive impact on patient care and service provision. This may well be the case but employers and professional bodies need to do far more in evaluating the impact of such roles, setting standards and generally establishing a more uniform approach to advanced practice. There is an urgent need to address the long-term future for those who become advanced practitioners so that they are empowered to continue as professional and clinical leaders, as role models for those who wish to develop clinical careers.

 Key questions for Chapter 15

In your field of practice:
(1) What contribution might an advanced practitioner make to patient care and service provision and why?
(2) How might the effectiveness of that contribution be evaluated and why?
(3) How might advanced roles develop in the long term and why?

References

Baer, E. (2003) Philosophical and historical bases of advanced practice nursing roles. Chapter 2 in *Nurse Practitioners. Evolution of Advanced Practice*, (eds M. Mezey, D. McGivern and E. Sullivan-Marz), 4th edn. pp 37–53. New York, Springer Publishing Company.

Ball, J. (2006) *Nurse Practitioners 2006. The Results of a Survey of Nurse Practitioners Conducted on Behalf of the RCN Nurse Practitioner Association*. Hove, Employment Research Ltd.

Booth, J. (2006) New nursing roles: the experience of Scotland's consultant nurse/midwives. *Journal of Nursing Managements* **14** (2) 83–9.

Department of Health (1994) *The Allitt Inquiry: Independent Inquiry Relating to Deaths and Injuries on the Children's Ward at Grantham and Kesteven General Hospital During the Period February to April 1991*. London, The Stationery Office.

Department of Health (1999) *Making a Difference. Strengthening the Nursing, Midwifery and Health Visiting Contribution to Health and Healthcare*. London, DH.

Department of Health (2007) *Trust, Assurance and Safety – The Regulation of Health Professionals in the 21st Century*. Norwich, HMSO.

Dimond, B. (2003) Legal and ethical issues in advanced practice. Chapter 15 in *Advanced Practice*, (eds P. McGee and G. Castledine), 2nd edn. pp 184–99. Oxford, Blackwell Science.

Keeling, A. and Bigbee, J. (2005) The history of advanced practice nursing in the United States. Chapter 1 in *Advanced Practice Nursing, An Integrative Approach*, (eds A. Hamric, J. Spross and C. Hanson). St Louis, Elsevier, Saunders.

McGee, P. and Castledine, G. (1999) A survey of specialist and advanced nursing practice in the UK. *British Journal of Nursing* **8** (16) 1074–8.

National Health Service Management Executive (1991) *Junior Doctors: The New Deal*. London, NHSME.

Nursing and Midwifery Council (2005) *Implementation of a Framework for the Standard of Post Registration Nursing*. Agendum 27.1C/05/160 December. Available at http://www.nmc-uk.org.

Nursing and Midwifery Council (2006) *Advanced Nursing Practice*. Update 4 July. Available at http://www.nmc-uk.org.

Phillips, S.J. (2006) Eighteenth annual update. A comprehensive look at the legislative issues affecting advanced nursing practice. *The Nurse Practitioner* **31** (1) 6–8, 11–7, 21–8, 31, 34–8.

Phillips, S.J. (2007) Nineteenth annual update. *The Nurse Practitioner* **32** (1) 14–7, 19–20, 22, 24–5, 27–40, 32–42.

Schober, M. and Affara, F. (2006) *International Council of Nurses. Advanced Nursing Practice*. Oxford, Blackwell Science.

Smith, M. (1995) The core of advanced nursing practice. *Nursing Science Quarterly* **8** (1) 2–3.

Tingle, J. (1998) Legal issues for advanced and specialist nurse practitioners. Chapter 4 in *Advanced and Specialist Nursing Practice*, (eds G. Castledine and P. McGee), pp 71–86. Oxford, Blackwell Science.

Woods, L. (1999) The contingent nature of advanced practice. *Journal of Advanced Nursing* **30** 121–8.

Woods, L. (2006) Evaluating the clinical effectiveness of neonatal nurse practitioners: an exploratory study. *Journal of Clinical Nursing* **15** (1) 35–44.

Chapter 16

An International Perspective of Advanced Nursing Practice

Madrean Schober

Introduction

Advanced nursing practice and the exploration of advanced practice nursing roles have become a global phenomenon. This rapidly emerging field is one of the most dynamic and exciting developments in nursing at present, capturing not only the attention of nurses and other health-care professionals but also key decision-makers and health-care planners. Issues of importance to new initiatives, which include the integration of innovative models of practice, and health-care workforce skills mix have increased the visibility and highlighted the importance of nursing's contribution to health-care provision worldwide.

This chapter aims to identify factors contributing to global attention in relation to advanced clinical nursing roles, to give details on the extent of interest in this development and to emphasise the role international organisations play as new schemes are introduced and progress. In addition, this chapter provides the International Council of Nursing's definition for advanced nursing practice, contrast examples of national definitions and give an account of progress towards international guidelines for use when defining scope of practice, standards and competencies. Finally, this chapter comments on issues arising in interaction with health professionals when introducing advanced roles concluding with speculation for future directions and challenges for advanced nursing practice. Country and regional illustrations are used to draw attention to the realities of promoting and implementing new nursing roles in various settings.

Factors contributing to the emergence of advanced nursing practice globally

Technological advances, the increasing complexities of providing health care, modifications in delivery of services and changing needs have drawn attention to conditions that require investigation into expanded health-care options for the world's populations. Nurses with advanced knowledge and skills provide possibilities for enhancing these choices. Current circumstances have highlighted the integral position nursing holds in the delivery of health-care services while promoting possibilities for groundbreaking developments. Discussions of nurse-led clinics, autonomous practice for nurses, advanced clinical nursing specialists as part of teams in hospitals and advanced practitioners in Primary Health Care (PHC) delivery are becoming increasingly common (Box 16.1).

Box 16.1   Reasons given for heightened global awareness

- Need for improved access to health-care services, especially in the community
- Continued technological developments requiring advanced knowledge for nurses and other health-care professionals
- Primary health care initiatives promoted by international organisations such as the World Health Organization (WHO), which highlight nursing roles
- Increasing needs to address rapidly escalating disease worldwide
- Growing requests for home care
- Increased rate of specialisation in nursing
- Advancement of the profession in general

Source: Summarised from Schober and Affara (2006).

Shaping and attaining the suitable mix of human resources and appropriate personnel is challenging health-care organisations and systems worldwide. There is an indication of unrealised possibilities in relation to the scope of practice and presence of nursing in the health-care workforce (Buchan and Dal Poz 2002). Research and anecdotal reports demonstrate the effectiveness and feasibility of integrating advanced roles into a variety of primary, secondary and tertiary health-care settings (World Health Organization 2002, Buchan and Calman 2004, Gardner *et al*. 2004, Schober and Affara 2006). Expansion of nursing responsibilities has the potential for improving accessibility to health-care services in addition to advancing quality of care for individuals, their families and the communities they live in.

Extent of international presence

The introduction of advanced nursing practice has been attributed to the successful presence of nurse practitioner and other roles in the United States (Sheer 2000, McGee 2003, Gardner *et al*. 2004). Even though it appears that new ventures have some degree of orientation to various aspects of advanced clinical practice in the United States, it is important to note that the introduction and implementation of new advanced nursing roles are extremely sensitive to the environment in which they evolve. The extent to which one country has contributed to or impacted the phenomenon of advanced practice globally is a topic worthy of study and analysis.

The International Council of Nurses was aware of the growing presence of advanced nursing practice in the United States and, from the early 1990s, noted similar developments in Australia, Canada, New Zealand and the United Kingdom. However, information related to advanced nursing roles in other countries was unclear. Various reports indicated promising development in areas of the world where there is a desperate need for health-care services and where the integration of expanded nursing roles is a viable consideration but there was little information to clarify the extent of advanced nursing practice (Schober and Affara 2006).

In an exploratory survey conducted by the International Council of Nurses (2001), 109 responses from 40 countries revealed wide-ranging interest in or the presence of advanced nursing practice. Roodbol (2004), in reporting results from a similar survey, found that over 60 countries were exploring, developing or implementing advanced roles but that the depth and extent of expansion was unclear. Schober and Affara (2006), in an effort to represent advanced practice worldwide, provided information from key informants, personal communications and site visits representing over 40 countries. Additional reports compared international developments with descriptions of activity mainly in Australia, Canada, New Zealand, the United Kingdom and the United States (Buchan and Calman 2004, Gardner *et al*. 2004).

There are circumstances where, out of necessity and often without physicians, nurses function as the only health-care providers, diagnosing and prescribing as the need arises. Countries and regions in conflict, with rural or remote areas and underserved populations provide examples of such activities (Schober and Affara 2006). Knowledge of the extent of advanced practice throughout the world remains mainly anecdotal, based on isolated surveys, literature reviews and personal experiences and most likely does not completely represent areas of the world where nursing roles elude research analysis but are in evidence at an advanced level.

An international presence marked by confusion

Respondents to the International Council of Nurses' (2001) survey replied to questions about the presence of advanced nursing roles in their countries, the characteristics of these roles, the educational preparation required, the scope of practice and regulatory processes. The analysis of this survey indicated ambiguity, vagueness and a sense of confusion as to what these roles are. Those answering survey questions commonly cited concerns or uncertainty related to appropriate education for and the evaluation of competence levels for advanced practice roles (Schober and Affara 2006).

Of the 40 countries that responded to this survey, 33 reported that there is a nursing role requiring education beyond that of a licensed or registered nurse. However, the level of education for these roles varied. In 30 countries formal educational programmes preparing individuals for advanced nursing roles existed, but in only 26 did the education lead to a recognised qualification such as a degree, diploma or certificate. Some kind of accreditation or approval process for educational programmes was cited in 31 countries. However, accrediting or approval agencies were different in nature ranging from national nursing boards or councils, departments or ministries of health or education to federations of nursing schools, universities, private accrediting bodies and local government. Thirteen countries had legislation or some other type of regulatory mechanism for nurse practitioners or advanced practice (Schober and Affara 2006).

Ambiguity was pronounced when it came to role characteristics. A relatively high number of respondents identified nurses working in advanced roles that included responsibilities related to programme planning, providing consulting services, doing research, acting as the first point of contact for patients and referrals to other professionals. However, such characteristics diminished significantly when they involved exercising autonomy and independence in practice; the authority to prescribe treatments and/or medicines; and the right to make a diagnosis; all areas likely to conflict with the traditional role of other health-care providers.

Lack of consistent titles for the advanced practice role(s) among countries and even within institutions of the same country appears to further add to the confusion. While the titles *nurse practitioner*, *clinical nurse specialist* and *nurse specialist* are often used, in some countries more than one title is used in reference to advanced practice roles although titles referring to a specific speciality or subspeciality are also used, for example, psychiatric/mental health, gerontologic or orthopaedic nurse. Titles used in one country do not necessarily refer to the same scope of practice when used in another country and variation occurs even in different institutions within the same country as well as from state to state or province to province (International Council of Nurses 2001, Buchan and Calman 2004, Gardner *et al.* 2004, Schober and Affara 2006).

In spite of the divergence in available information, the details are noteworthy not only because of the multiple factors contributing to the emergence of advanced clinical nursing but also the extent to which advanced practice is becoming a worldwide trend. Further data would be useful in gaining a clear understanding and for comparing the developmental stages and progress of countries with an established advanced nursing presence. International consensus on issues defining and describing the parameters of advanced practice along with effective practice models would be helpful in focusing dialogue and research.

Advanced nursing practice defined: an international view

The International Council of Nurses regards clear definitions as an essential part of identifying and introducing a new nursing role (Styles and Affara 1997). Definitions are key to distinguishing who a health-care worker is and to providing boundaries for practice. Role definitions can be viewed as a brief method to convey what services to expect from a specific health-care provider and under what conditions these services will be offered (Schober and Affara 2006).

To contribute to a common understanding and guide additional development of advanced practice roles the International Council of Nurses, through the expertise of its International Nurse Practitioner/Advanced Practice Nursing Network, developed a definition and characteristics of *nurse practitioner* and *advanced practice nursing* roles. This definition and these characteristics reflect the International Council of Nurses' official position and are meant to represent current and potential roles worldwide. The intent and purpose is to promote an exchange of ideas that lead to models and frameworks that are usable and responsive to the needs of a specific country or region (Box 16.2).

Box 16.2 Definition of advanced practice

'A Nurse Practitioner/Advanced Practice Nurse is a registered nurse who has acquired the expert knowledge base, complex decision-making skills and clinical competencies for expanded practice, the characteristics of which are shaped by the context and/or country in which she/he is credentialed to practice. A Masters degree is recommended for entry level'.

Source: Summarised from ICN (2002); retrieved from http://www.icn-apnetwork.org 15 November 2006.

Characteristics

The characteristics of advanced nursing, as contained in the council's official position, refer to educational preparation (Box 16.3), nature of practice (Box 16.4) and regulatory mechanisms recommended to be in place to support and identify the advanced practice nurse (Box 16.5).

Box 16.3 Educational preparation

- Educational preparation at advanced level
- Formal recognition of educational programmes preparing nurse practitioners/advanced nursing practice roles accredited or approved
- Formal system of licensure, registration, certification and credentialing

Source: Summarised from ICN (2002); retrieved from http://www.icn-apnetwork.org 15 November 2006.

Box 16.4   Nature of practice

- Integrates research, education, practice and management
- High degree of professional autonomy and independent practice
- Case management/own caseload
- Advanced health assessment skills, decision-making skills and diagnostic reasoning skills
- Recognised advanced clinical competencies
- Provision of consultant services to health providers
- Plans, implements and evaluates programmes
- Recognised first point of contact for clients

Source: Summarised from ICN (2002); retrieved from http://www.icn-apnetwork.org 15 November 2006.

Box 16.5   Regulatory mechanisms

- Right to diagnose
- Authority to prescribe medication
- Authority to prescribe treatment
- Authority to refer clients to other professionals
- Authority to admit patients to hospital
- Legislation to confer and protect the title 'Nurse Practitioner/Advanced Practice Nurse'
- Legislation or some other form of regulatory mechanism specific to advanced practice nurses
- Officially recognised titles for nurses working in advanced practice roles

Source: Summarised from ICN (2002); retrieved from http://www.icn-apnetwork.org 15 November 2006.

National approaches to shaping a definition and characteristics include the use of *advanced practice nursing* or *advanced nursing practice* as an all-inclusive term for all advanced practice nurses and advanced nursing specialities. In the United States, this approach includes clinical nurse specialists, nurse practitioners, nurse anaesthetists and nurse midwives. The American Nurses Association offers a definition that recommends a high level of expertise in the assessment, diagnosis and treatment of individuals, families or communities; a master's or doctoral degree in a specific area of advanced nursing practice; supervised practice during graduate education and ongoing clinical experiences.

The American definition emphasises that the difference in practice between a generalist and an advanced nurse relates to a greater depth and breadth of knowledge, synthesis of data and complexity of skills and interventions (ANA 1996). It is worth noting that this definition is provided by one professional organisation in a country where other nursing organisations offer definitions based on speciality or subspeciality. In practice, each of the 50 states has legislative authority to adopt state-specific definitions, scopes of practice and related legal boundaries for advanced practice nursing under state designated governing bodies.

Canada regards *advanced nursing* as an all-inclusive term that 'describes an advanced level of nursing practice that maximizes the use of in-depth nursing knowledge and skills in meeting the health needs of clients (individuals, families, groups, populations, or entire communities). In this way, advanced nurse practitioner (ANP) extends the boundaries of nursing's scope of practice and contributes to nursing knowledge and the development and advancement of the profession' (Canadian Nurses Association 2002, p. 4). The *clinical nurse specialist* and *nurse practitioner* roles in acute and primary health-care settings have developed under the auspices of advanced nursing practice with each province and territory following different approaches to education, licensure and scope of practice. A current government-funded initiative aims to create a pan-Canadian framework for the sustained integration of nurse practitioners.

The Nurse Practitioner Standards Project (Gardner *et al.* 2004) conducted for the Australian and New Zealand Nursing Councils recommends that a standard *nurse practitioner* definition, standards and competencies be adopted for these two countries in accordance with the Trans-Tasman Mutual Recognition Agreement (Gardner *et al.* 2004). If agreed to, this would be the first bilateral definition for advanced nursing practice. Currently, New Zealand defines *nurse practitioners* as 'registered nurses with Masters degrees and at least four years experience working in their chosen clinical area' (Nursing Council of New Zealand 2002). The Australian approach to the development of *nurse practitioners* has followed a state-by-state process towards definition, education, scope and regulation (Schober and Affara 2006).

Primary health-care authorities in Skaraborg, Sweden, worked with the University of Skovde to develop a definition that met the requirement of the National Board of Health and Welfare, key stakeholders and the Swedish health system:

> An Advanced Nurse Practitioner in Primary Health Care is a registered Nurse with a special education as a district nurse with the right to prescribe certain drugs, and with a post graduate education that enables [the advanced nurse practitioner] an increased and deepened competence to be independently responsible for medical decisions, diagnosing, prescribing of drugs and treatment of health problems within a certain area of health care. (Schober and Affara 2006, p. 7)

Ireland furnishes a national framework that provides a definition for the ANP and advanced midwife practitioner: 'Advanced nursing and midwifery practice is carried out by autonomous, experienced practitioners who are competent, accountable and responsible for their own practice' (National Council for the Professional Development of Nursing and Midwifery 2001, p. 1). This definition introduces the idea of nursing and midwifery as separate disciplines functioning at an advanced level.

Singapore has developed a hybrid advanced practice role based on that of the clinical nurse specialist and the nurse practitioner roles in the United States while adopting a definition based on that of the International Council of Nurses (Premarani 2006). The Western Pacific Region speaks of nurse practitioners as nurses who have advanced clinical curative and preventive primary care skills following advanced training and who are at times designated as mid-level practitioners (WHO – WPR 2001).

In comparing various approaches to defining advanced practice there appears to be a consensus that it requires a level of education beyond the generalist nurse level and makes clear that the nurse is accountable and responsible at an advanced level for decision-making based on an in-depth knowledge base. The specifics of this, however, vary from country to country and among states and provinces within countries. Additionally, in countries where nursing as a profession is unclear and where nurses respond in an advanced capacity to the necessities of care, the requirements of master's level education and a precise definition with clear legislative authority may appear to be as much of a threat as an assurance of quality for the discipline.

Country illustrations of development

There does not seem to be one common starting point in the promotion, introduction and implementation of advanced nursing practice. Roles may evolve in response to a need for health-care services, as part of a country scheme to enhance or improve service delivery or as part of an institutional plan to expand and enhance nursing programmes and education. An enthusiastic agency or institution may independently proceed to incorporate advanced nursing principles. A countrywide scheme may be the result of exploration by a task force or a multi-disciplinary committee.

The Cayman Islands provides an example of how nurse practitioner-like services evolve and develop in response to the needs of the people and the geographical circumstance but without the official titling of nurse practitioner or advanced practice nurse. As early as 1930, a local midwife responded to the scarcity of physician services and insufficient community health services. Services progressed to the official employment of a nurse in 1990. Expansion of services occurred rapidly with the nurse as the main health-care provider treating 'whatever walked in through the door' (Schober 2004, p. 80). The nurse diagnoses, treats, prescribes and dispenses what is viewed to be necessary. Assistance and consultation are provided by a call to the nearest hospital or physician (Schober 2004).

Development of advanced practice in Botswana has focused on the family nurse practitioner (FNP) role. The need for a defined educational programme surfaced as the result of the establishment and development of national primary health care following independence in 1966. A severe shortage of doctors mandated that nurses make not only nursing decisions but were also required to make medical decisions. It became evident that basic nursing education was not adequate to support the level to which the nurses' role had evolved. In response to the needs of the communities and requests from the nurses the Ministry of Health, in collaboration with the National Health Institute, established an FNP programme (Schober 2004).

At the Aga Khan University in Pakistan, the School of Nursing developed a master's level education programme with an ANP focus in mind while emphasising the advancement of professional nursing in the country. A clinical advanced practitioner role has yet to emerge but the educational programme continues to grow. The Institute of Nursing Science at the University of Basel in Switzerland developed advanced nursing practice through a master's degree in nursing in response to a potential physician shortage and an expected need for nurses with higher-level skills to cope with this change. Similar situations have stimulated exploration and development of advanced practice in France and the Netherlands (Schober and Affara 2006).

In the Philippines and Singapore, national task forces were formed with designated time lines to explore, evaluate and consider advanced nursing practice as a possibility. Both countries are in the early stages of development; therefore, it is premature to completely assess the success of these new ventures. The United Kingdom is often viewed as a homogeneous entity; however, in reference to nurse practitioner or advanced practice nurse, the presence and definition of these roles vary among the four countries of England, Northern Ireland, Scotland and Wales with all four countries moving at a different pace towards master's and clinical doctorate education (Schober and Affara 2006).

The role of international organisations

International organisations promoting nursing at different levels of health-care provision provide the authority a country or a new initiative may need to convince decision-makers of the usefulness of expanding the roles and presence of nurses. International backing offers a level of credibility to key health-care planners when a scheme is viewed as part of global advancement versus a local or even a national directive. International organisations provide influence in various ways.

Recognising the growth in advanced nursing practice, the International Council of Nurses launched the International Nurse Practitioner/Advanced Practice Nursing Network (INP/APNN) in 2000 to better follow trends and new developments in the field. This network acts as a resource for the international nursing community providing and disseminating comprehensive up-to-date information on advanced nursing practice worldwide. In addition, the network provides periodic conferences to facilitate networking and sharing of research and clinical topics of interest as well as actively supporting a website resource for advanced practice issues (http://www. icn-apnetwork.org). International guidelines for scope, standards and competencies for advanced nursing practice are in the final stages of development and plans are under way to promote, facilitate and conduct multinational research on advanced nursing practice issues.

The International Council of Nurses' decision to take an official position on nurse practitioner and advanced nursing roles provides a basis from which member countries and others can utilise this definitive information and adapt pertinent sections for country-specific development. In addition, the council actively represents nursing in such arenas as the WHO's governing body and the World Health Assembly and provides representation to other international organisations to further ensure that nursing participates in discussions of cost-effective and quality health-care programmes for the world's populations.

As an agency of the United Nations, the WHO works to further international cooperation aimed at improving health conditions. WHO has a broad mandate to promote the attainment of the highest possible level of health for all people (retrieved from http://www.who.int/ 15 November 2006). The approach of this international organisation is not specific to nursing but can influence the amount of attention given to nursing roles. *Strategic Directions for Strengthening Nursing and Midwifery Services, 2002–2008* (WHO 2002) provides a framework for collaborative action to support countries in enhancing the capacity of nursing and midwifery services to contribute to national health goals. By taking a leading role in encouraging governments to address emergent issues, WHO acts as a catalyst for debate over urgently needed restructuring and inclusion of nursing and midwifery services.

WHO advocacy occurs more directly under the guidance of its regional offices and Regional Directors of Nursing. For example, the WHO Regional Nursing Director for the Eastern Mediterranean Region (EMRO) has supported a proactive position to promote exploration of advanced nursing in the region. In 2001, 14 member nations of EMRO gathered to discuss, explore and offer recommendations for the promotion of and assistance in establishing advanced practice nursing roles (WHO 2001). An action plan and documents supporting advanced nursing practice and nurse prescribing were created as a result. Following this regional meeting, the Sultanate of Oman, a member country of EMRO, with support from the WHO regional office, is currently in the process of developing educational requirements and scope of practice anticipating implementation of community nurse practitioners to enhance primary health-care services. If successful, this country will provide a model for the rest of the region.

International organisations, when effective, provide the ability and influence to conduct forums for discussion, convene meetings or conferences to share ideas and initiate research at a global level. Specific units functioning within the organisational structures act as a resource to provide guidance for interested factions who wish to collaborate in these discussions and consider options for implementing country-specific schemes.

Scope of practice, regulation and standards

Advanced nursing practice is not only emerging as a global phenomenon but also struggling to establish legitimacy and authority in relation to recognised scopes of practice, standards and competencies. It is not the intention of this section to explore these topics in depth but to introduce the significance of these issues for advanced nursing practice and to remark on the work currently under way by the International Council of Nurses to provide international guidelines. Establishing scope of practice is important because it 'describes the range of activities associated with recognised professional responsibilities that are in keeping with the limitations imposed by regulatory provisions in the setting where practice occurs. Specifically, the scope describes what an APN can do, what population can be seen or treated, and under what circumstance or guidance the APN can provide care. Ethical and cultural conduct, educational requirements, along with aspects of accountability for professional actions, form components of scope of practice' (Schober and Affara 2006, p. 26).

Scope statements tend to be broad and flexible in order to promote safe, good quality health care while also reflecting the settings in which the advanced practitioner will practice. A challenge in developing consensus for scope of practice at national or international levels is to define a scope of practice supportive of advanced roles while avoiding the temptation to designate nurses in a way that is too limiting and that might result in fragmented rather than collaborative health-care services.

Standards being identified in the international guidelines will be based on the assumption that core competencies will arise from the three pillars of nursing articulated by the International Council of Nurses, namely, the standards for regulation, practice and socio-economic welfare. Essential standards for education, regulation and core competencies of the advanced practice nurse are intended to assist countries during decisive periods of expansion of advanced roles. The aim is that policies will be refined and adapted as roles emerge to reflect the relevant scope of practice and demographic environment (retrieved from http://www.icn-apnetwork.org 15 November 2006).

To 'endure and evolve, advanced nursing practice needs a regulatory/legislative framework' (Schober and Affara 2006, p. 82). Educators, clinicians, nursing leaders and health-care planners must become aware of and understand the milieu in which regulation occurs in order to influence the structure of the related system. The process involves credentialing of nurses for advanced practice roles and the accreditation of institutions and programmes offering education. Standards and competencies are positioned as the focal point of a credentialing system. 'Standards set the level of education and performance and entry into practice for renewal of credentials. Competencies define the level and quality of performance the credentialee is expected to demonstrate as a practising APN' (Schober and Affara 2006, p. 97). Legislation and regulation, when in place, should grant identity and legitimise the advanced practice role.

Practice settings

Debate and discussion arises in attempting to clarify whether advanced practice is or should be focused on nursing function in a clinical speciality or within a broader and more comprehensive framework. One way to express possibilities is to identify domains of practice within the institution, site or environment where the advanced practice role will be present. In describing domains of practice, Read and Roberts-Davis (2000), in their study of clinical nurse specialist and nurse practitioner models present in the United Kingdom, conclude that the *nurse practitioner* is a generalist clinician who makes an assessment and diagnosis in undifferentiated conditions; a *clinical nurse specialist* provides care in a specialist area where the initial diagnosis has already been decided. This provides a means to compare the two roles, or contrast hospital-based versus primary health care-based care. However, difficulty arises when the *clinical nurse specialist* and *nurse practitioner* titles refer to different clinical capacities or when similar clinical roles exist under an array of titles. The confusion over titling also makes it difficult to accurately assess the presence of an advanced nurse practitioner in work settings when there is simply a change in titling of the nurse with little or no change in the scope of clinical practice (Schober and Affara 2006).

The potential for advanced nursing practice exists wherever health-care services are provided or needed. Convenience, access to care, human resources and funding drive the exploration and implementation of advanced practice roles in a variety of settings throughout the world. Restrictions will more likely come from the health-care systems or structures in which the roles are developing than from the needs of the world's populations or the ability of nurses to provide the services. Clinically based options can range from acute care to palliative care; paediatric to geriatric; and include specialities based on body systems, educational settings, substance abuse, mental health and immigrant populations. Flexibility and innovative thinking will contribute to reasonable options. Settings such as mobile clinics and services within pharmacies or shopping malls currently provide resourceful examples of convenient care centres and potential for advanced practice.

Interaction with health professionals

A change in the definition and scope of practice for nurses will impact on an entire health-care structure and, subsequently, interaction among all professionals providing care. The most written about interactions, those that cause the most conflict, appear to be rooted in relationships between advanced practitioners and other nurses, physicians and to a lesser degree with pharmacists. In a scope of practice where duties cross over, or overlap with another professional's scope, attempts to block or sabotage advanced practice can become heated. In the United States with a 40-year history of nurse practitioners, longer than any other, combative issues continue to mar the success of nurses in providing cost-effective quality care.

Nurses themselves voice concern that the new advanced practice roles are not really nursing and follow too closely a medical model approach to health care, consequently leaving behind the core principles of nursing education. The reality is that medical and nursing scopes of practice do overlap, thus raising concerns among advanced practitioners themselves as to how their roles are viewed in the health system structure. Marshall and Luffingham (1998) report this concern in relation to poor working relationships among nurses. Roodbol (2005) cites reported beliefs that advanced practitioners lack a respectful attitude to nurses who competently function in other nursing capacities, thus contributing to dissension among nurses expected to work together. In this study, nurses did not share the physician's view of a positive identity for advanced nursing practice and the nurse practitioners felt conflict about role expectations. On the one hand, the nurse practitioner is expected to be a nurse; on the other hand, the scope of practice overlaps with medical practice.

Physicians are often placed in a position of authority and supervision over other professionals and as designated gatekeepers for health-care services. Hierarchical role definitions can occur where a collaborative inter-disciplinary or multi-disciplinary approach benefits individuals, families and communities. When the scope of practice for the advanced practitioner overlaps areas of jurisdiction traditionally claimed by physicians, the competency or authority of a nurse to function in an advanced capacity will be challenged. On the other hand, a physician who understands the value of advanced nursing roles is often the pivotal, most supportive champion.

In the beginning of a new initiative, professionals, time and again, do not comprehend the educational background, scope of practice or regulations underpinning advanced practice and thus either do not understand or misunderstand the competencies and capabilities of a nurse in this role. These misunderstandings, if left unexplained, can lead to fragmented care and gaps in service delivery unless they are addressed clearly and openly. In effect, a cautious renegotiation of professional boundaries within the health-care structures and settings is beneficial in acknowledging variations in service delivery and to better ensure that providers and the public are aware of the benefits of a new model of service delivery.

Future directions in advanced nursing practice

In speculating on future directions for advanced nursing practice, Schober and Affara (2006) propose that, as a profession, nursing is in a position to develop alternatives suitable and beneficial for the needs and requests of populations worldwide. The complexity of health problems in the world today provides an opportunity for nurses to demonstrate competence and capability in roles that are identified with advanced clinical practice (Box 16.6). Nurses with advanced skills practising at an advanced clinical level are in a decisive position to play a part in health workforce strategies (Box 16.7).

Box 16.6 Opportunities for advanced nurses to demonstrate competence

- Involvement in health-care systems worldwide without losing core nursing characteristics
- International consensus on scope of practice based on core values of nursing
- Demonstrating consistency across clinical and educational models
- Providing evidence that advanced practice nurses are valued health-care providers
- Offering leadership, strategic thinking and action plans to move advanced nursing practice into the position of an accepted health-care team member

---

Box 16.7 The potential for advanced practitioners to participate in health workforce strategies

- PHC services are getting more and more attention internationally. The future calls for nurses to work collaboratively and effectively in community and PHC settings
- Increasing demands to meet the escalating requirements for care associated with chronic conditions worldwide provides diverse opportunities for skilled advanced practice nurses
- Advanced practice nurses of the future will be mandated to integrate advanced knowledge and clinical skills with effective and practical telehealth and health-care technologies

---

- As the level of confidence and expertise experienced by some advanced practice nurses takes shape, there will likely be a tendency to move towards a more independent entrepreneurial model of practice. Although the numbers may be small, these nurses will need to take on additional roles related to business, risk management and regulatory aspects of practice in addition to clinical services

Source: Summarised from Schober and Affara (2006).

The future for advanced nursing practice includes opportunities along with significant challenges. In countries where nursing is in its infancy, capacity building and transitioning from current levels of practice, competency and education to advanced levels will take well thought-out consideration to meet a minimal standard for practice while taking care to avoid dampening enthusiasm for new roles. Balancing cost-effective options appropriate to populations, requesting and requiring services will increasingly impact on choices for advanced nursing practice services. An adequate supply of qualified educators is central to ensuring that practitioners competently develop skills necessary for practice. Appropriate legislation and credentialing will better ensure that an advanced practitioner or nurse practitioner can practice at a level to which they are educated.

Conclusion

Beneficial models for advanced practice will continue to be analysed and best practices identified as options for delivery of health-care services throughout the world. A proactive voice on behalf of nursing is pivotal in order to demonstrate the value and diversity of advanced practice roles. Nurses will be obliged to attain the outlook, knowledge and skills to respond and adapt to current and future health-care needs and requests. Health-care planners, key decision-makers and other professionals are in positions to determine what strategies will best move the world's health-care agenda forward. Nursing advocacy, strong leadership and a sound evidence base will aid decision-makers in their choice of options that facilitate the provision of innovative, cost-effective, high-quality advanced nursing services.

 Key questions for Chapter 16

In your field of practice:
(1) What factors have contributed to the heightened awareness and interest in advanced nursing practice globally?
(2) What is the official position of the International Council of Nurses as it relates to a definition and the characteristics for advanced nursing practice?
(3) How do international organisations and the authority associated with them influence new and advanced nursing roles worldwide?

Acknowledgements

Much of the material in this chapter is adapted from Schober, M. & Affara, F. (2006) *Advanced Nursing Practice*. Oxford, Blackwell Publishing. Reproduced with permission from Wiley-Blackwell and the International Council of Nurses.

References

American Nurses' Association (1996) *Scope and Standards of Advanced Practice Registered Nursing.* Washington, DC, ANA.

Buchan, J. and Calman, L. (2004) *Skill-Mix and Policy Change in the Health Workforce: Nurses in Advanced Practice Roles.* OECD Working Paper No 17, DELSA/ELSA/WD/HEA, 8.

Buchan, J. and Dal Poz, M.R. (2002) Skill mix in the health care workforce: reviewing the evidence. *Bulletin of the World Health Organization* **80** (7) 575–80.

Canadian Nurses Association (2002) *Advanced Nursing Practice. A National Framework.* Ottawa, Author.

Gardner, G., Carryer, J., Dunn, S.V. and Gardner, A. (2004) *Nurse Practitioner Standards Project.* Queensland University of Technology, Australian Nursing Council, Queensland, Australia.

International Council of Nurses (2001) *Update: International Survey of Nurse Practitioner/Advanced Practice Nursing Roles.* Retrieved 15 November 2006 from http://www.icn-apnetwork.org.

Marshall, Z. and Luffingham, N. (1998) Does the specialist nurse enhance or deskill the general nurse? *British Journal of Nursing* **7** (11) 658–61.

McGee, P. (2003) International perspectives on advanced practice. In *Advanced Nursing Practice*, (eds P. McGee and G. Castledine), 2nd edn. pp 144–56. Oxford, Blackwell Publishing.

National Council for the Professional Development of Nursing and Midwifery (2001, 2004) *Framework for the Advanced Nurse Practitioner and Advanced Midwife Practitioner Posts*, 2nd edn. Dublin, Author.

Nursing Council of New Zealand (2002) *The Nurse Practitioner: Responding to Health Care Needs in New Zealand*, 3rd edn. Wellington, Author.

Premarani, K. (2006) How do we access education when we have to create our own? *Presentation Sandton, South Africa for the 4th ICN International NP/APN Network Conference*, http://www.icn-apnetwork.org Accessed 19 February 2009.

Read, S. and Roberts-Davis, M. (2000) *Preparing Nurse Practitioners for the 21st Century. Executive Summary from the Report of the Project Realizing Specialist and Advanced Nursing Practice: Establishing the Parameters of and Identifying the Competencies for 'Nurse Practitioner' Roles and Evaluating Programmes of Preparation (RSANP).* University of Sheffield, Author.

Roodbol, P. (2004) *Survey Carried Out Prior to the 3rd ICN-International Nurse Practitioner/Advanced Practice Nursing Network Conference.* Groningen, The Netherlands.

Roodbol, P. (2005) *Willing o'-the-Wisps, Stumbling Runs, Toll Roads and Song Lines: Study into the Structural Rearrangement of Tasks Between Nurses and Physicians.* Summary of doctoral dissertation. Unpublished.

Schober, M. (2004) Global perspective on advanced practice. In *Advanced Practice Nursing*, (ed. L.A. Joel). Philadelphia, F.A. Davis.

Schober, M. and Affara, F. (2006) *Advanced Nursing Practice.* Oxford, Blackwell Publishing.

Sheer, B. (2000) International collaboration: initial steps and strategies. *Journal of the American Academy of Nurse Practitioners* **12** (8) 303–8.

Styles, M.M. and Affara, F.A. (1997) *ICN on Regulation: Towards a 21st Century Model.* Geneva, International Council of Nurses.

World Health Organization – Eastern Mediterranean Region (2001) *Fifth Meeting of the Regional Advisory Panel on Nursing and Consultation on Advanced Practice Nursing and Nurse Prescribing: Implications for Regulation, Nursing Education and Practice in the Eastern Mediterranean.* WHO-EM/NUR/348/E/L. Cairo, Author.

World Health Organization – Western Pacific Region (2001) *Mid-Level and Nurse Practitioners in the Pacific: Models and Issues.* Manila, Author.

World Health Organization (2002) *Nursing and Midwifery Services: Strategic Directions 2002–2008.* Geneva, WHO.

Chapter 17

The Future for Advanced Practice

Paula McGee

Introduction

The concept of advanced practice is now well established in nursing and is gradually developing in allied health professions. The focal point of advanced practice, in any health profession, is direct practice. This can take many different forms but it must involve regular contact with patients and the delivery of expert care based on a wide repertoire of knowledge, skills and experience. These are expressed as competencies and include leadership, teaching and guiding, working collaboratively, acting as a consultant and ethical practice. Exercising these competencies requires the advanced practitioner to be a professionally mature individual whose interpersonal skills and practice are easily adapted to meet the communication styles of patients from diverse backgrounds. Practitioners who do not engage regularly with patients cannot be considered advanced, no matter what strengths they bring to health care generally.

As a senior professional and leader, the advanced practitioner is expected to challenge professional boundaries and pioneer innovations, indirect care activities that require the application of other skills. The advanced practitioner approaches practice from a critical standpoint, evaluating what is going well and identifying what should be changed. It is the advanced practitioner's responsibility to ensure that practice within the workplace is based on the best available evidence and to systematically investigate those aspects of care that give cause for concern. This type of indirect care activity requires the expertise of an advanced practitioner who understands the structures and processes through which the health-care organisation functions, and how to get something done. National and international links provide useful insight into the world outside the organisation and enable the advanced practitioner to ensure that innovations reflect current policy, practice and research.

Advanced practice is, therefore, a highly skilled and demanding role but one which, as this book has demonstrated, continues to evolve. Each health profession must determine what it wishes advanced practitioners to be able to do, the competencies they must attain and the type and level of preparation they require. Inevitably, research is needed to address these issues in order to identify what is desirable and achievable. This chapter presents an agenda for that research with a view to enabling advanced practitioners, professionals and others, such as policy-makers and those responsible for service commissioning, to facilitate the development of advanced practice over the next few years. The agenda presented draws on that of the previous edition of this book but has been expanded to include allied health professions.

An agenda for research

Direct practice

The essence of advanced practice is direct engagement with patients within the context of providing care. The nature of this engagement may vary but it must occupy a significant proportion of working time so that patients can benefit from the advanced practitioners' expertise. Advanced practitioners who have been prepared at master's level are now equipped to meet the everyday health needs of patients: to assess, diagnose and treat people with a variety of conditions and problems. Advanced practitioners can provide a single point of contact for service users, thus allowing other practitioners more time and resources to devote to those with more challenging difficulties. However, direct care roles require more exploration. Certain types of direct care may prove more appropriate and cost-effective than others. For instance, in some settings, such as intensive care or secure mental health units, an advanced practitioner may be necessary to provide care on a continuous basis. This may not be suitable in other situations, for example, those involving challenging behaviour from people with severe learning disabilities. The problem is that, at present, service planners can only guess at what may be needed; research would help to clarify the types of advanced practice activity that are best suited to particular care settings.

In addressing this issue, researchers may find it useful to consult recommendations made recently to the Department of Health (DH 2008a). These focus on enabling people to stay healthy and the provision of more personalised care, especially for those with long-term conditions (Table 17.1). Health service regions have developed models of care, 'based firmly on the best available clinical evidence and the needs and preferences of local users' as a basis from which to implement the Department of Health's recommendations (DH 2008b, p. 1). These recommendations emphasise the need for treatment and care to be given at, or close to, patients' homes whenever possible, 'clearer and simpler routes to finding the right care' and improvements in patient's lives (DH 2008b, p. 2).

Table 17.1   High-quality care for all.

Recommendation	Strategies for achieving high-quality care
Create a National Health Service (NHS) that helps people stay healthy	Preventative services that meet local and personal needs that include staying healthy at work, reducing the risks of vascular disease and ensuring that people with long-term conditions have personalised care plans Examining the possibility of personal health budgets Increasing choice in general practitioner (GP) practice and helping GPs to promote health Access to the most clinically and cost-effective drugs and treatments
High-quality care	Getting the basics right first time, every time Linking hospital funding to the quality of care Introducing measures for continued improvements in quality, best practice and priority setting. These will include enabling staff to have access to information and further developing the Clinical Excellence Awards Scheme for senior doctors Measuring and publishing information about the quality of care Introducing new responsibilities, funds and prizes to support and reward innovations and implementing those shown to be clinically and cost-effective
Fostering innovation	New partnerships among the NHS, universities and industry
Working in partnership with staff	Improving NHS education and training and investing more in providing opportunities for staff to undertake professional development and updating Investing more in nurse and midwife preceptorships

Source: Summarised from Department of Health (2008a) *High Quality Care for All. NHS Next Stage Review Final Report*. London, DH.

The intention is to improve the quality of care by linking it with funding, introducing new responsibilities such as a legal duty to promote innovation and the creation of partnerships among the NHS, universities and industry (DH 2008a). Advanced practitioners are well equipped to implement recommendations about health promotion, for example, by working with patients to reduce their weight and alcohol consumption. They are also able to assess patients and use their collaborative working skills to negotiate effective personalised care plans that empower patients to take control of their health problems (DH 2008c).

Collaboration with service users

One of the cornerstones of recent health service reforms has been the emphasis placed on patient and public involvement at every level. The key message is that the National Health Service (NHS) belongs to everyone and so service users and providers should work together to provide accessible, appropriate treatment and care (DH 2005a). Inherent in this aspect of reform is a comprehensive cultural shift in values, attitudes and working practices. Service providers and practitioners have had to abandon the idea that they always know what is best for patients. Policies and procedures have had to be redrafted as established, and perhaps cherished, ways of doing things are no longer appropriate. Patients now have a far wider choice about their treatment and are more aware of their rights, especially with regard to the management of long-term conditions. People with diabetes, epilepsy, asthma and other problems are now to be considered as experts on their own health. The practitioner's role is to support such individuals in managing their symptoms within the context of their daily lives and to provide care that enables them to avoid hospital admissions (DH 2005b, 2007a).

This cultural shift in health care has engaged patients and the public in new ways that have moved well beyond the initial attempts at measuring patient satisfaction, although that remains important. The Next Stage Review has 'actively engaged, involved and solicited the views of patients, service users and the public, staff and stakeholders through a number of different channels. We have used new and innovative ways to engage them, as well as tried and tested more traditional methods' (DH 2008d, p. 5) (Box 17.1).

Box 17.1   Strategies used in the Next Stage Review to engage with patients, the public and NHS staff

Visits to strategic health authorities
Stakeholder forum attended by organisations
Two deliberative events with over 1000 patients, members of the public and
    NHS staff at each session
An international clinical summit
Existing Department of Health forums, e.g. Social Partnership Forum
Regionally based events for service users and staff
Ten thousand interviews in service users' homes
Surveys of marginalised groups such as travellers
Online web chats
Questionnaires to the public and NHS staff

Source: Summarised from Department of Health (2008g) *Engagement Analysis. NHS Next Stage Review What we heard from the Our NHS, our future process*. London, DH.

Involvement in direct practice provides opportunities for advanced practitioners to work with patients, families, carers and associations to elicit their views on the care and services that best suit their needs. Collaborative working skills enable advanced practitioners to take the lead in promoting dialogue among service users, practitioners and service providers at different levels in the organisation and the health service as a whole. There is ample scope for advanced practitioners to pioneer new ways of achieving this, for instance, by using chat rooms, message boards, local radio, the local press and focus groups.

Examples of national developments include the NHS National Centre for Involvement, which provides tools and methodologies for supporting patient involvement (http://www.nhscentreforinvolvement.nhs.uk.). Among the many initiatives it has established is a People Bank of patients and members of the public, who have been trained to work with professionals, to facilitate the work of the centre. This development demonstrates that patients and the public cannot be expected to automatically know how the health service functions; they need training and support if they are to make meaningful contributions. One source of support is the National Library for Health, which has set up a specialist library for patient and public involvement with a view to supporting involvement with the NHS; medical conditions are not included on the site (http://www.library.nhs.uk/ppi/).

At regional levels there are numerous examples of strategies for patient and public involvement (see, e.g. the York Cancer Network 2006, available at http://www.ycn.nhs.uk and Waltham Forest NHS Trust 2004, available at http://www.walthamforest-pct.nhs.uk.). Advanced practitioners, service providers and the professionals need to investigate ways of engaging with patients and the public locally, ensuring that they gain representative views from across the community, including groups that might not normally participate. For example, Egan *et al.* (2006) used e-mail to elicit the views of people who had experienced traumatic brain injury in adult life and who were unable to cope with the stress generated by face-to-face encounters.

Such examples highlight the importance of organisational support in terms of providing resources. These may include software and possibly legal advice where some communities are concerned. For example, Hains and McGee (2006) recommended that using chat rooms to reach sex workers requires clear protocols to protect practitioners. Employers have a responsibility to make sure that they understand what innovation involves and take appropriate steps to provide constructive support rather than just leaving the individual practitioner to cope alone.

Engaging with service users is a new and relatively untapped field for research activity and one that could attract rewards for fostering innovation (DH 2008a) (Table 17.1). It has brought about changes in the ways in which patients and professionals relate to one another, just as advanced practice has challenged the boundaries of practice. Advanced practitioners and patients have much to gain from working together in exploring new approaches to care and services. A collaborative approach to research is essential if the health service is to be truly patient centred and patient led (DH 2005c). Advanced practitioners should be able to participate in or lead such an approach.

Diversity and inclusiveness

Access to health care is a human right that is made evident in the United Kingdom's NHS, which, despite numerous difficulties, remains free at the point of delivery. Professional codes of conduct emphasise this right and prohibit discrimination against any patient on the grounds of gender, religion, ethnicity, culture, sexual orientation or any other distinguishing characteristic. Recent developments in legislation, such as the Equality Act 2006 and the Race Relations (Amendment) Act 2000, have brought equality issues to the forefront of service delivery. Chapter 11 of this book examined the implications of cultural competence for advanced practitioners. Their role as professional and clinical leaders extends to demonstrating and modelling appropriate engagement with cultural diversity and facilitating similar abilities in others. Current health policy is directed towards tackling institutional racism through race equality action plans and schemes such as Pacesetters and Race for Health (Home Office 1999, DH 2007b, 2008d).

However, culture, race and ethnicity are only one aspect of promoting equality. Many other individuals and groups have also been socially marginalised: the homeless, transgender people, children, the poor and those with physical or intellectual disabilities. Asylum seekers are a particular case in point. Socially marginalised and made to feel distinctly unwelcome, they were not entitled to health care except in emergencies according to a ruling of the UK government; this ruling was overturned by the High Court in April 2008 (Boseley 2008).

The advanced practitioner needs to find ways of engaging with people whose social status is very low or who have limited opportunities to make their voices heard. For example, people with learning disabilities find it very hard to access treatment for everyday health problems. Health services do not adapt to meet their needs. Parents and carers are often ignored or belittled by professionals with limited knowledge of learning disabilities and who refuse to pay attention to what they say (DH 2008e). Despite legislation to promote equality for people with disabilities, monitoring for compliance is poor, which suggests that little has changed since the introduction of Valuing People (DH 2001, http://valuingpeople.gov.uk/index.jsp). People with learning disabilities remain invisible in the health service and commitment to changing this situation appears to be weak. Advanced practitioners, service commissioners and policy makers working outside the field of learning disabilities are in positions to bring about change, beginning by investigating what happens to such people within their services (DH 2008e). They each have an ethical and legal responsibility to ensure that patients receive care that is appropriate to their needs, on the same basis as everyone else; advanced practitioners have a key role in ensuring that this happens.

Professional regulation and control

A major concern in the development of advanced practice must be that of public protection. People have a right to know that those who treat and care for them are appropriately qualified; that the fact that patients might not see a doctor does not mean that they are being fobbed off with inferior services. Thus patients and the public need to know what advanced practitioners are, what they can do and that they are competent to do it. This is, in itself, an opportunity for research and marketing through multiple channels, including the popular media. As Chapter 14 has shown, competence eludes precise definition but professionals will have to determine what they each regard as advanced, competent performance and how this will translate into professional regulation. It is clear that initial registration is not enough; some additional form is needed. Job titles, often lengthy and meaningless beyond the immediate work setting, do not help to clarify advanced status or convey it to patients. What is needed is a legally protected, registerable title. This may be specific to each profession or generic, for example, *advanced nurse practitioner* or *advanced practitioner (nursing)*.

Professional organisations, policy makers and other relevant bodies should address this as a matter of some urgency but, as noted in Chapter 14, their progress appears to be extremely slow. This situation is very frustrating for those who are involved in trying to provide day-to-day services but it highlights the difficulties of trying to position a new role within the context of a multi-professional service. To explain this more clearly, advanced practice challenges traditional professional boundaries. Initially these were conceptualised in terms of nursing and medicine but, as advanced practice has developed in other professions, all the certainties about what a doctor, a nurse or a physiotherapist does have come under scrutiny (Litchfield 1998, Hanrahan *et al.* 2001, Gidlow and Ellis 2003). Professions, policy makers and society as a whole are having to address fundamental questions about what nurses, doctors, physiotherapists and others are required to do, whether, at advanced levels, there are generic competencies. If such competencies exist, then it may be that advanced practice is emerging as truly a new profession altogether and it will take time to clarify its position in relation to those already established. It may even, eventually, lead to a reconsideration of the need for separate professions at all if a new, generic role can fulfil what is required.

Inevitably the development of advanced practice creates a sense of threat among established professionals. People at the forefront of change are apt to be rather impatient with those they see as reactionaries. For example, Freudmann (2006) has criticised the introduction of surgical practitioners. He admits that his views are based on anecdote but, nevertheless, he makes some useful points. 'They have no regulatory body, and so there are no rules governing what they can do,' he says and, if they are trained to perform the simpler surgical procedures, this will seriously affect the training of surgeons. This idea that advanced forms of practice will leave doctors without training, or even nothing to do, is a common complaint.

Experience elsewhere is instructive in dealing with such situations. Advanced practice literature shows that individual doctors have been very influential, often providing a vision of what can be achieved. For example, in 1957, a Dr Eugene Stead envisaged a role that was between nursing and medicine, found a nurse to share this but was opposed by both the dean of nursing and the National League for Nursing, which refused to accredit the necessary training course. Loretta Ford, a nurse, worked with Dr Silver, setting up a postgraduate course in paediatric care for poor rural children in Colorado but the American Nurses' Association would not support this. In both examples, the nurse and the doctor produced something new that met particular local health needs; it was the professional bodies that appeared to have difficulties (Dunphy *et al.* 2004). Professional medical bodies must also share some of the blame. While individual medical practitioners have been influential, the American Medical Association has mounted 'an intensive on-line advocacy campaign to help medical societies defeat state and national legislation that increases the professional autonomy of APNs and other providers. The AMA's goal is to kill legislation that does not allow ultimate physician control' (Pearson 2001, p. 7). In the United States, doctors' associations continue to form the main opposition to advanced practice (Pearson 2003, 2004).

Thus it would seem that professional bodies, senior professionals and policy makers need to take a long, hard look at how they react to new ideas and developments. It is too easy to react defensively and reject change rather than maintain an open mind and examine a proposal logically. Many of the professions currently featured in health are of quite recent origin. The Society of Physiotherapists was founded in 1894 (http://www.csp.org.uk.) and the British Association of Occupational Therapists was not formed until 1974 (http://www.cot.co.uk.). Thus the introduction of new roles is not without precedent.

Overall the interface with medicine remains the most crucial element in the success of advanced practice in nursing and all allied health professions. Research is needed to establish clear scopes of practice for advanced roles that are supported by appropriate education (Schober and Affara 2006). The involvement of senior medical professionals, including some sceptics, will help to provide leadership for doctors to become involved in new developments. In doing so, they may come to appreciate the ways in which new developments can enhance patient care and to recognise that, far from losing work, they are better able to concentrate on patients who really need their expertise.

Education and assessment

Education is an essential consideration in the development of advanced practice. Although master's level study is thought desirable, many countries face difficulties in making it mandatory because their postgraduate education sectors are underdeveloped or they have yet to decide on other aspects of professional education. There are, as yet, no clear guidelines on whether student advanced practitioners should follow a core curriculum or whether separate courses provide better preparation. A great deal of work is needed to determine the most appropriate level and type of education for advanced practice; this should include consideration of the potential benefits of clinical doctorates (The American Association of Colleges of Nursing 2004). It should also include attention to the preparation of teachers. In time, some advanced practitioners may move into education and become course leaders and tutors but, in the meantime, as the Fijian experience demonstrated, it is no use trying to provide advanced levels of education if teachers themselves are not adequately prepared. Research is needed to clarify the type and level of preparation that is most beneficial to teachers and how best to enable them to maintain or further develop their skills (Downes 2007).

Recording developments

The development of advanced roles is marked by a period of rapid and constant change at all levels in the health service. Current policies and reforms bring new directions in service development with many implications for commissioners and practitioners further down the line. Working directly with patients, in posts that may have no precedent within the organisation concerned, poses many challenges. These posts evolve over time and so post holders and managers need to meet and review developments at regular intervals.

The author's own experience in new posts suggests that these intervals should be no longer than 6 months. This is sufficient time for both parties to identify where they began, where they are now and where they would like to be. Short-term action plans allow a period of time, 6 months, in which to work towards desired goals and then re-review the situation. This approach allows for regular consultation with other personnel, such as the organisation's human resources department and legal advisors, and the practitioner's professional association. The aim is to meet the multiple demands of the patients, services, commissioners, law, organisation and the profession concerned. Allied to this is the need to consider professional development. The direct care element of their role means that advanced practitioners will always be busy and they may feel they cannot spare the time to undertake further development. Managers charged with responsibility to ensure that targets are achieved may lose sight of the advanced practitioner's educational needs, especially if other, less experienced members of staff are also seeking to develop.

Addressing all these issues requires some form of record keeping, which documents, from the beginning, how the advanced role was developed within a particular post and why: the decisions that were taken, the work that was done and the outcomes. This should not require a great deal of effort. All practitioners keep records of their work with patients and it should be easy to establish a similar record of the development of advanced practice within a post. This record could have two dimensions: professional and managerial. The managerial section could be used for reporting within the organisation and the professional section could take a more reflective approach.

Records of this nature would be invaluable in several ways. First, they would provide an account of each advanced practice post and enable the individual post holder to put forward a case for regrading, pay enhancement, professional or career development. Second, analysis of records could be useful to organisations and professions in developing future advanced roles, deciding on the work activities that practitioners will undertake, the preparation required for these and the necessary regulatory systems that should be set in place. Finally, these records would form a comprehensive record of advanced practice. This is notably lacking, particularly in the United Kingdom. The historical account of advanced nursing in Chapter 1 and chapters in previous editions of this book (Castledine 1998a–2003) have been pieced together from fragments of information. They probably form the most comprehensive narrative of the history of advanced nursing practice in the United Kingdom and, to date, nothing similar has emerged for any of the allied health professions. Record keeping is essential if future generations of practitioners are to understand how their professions have developed, what worked well, what did not and why. History is far more than a set of stories; it provides an instructional account of what took place so that mistakes are not repeated and achievements can be celebrated.

Conclusion

This chapter has proposed a number of pathways for research and development in advanced practice. The findings will facilitate the continued development of expert practitioners as clinical and professional leaders in their respective fields. Inherent in this leadership will be:

- valuing direct and critical practice so that patients receive expert treatment and care, on an equal basis, irrespective of any distinguishing characteristics they may have
- collaborative working that brings together patients, families and carers with different forms of professional expertise, so that health care becomes truly patient led and patient centred
- critical appraisal of developments and their impact on patient care, services and staff as a basis for ethical, research and evidence-based practice
- focused professional development at an agreed level, based on clear, generic and specialist competencies and governed by a regulatory framework
- clear titles, for advanced practitioners, that are protected by law
- contributions to the theoretical development of advanced practice in nursing and allied health professions, both nationally and internationally

Most importantly, advanced practitioners will continue to be with patients, enabling them to stay well and manage their health problems. Advanced practitioners will do their best to alleviate distressing symptoms, pain and suffering, providing care that maintains each patients' dignity and, where appropriate, enables them to achieve a peaceful death. These activities reflect their professional values and are in line with the proposed new constitution for the NHS, which, it is anticipated, will bring together the rights and responsibilities of patients and staff with clear pledges relating to both (DH 2008f) (Table 17.2). Advanced practitioners must make sure that they are equipped to make the ideals behind this constitution a reality.

Table 17.2 Pledges to patients and staff in the draft NHS Constitution.

Pledges to patients are concerned with	Pledges to staff
Access to services	Providing well-designed and rewarding jobs
Quality of care and environment	Providing personal development, access to appropriate training and management support to succeed
Nationally approved treatments, drugs and programmes	Providing support and opportunities for staff to keep themselves healthy and safe
Respect, consent and confidentiality	Engaging staff in decisions that will affect them and the services they provide. All staff will be empowered to put forward ways to deliver better and safer services
Informed choice Patient and public involvement in health care Complaints and redress	

Source: Summarised from Department of Health (2008f) *Handbook to the draft NHS Constitution.* London, DH.

References

The American Association of College of Nursing (2004) *AACN Position Statement on the Practice Doctorate in Nursing*. October 2004. Available at http://www.aacn.nche.edu/DNP/DNPPositionstatement.htm.

Boseley, S. (2008) Asylum seekers have right to full NHS care, high court rules, but Government considers appeal. *The Guardian*, April 12. Available at http://www.guardian.co.uk/uk/2008/apr/12/immigration.publicservices

Castledine, G. (1998a) Clinical specialists in nursing in the UK: the early years. Chapter 1 in *Advanced and Specialist Nursing Practice*, (eds G. Castledine and P. McGee), pp 3–32. Oxford, Blackwell Publishing.

Castledine, G. (1998b) Clinical specialists in nursing in the UK: 1980s to the present day. Chapter 2 in *Advanced and Specialist Nursing Practice*, (eds G. Castledine and P. McGee), pp 33–54. Oxford, Blackwell Publishing.

Castledine, G. (2003) The development of advanced nursing practice in the UK. Chapter 2 in *Advanced Practice*, (eds P. McGee and G. Castledine), 2nd edn. pp 8–16. Oxford, Blackwell Publishing.

Department of Health (2001) *Valuing People: A New Strategy for Learning Disability for the 21st Century*. Available at http://www.archive.official-documents.co.uk/document/cm50/5086/5086.htm.

Department of Health (2005a) *Creating a Patient-led NHS – Delivering the NHS Improvement Plan*. London, DH.

Department of Health (2005b) *Supporting People with Long Term Conditions, an NHS and Social Care Model to Support Local Innovation and Integration*. London, DH.

Department of Health (2005c) *Research Governance Framework*, 2nd edn. London, DH.

Department of Health (2007a) *Generic Choice Model for Long Term Conditions*. London, DH.

Department of Health (2007b) *Race Equality Action Plan*. Available at http://www.dh.gov.uk/en/Publicationsandstatistics/Bulletins/DH_4072494.

Department of Health (2008a) *High Quality Care for All. NHS Next Stage Review Final Report*. London, DH.

Department of Health (2008b) *NHS Next Stage Review: Impact and Equality Impact Assessments*. London, DH.

Department of Health (2008c) *NHS Next Stage Review: Our Vision for Primary and Community Care*. London, DH.

Department of Health (2008d) *Making the Difference. The Pacesetters Beginner's Guide to Service improvement for Equality and Diversity in the NHS*. Available at http://www.dh.gov.uk/en/publications.

Department of Health (2008e) *Healthcare for All. Report of the Independent Inquiry into Access to Healthcare for People with Learning Disabilities*. London, DH. Available at http://www.dh.gov.uk/en/Publicationsandstatistics/Bulletins/theweek/DH_086590.

Department of Health (2008f) *Handbook to the Draft NHS Constitution*. London, DH.

Department of Health (2008g) *Engagement Analysis. NHS Next Stage Review. What We Heard from Our NHS, Our Future Process*. London, DH.

Downes, E. (2007) *Fiji*. ICN/ICP Network Bulletin Issue 7 May available at http://www.icn.org.

Dunphy, L.M., Youngkin, E. Q. and Smith, N. K. (2004) Advanced practice nursing: doing what had to be done – radicals, renegades and rebels. Chapter 1 in *Advanced Practice Nursing. Essentials for Role Development*, (ed. L.A. Joel), pp 3–30. Philadelphia, F.A. Davis.

Egan, J., Chenoweth, L. and McAuliffe, D. (2006) Email-facilitated qualitative interviews with traumatic brain injury survivors: a new accessible method. *Brain Injury* **20** (12) 1283–94.

Freudmann, M. (2006) Surgical care practitioners are having a detrimental effect on surgical training. *British Medical Journal* 09 September 2006. Available http://careers.bmj.com/careers/advice/bmj.333.7567.s97.xml.

Gidlow, A. and Ellis, B. (2003) Advanced nursing practice and the interface with nursing in the UK. Chapter 13 in *Advanced Practice*, (eds P. McGee and G. Castledine), 2nd edn. pp 157–68. Oxford, Blackwell Science.

Hains, M. and McGee, P. (2006) The working men's project. *Diversity in Health and Social Care* **3** (1) 43–5.

Hanrahan, C., Way, C., Housser, J. and Applin, M. (2001) *The Nature of the Extended/Expanded Nursing Role in Canada*. Report of a project undertaken and published by the Centre for Nursing Studies, McMaster University and the Institute for the Advancement of Public Policy, Canada. Available at http://www.cns.nf.ca/research/execsum.htm.

Home Office (1999) *The Stephen Lawrence Inquiry. Report of an Inquiry by Sir William Macpherson of Cluny*. London, The Stationery Office.

Litchfield, M. (1998) The scope of advanced practice. *Nursing Praxis in New Zealand* **13** (3) 13–24.

Pearson, L. (2001) Annual legislative update. How each state stands on legislative issues affecting advanced nursing practice. *The Nurse Practitioner* **26** (1) 7, 11–5, 17–8, 21–7, 28, 31–8, 47–54, 57.

Pearson, L. (2003) Fifteenth annual legislative update. How each state stands on legislative issues affecting advanced nursing practice. *The Nurse Practitioner* **28** (1) 26–7, 31–2, 35–6, 38, 41–4, 46–50, 52–8.

Pearson, L. (2004) Sixteenth annual legislative update. How each state stands on legislative issues affecting advanced nursing practice. *The Nurse Practitioner* **29** (1) 26–7, 30–51.

Schober, M. and Affara, F. (2006) *International Council of Nurses, Advanced Nursing Practice*. Oxford, Blackwell Science.

Index